The First Interview

The FIRST INTERVIEW

Third Edition

James Morrison

THE GUILFORD PRESS
New York   London

© 2008 The Guilford Press
A Division of Guilford Publications, Inc.
72 Spring Street, New York, NY 10012
www.guilford.com

Printed in the United States of America

This book is printed on acid-free paper.

Last digit is print number: 9 8 7 6 5 4 3 2 1

Library of Congress Cataloging-in-Publication Data

Morrison, James R.
    The first interview / by James Morrison.—[3rd ed.].
      p. ; cm.
    Includes bibliographical references and index.
    ISBN-13: 978-1-59385-636-6 (hardcover : alk. paper)
    ISBN-10: 1-59385-636-9 (hardcover : alk. paper)
    1. Interviewing in psychiatry. I. Title.
    [DNLM: 1. Interview, Psychological. 2. Mental Disorders—
diagnosis. WM 141 M879f 2008]
    RC480.7.M67 2008
    616.89—dc22

                                 2007036140

For Jason

You've taught me more than I could ever imagine.

About the Author

James Morrison, MD, graduated from Reed College and earned his MD at Washington University in St. Louis, where he trained in psychiatry. He is currently Professor of Clinical Psychiatry at Oregon Health and Science University in Portland. Dr. Morrison's other books for professionals include *Diagnosis Made Easier, DSM-IV Made Easy, When Psychological Problems Mask Medical Disorders,* and *Interviewing Children and Adolescents.* In 2002 he wrote a comprehensive guide for patients and their relatives, *Straight Talk about Your Mental Health.*

Preface

The First Interview resulted from my desire to write, as much as possible, a manual on interviewing mental health patients that was based on objective research and best-practice principles. Of course, that was a pretty tall order when the first edition was published over a decade ago, and it remains so today—there isn't yet nearly enough controlled research to guide interviewers through the process of evaluating mental health patients. That's why, though I've updated the text with every scrap of new information I've been able to collect, the text still embodies a synthesis of the best techniques I've been able to cull from both the science and art of interviewing patients.

Any published book is really the work of more than one person, and I remain grateful to all those who have helped me over the years. They remain too many to name them all. But there are several people to whom I owe a special, ongoing debt of gratitude.

Matt Blusewicz, PhD, Rebecca Dominy, LCSW, Nicholas Rosenlicht, MD, Mark Servis, MD, and Kathleen Toms, RN, all contributed to the first edition. James Boehnlein, MD, generously read and provided a critique for this most recent edition. As always, Mary Morrison provided insightful and relevant comments at various stages of the preparation of the manuscript. I'll be forever grateful to the crew at The Guilford Press, especially my long-time editor, Kitty Moore, for her continuing wisdom and support. Marie Sprayberry, probably the best copy editor in the world, has immeasurably enhanced the looks and readability of this book with her close attention to detail. And Anna Brackett, once again my editorial project manager—thanks again for your diligence and skill in the face of too many author's requests for change.

Contents

Introduction

What Is Interviewing?

You'll probably never forget your first interviewing experience; I know I'll never forget mine. The patient, a young woman hospitalized with a thought disorder that turned out to be early schizophrenia, spoke vaguely and often wandered off the topic. She'd occasionally make sexual references that I, a young student in that more innocent era, had never before encountered. I wasn't sure what to talk about, and I spent more time planning what to ask next than I did considering what the previous answer meant. For some reason this patient seemed to like me, which was a good thing; I needed three more trips to the ward that weekend just to get the entire history.

I now realize that my early experience was about par for the course. No one had told me that most novice interviewers have trouble thinking up questions, or that many feel uncomfortable with their first few patients. I wish someone had pointed out what I now know: that mental health interviewing is usually easy and almost always quite a lot of fun.

It should be both. After all, clinical interviewing is little more than helping people talk about themselves, which most people love to do. In the field of mental health, we ask patients to reveal something of their emotions and their personal lives. Practice teaches us what to ask and how to direct the conversation to give us the information we need to help the patient best. Developing this ability is important: In a survey of practicing and teaching clinicians, comprehensive interviewing was ranked the highest of 32 skills needed by mental health practitioners.

If interviewing only involved getting patients to answer questions, clinicians could assign the task to computers and spend more time drinking coffee. But computers and paper questionnaires cannot begin to perceive the nuance of feeling, or assess the hesitation or the moist eye, that alerts a live clinician to yet another fruitful line of inquiry. A good interviewer must know how to work with a range of different personalities and problems: to give free rein to the informative patient, to guide the rambling one, to encourage the silent one, and to mollify the hostile one. Nearly anyone can learn these skills. There is no single kind of interviewing personality, and you can succeed with a variety of interviewing styles. Still, you will need guidance and practice to develop a style that works well for you.

Clinical interviews are used to accomplish various goals, of course, and professionals from diverse fields have different agendas. But all interviewers—psychiatrists, psychologists, family practitioners, social workers, nurses, occupational therapists, physicians' assistants, pastoral counselors, and drug rehabilitation specialists—must first obtain basic information from each patient they encounter. The similarities in the sort of data they need far outweigh any differences that might be expected from their different kinds of training and perspectives.

Good interviewers share three features. They

1. obtain the greatest amount of accurate information relevant to diagnosis and management,
2. in the shortest period of time,
3. consistent with creating and maintaining a good working relationship (rapport) with the patient.

Of these three components, (1) the database and (3) rapport are crucial. If you ignored time constraints, you could provide good care, although you might have difficulty coping with more than a very few patients at one time.

Your first contact with any patient could be for a variety of reasons—a brief screening, an outpatient diagnostic intake, an emergency room visit, a hospital intake, or a consultation for medication or psychotherapy. A nurse clinician might need to develop a nursing treatment plan based on several behavioral diagnoses. Forensic reports and research interviews have very different goals, but their methods and content have much in common with all the other types of interviews I've mentioned—each of which is a specialized use of the basic, comprehensive initial interview. Whatever your interview goals, this book aims to outline the information you should try to obtain for all patients, and to recommend techniques that will help you during the different stages of your interview.

While doing research for this edition, I was impressed by how much we have learned even recently about the interview process. However, in my everyday evaluations of young mental health professionals, I am often disconcerted at how little this knowledge is being used in the training process. Clinicians often use far less than the time allotted for an interview; fail to ask about suicidal ideas; and forget that many,

many mental health patients also have substance use issues. In short, much of what we know about the processes of interviewing and evaluation is being ignored. *The First Interview* attempts to remedy this deficit. Addressed primarily to beginners, it emphasizes the basic material that clinicians of all mental health disciplines need to know. I hope that practiced clinicians will also find it helpful for review.

THE NEED FOR COMPREHENSIVE INFORMATION

Clinicians can view a patient in an astonishing variety of ways. Indeed, all clinicians should be able to view each patient from biological, dynamic, social, and behavioral perspectives, because a single patient may need the treatment implied by any or even all of these theoretical perspectives. For example, the problems of a young married woman who drinks too much alcohol might be determined by a combination of factors:

> *Dynamic.* Her overbearing husband resembles her father, who also drinks.
> *Behavioral.* She associates drinking with relief from the tensions induced by these two relationships.
> *Social.* Several girlfriends drink; drinking is accepted, even encouraged, in her social milieu.
> *Biological.* The genetic contribution from her alcoholic father needs to be considered.

A comprehensive evaluation brings out the contributions of each of these points of view. Each is folded into the treatment plan.

Throughout the book I emphasize the need to hold all perspectives when conducting a comprehensive interview. Unless you do a complete evaluation, you are likely to miss vital data. You might not learn, for example, that a patient who seeks help for a "problem of living" actually has an underlying psychosis, a depression, or substance misuse. Even if your patient turns out to have no actual mental disorder, you need to learn how past experiences contribute to the current problems. Only a complete interview can satisfactorily give you this information.

Needless to say, you will obtain much more additional information as treatment progresses. You may even find that you must revise certain of the opinions you formed during your first meeting. But you can plan rationally for management only if you first carefully elicit the relevant data during the initial interview.

Your success as a mental health interviewer will hinge on several different skills. How well can you elicit the entire story? Can you probe deeply enough to obtain all the relevant information? How quickly can you teach your patient to tell you accurate, pertinent facts? How adequately do you evaluate and respond to your patient's feelings? Can you, when necessary, stimulate your patient's motivation to reveal embarrassing experiences? All of these skills are needed by anyone who must obtain mental health histories. The time to learn them is early in your training, before ineffective—or even maladaptive—interviewing habits become a fixed part of your style. The benefits of early training should persist for a lifetime.

More than half a century ago, two volumes set the tone for interviewing style: *The Initial Interview in Psychiatric Practice* by Gill, Newman, and Redlich, and *The Psychiatric Interview* by Harry Stack Sullivan. Although a number of other books on interviewing have appeared over the years, most have followed the models established by these two volumes. But taste and needs have changed over the decades, and such venerable works no longer adequately serve the mental health interviewer. Over the past several decades, a number of research papers—most notably those by Cox and associates—have provided a scientific basis for modern interviewing practice. I have based much of this book on these sources. I have also consulted nearly every available relevant monograph and research article on interviewing published during the past 50 years. Citations for the more important of these are provided in Appendix F.

In their monograph, Cannell and Kahn (1968) stated, "The people who write instructions and books for interviewers are not themselves given much to interviewing." At least in the case of *The First Interview*, that assertion is dead wrong. A significant part of what has gone into this volume comes from my own interviews over the years with more than 15,000 mental health patients. The interviewing approach I recommend is an amalgam of clinical research, the experience of others, and my own perception of what works. If it sometimes seems formulaic, it's a formula that works well. Once you have learned the basics, you can adapt and expand it to create your own interviewing style.

THE IMPORTANCE OF PRACTICE

When I was in training, my professors often said that a student's best textbook is the patient. Nowhere is this more true than in learning to do a mental health interview. Indeed, no textbook can be more than a supplement—a guide to the real learning that comes through experience. I therefore urge you to practice early and often.

First, read Chapters 1 through 5 quickly. Don't try to memorize this material; the amount may be daunting, but it is presented in sequence to help you learn it a bit at a time. (Appendix A provides a concise outline of the information you need and strategies you can use at each stage of the typical initial interview.) Then find a patient who will help you learn.

For the beginning interviewer, patients hospitalized in a mental health unit are an excellent resource. Many of them have been interviewed before (some are highly experienced), so they have a good idea of what you expect of them. Even in modern hospitals with many scheduled activities, they usually have time available. Many patients appreciate the chance to ventilate, and most enjoy the feeling that from their own difficulties some good can come—in this case, the training of a mental health professional. Sometimes an interview by a fresh observer, even a trainee, reveals new insights that can help redirect therapy.

So enlist the aid of a cooperative patient and start to work. Don't worry about trying to find a "good teaching patient"; for your purposes, any cooperative patient will do. And all lives are inherently interesting. Don't try to follow an outline too closely, especially in the early going. Relax and try to give both yourself and the patient an enjoyable experience.

After an hour or so—a longer session will be too tiring for both of you—break it off with the promise that later you'll come back for more. Return to *The First Interview* to read about any areas of interview management that gave you trouble. Carefully compare the personal and social information you have obtained with the recommendations in Chapter 8 (which are also outlined in Appendix A). How complete is your mental status exam? Compare your observations with the suggestions in Chapters 11 and 12.

A student might reasonably ask, "How can I interview about mental disorders when I know so little?" Doing a complete interview does imply knowing the symptoms, signs, and course typical of various mental disorders, but you can study these while you learn interview technique. In fact, learning about disorders from patients who have experienced them will fix the characteristics of these diagnoses in your mind forever. In Chapter 13 you will find listed the features that you should cover in your interview, broken down by the areas of clinical interest your patient presents.

Armed with a list of the questions you forgot to ask the first time through, return for another session with your patient. As I learned that weekend as a medical student and beginning interviewer, there is no better way to learn what to ask than by going back to correct your own omissions. The more patients you interview, the less you will forget. When you have completed your interview, any of several standard textbooks (see Appendix F for an annotated list) can help you with the differential diagnosis of your patient's disorder.

You will become skilled faster if you have feedback from an experienced interviewer. It could be direct, as when an instructor sits with you while you interview your patient. Numerous studies have demonstrated the effectiveness of videotape or audiotape recordings, which can be played back while you and your instructor discuss the facts you have omitted and the interview techniques you could have used to better effect. You will probably find that you can learn a lot just by listening in private to audiotapes of your own early interviews. I've provided a score sheet in Appendix E to help you evaluate the content and process issues of your interviews.

Chapter 1

Openings and Introductions

By the time you have completed an initial interview, you should have (1) obtained information from your patient and (2) established the basis for a good working relationship. The information includes various types of history (a history is a detailed account that includes current symptoms, previous illnesses, medications, family and social relationships, health risk issues—in short, everything that bears on your patient's life and mental health problems) and a mental status examination, which is an evaluation of your patient's current thinking and behavior.

In the course of this book, I will take you through each section of the history and mental status exam, in more or less the chronological order you would use when talking with your patient. In separate chapters, I'll discuss the content of the information you should expect to obtain and the interview techniques that are most appropriate to that content. Where it seems appropriate, I will also discuss issues of rapport.

TIME FACTORS

In the first few moments of an initial interview, you will need to accomplish several tasks.

- You should indicate what form your interview will take—how much time it will take, what sort of questions you will ask, and the like.
- You should convey some idea about the sort of information you expect your patient (or other informant) to give you.
- You must create a comfortable and secure environment that will allow your patient as much control as possible, under the circumstances.

Table 1 lists the basic material that should be covered by the time you complete your interview. An experienced clinician usually takes about an hour to examine the average patient. A student will probably require several hours to obtain all the relevant information. Regardless of your level of experience, your emphasis should be on collecting the most information possible.

Even a seasoned interviewer occasionally requires more than one session for an initial evaluation, and anyone needs more time for a patient who is unusually talkative, vague, hostile, suspicious, or hard to understand, or for one who has a complicated story to tell. Some patients simply cannot tolerate a lengthy interview, and even those who are hospitalized may have other appointments to keep. Multiple interviews also give a patient time to reflect and to recall material that might have been initially omitted. Of course, if you interview relatives or other informants, you will need additional sessions, plus time to integrate the information from all of your sources.

I realize that with the rush of modern health care, time available is constantly shrinking. That's why I've expressed as percentages the amounts of time you should plan to devote to the various portions of an average initial interview:

15%: Determine the chief complaint and encourage free speech.
30%: Pursue specific diagnoses; ask about suicide, history of violence, and substance misuse.
15%: Obtain medical history; conduct review of systems; obtain family history.
25%: Obtain rest of personal and social history; evaluate character pathology.
10%: Conduct mental status exam.
5%: Discuss diagnosis and treatment with patient; plan next meeting.

Your own professional needs may change the focus somewhat. For example, social workers may spend additional time on the personal and social history. (Some institutions and agencies used to assign to social workers the responsibility for obtaining the entire social history. Today, most authorities would hold that all aspects of the entire history should be gathered by at least one clinician, who can then synthesize this information into a coherent clinical picture.)

Regardless of your profession, I recommend that you try to get the whole story early in the relationship with your patient. After the first few sessions, even experienced clinicians sometimes assume that they know a patient well and ignore certain vital information that may have escaped them.

TABLE 1. Outline of the Initial Interview

Chief complaint
History of present illness
  Stressors
  Onset
  Symptoms
  Previous episodes
    Treatment
    Consequences
  Course
  Treatment so far
  Hospitalizations?
  Effects on patient, others
Personal and social history
  Childhood and growing up
    Where born?
    Number of siblings and
      position
    Reared by one or both
      parents?
    Relationship with parents
    If adopted:
      What circumstances?
      Extrafamilial?
    Health as child
    Problems related to puberty
    Abuse (physical or sexual)?
    Education
      Last grade completed
      Scholastic problems?
      Overly active?
      School refusal?
      Behavior problems?
      Suspension or expulsion?
    Sociable as child?
    Hobbies, interests
  Life as an adult
    Current living situation
      Lives with whom?
      Where?
      Ever homeless?
      Support network
      Mobility
      Finances
    Marital history
      Age(s) at marriage(s)
      Number of marriages
      Age(s) at termination(s)
        and how ended
      Number, age, sex of
        children
      Stepchildren?
      Marital problems?
    Sexual preference, adjustment
      Problems with intercourse?
      Birth control methods
      Extramarital partners?
      Physical, sexual abuse?
    Work history
      Current occupation
      Number of jobs
      Reason(s) for job
        change(s)
      Ever fired?

Life as an adult (*cont.*)
  Leisure activities
    Clubs, organizations
    Interests, hobbies
  Military service
    Branch, rank
    Years served
    Disciplinary problems?
    Combat?
  Legal problems ever?
    Criminal record?
    Litigation?
  Religion
    Denomination
    Interest
Medical history
  Major illnesses
  Operations
  Nonmental medications
  Allergies
    Environmental
    Food
    Medications
  Nonmental hospitalizations
  Physical impairments
  Risk factors for AIDS?
  Adult physical or sexual
    abuse?
Review of systems
  Changes in appetite
  Head injury
  Seizures
  Chronic pain
  Unconsciousness
  Premenstrual syndrome
  Review for somatization
    disorder
Family history
  Describe relatives
  Mental disorder in relatives?
Substance misuse
  Type(s) of substance(s)
  Duration of use
  Quantity
  Consequences
    Medical problems
    Loss of control
    Personal and
      interpersonal problems
    Job difficulties
    Legal consequences
    Financial problems
  Misuse of medications
    Prescription
    Over-the-counter
Personality traits
  Lifelong behavior patterns
  Violence
  Arrests
Suicide attempts
  Methods
  Consequences
  Drugs or alcohol associated?

Suicide attempts (*cont.*)
  Seriousness
    Psychological
    Physical
Mental status exam
  Appearance
    Apparent age
    Race
    Posture
    Nutrition
    Hygiene
    Hairstyle
    Clothing
      Neat?
      Clean?
      Type/fashion?
  Behavior
    Activity level
    Tremors?
    Mannerisms and
      stereotypies
    Smiles?
    Eye contact
  Mood
    Type
    Lability
    Appropriateness
  Flow of thought
    Word associations
    Rate and rhythm of speech
    Accent in speaking
  Content of thought
    Phobias
    Anxiety
    Obsessions, compulsions
    Thoughts of suicide
    Delusions
    Hallucinations
  Language
    Comprehension
    Fluency
    Naming
    Repetition
    Reading
    Writing
  Cognition
    Orientation
      Person
      Place
      Time
    Memory
      Immediate
      Recent
      Remote
    Attention and concentration
      Serial sevens
      Count backwards
    Cultural information
      Five presidents
    Abstract thinking
      Similarities
      Differences
    Insight and judgment

Of course, just as no one has unlimited time, no evaluation can ever be considered complete. As long as you continue to care for your patient, you will be adding new facts and observations to your original database. But if you have done your job well in the beginning, these will largely be matters of corroborative detail that won't substantially affect diagnosis or treatment.

Patients seek help for serious problems that they find frightening, overwhelming, or even life-threatening. You should elicit their stories in such a way that they feel they have received a complete, fair, professional evaluation. If your patient is unusually dramatic, slow, or discursive, try to understand this behavior in the light of the stresses and anxieties any mental patient faces, and allow additional time.

SETTINGS

The first moments any professional person spends with a new patient set the tone for all subsequent interactions. Careful attention to such simple matters as introductions and the patient's comfort and sense of control helps establish a relationship grounded in respect and cooperation. If you have your own private office, you can decorate it as nicely as you choose, but institutional offices are often less than regal. Fortunately, the effectiveness of the interview is not related to the elegance of the surroundings. I have seen excellent interviews done at the bedside, or even in a corner of a busy hospital day room (though a measure of privacy will yield the most information). What is paramount is your concern for the patient's comfort and privacy.

Make the best of what you have available. Sitting across a desk from the patient, as is traditional in so many offices, creates an inflexible barrier between the two of you. It doesn't allow much leeway to give more space to the suspicious patient or to draw nearer someone whose depression requires the close comfort of another human being. Try instead to arrange your chairs so you can face the patient across the corner of a desk or table. That way, you can vary the distance between the two of you, as the needs of the moment indicate. If you are right-handed, you can more comfortably take notes if the patient sits to your left. Of course, two chairs that directly face one another will work well, too.

At the same time, you have another task to fulfill—one whose importance I won't have to spend any time at all trying to sell. That task is maintaining your safety. Now the vast majority of mental health encounters are completely risk-free, but in rare cases something happens and harm comes to the clinician, the patient, or both. (In 2006 Wayne Fenton, a psychiatrist who specialized in the management of schizophrenia at the National Institute of Mental Health in Bethesda, Maryland, was beaten to death by one of his patients—an attack that made headlines across the country.) It must become instinctive with you that at the beginning of every patient interview, you check to ensure your own safety and that of others. Practically speaking, this means following three principles: (1) Interview in a place where there are others nearby; (2) have available an easily triggered emergency alert system, such as an alarm bell; and (3) when you are conducting an interview in a closed office, seat yourself so that you are closer to the door than the patient is, with no furniture (such as a desk) that could serve as an obstacle if a speedy exit should become necessary.

Regardless of where you interview, your own appearance can affect your relationship with the patient. What's considered professional may depend somewhat upon the region of the country and the customs of the particular clinic or hospital where you work. This observation may seem obvious, but it bears repeating: You will be perceived as more professional if you pay attention to your dress, grooming, and manner.

In general, patients readily accept conservative clothing and hairstyles; excessively casual dress or manners may suggest nonchalance about the importance of your meeting. Indeed, a 2005 survey revealed that by huge margins, patients preferred physicians to be formally dressed and were more inclined to reveal personal information to those who wore white coats than to those who were casually attired. Most of the patients also stated that they were more likely to follow the advice of someone who was professionally dressed. The patients surveyed were on average middle-aged; although teenagers and children could yet prove to be significant exceptions to this rule, the report bears careful consideration (it is probably relevant to other health care personnel as well). Limit your jewelry to something modest; don't antagonize someone whose cooperation you need with adornments that suggest wealth or status beyond what the patient could hope to achieve. If you wear pins, pendants, or items of clothing that indicate a religious affiliation, consider whether any of your prospective clients might regard it as a barrier to an effective relationship. Observe how other professionals in your setting dress and behave. Let their examples guide your judgment as to what is appropriate.

BEGINNING THE RELATIONSHIP

Introduce yourself, offer to shake hands, and indicate the seating arrangement you prefer. (At a patient's bedside, always sit down, even if you intend to stay for only a few minutes. Even if you have a plane to catch, you don't want to appear too hurried to take time with the patient.) If you happen to be late for the interview, acknowledge it with an apology. Is your patient's name an uncommon one? Be sure that you have pronounced it correctly. If this is the first time you have met, explain your status (student? intern? teaching supervisor?) and the purpose of this interview. What do you hope to learn? What information do you have already? Give your patient an estimate of how much time you expect to spend together.

Often you will already know something about the patient from case notes of previous workers, from a hospital chart, or from a physician's referral. You can save time and increase the accuracy of your assessment by reviewing this material before you begin. However, for the purposes of this book, we'll assume that you have no access to such information.

Although some interviewers try to ease into a relationship with small talk, I recommend against it. In most cases your patient has come for treatment because of troubling problems. Comments about the weather, baseball, or television shows may seem at best a distraction, or at worst an expression of unconcern on your part. It is usually better to go right to the heart of the matter.

Should you feel that you *must* start with small talk, ask a question that demands more than a yes–no response. For example:

"How was the traffic coming here?"

"How have you been enjoying the summer months?"

If nothing else, such a question shows that you expect the patient to participate actively. Especially during the early part of your interview, you want to encourage the patient to elaborate, not to answer with "yes" or "no" while you do most of the work. (We'll further consider this and other aspects of interview control in Chapters 4 and 10.)

Occasionally, a relative or close friend will want to accompany the patient into the interview room—a situation to which you can respond in either of two ways. I prefer to see the patient and informant separately, because doing so maximizes the amount of information obtained. To reinforce the patient's sense of autonomy, I almost always start with the patient, advising the informant that "you'll be next." Occasionally, however, you may need to take the other tack and see patient and informant together. That's usually the case when the patient is severely impaired, such as with an advanced dementia. Then having the relative in the room can be a real time saver. Another occasion on which you'll need the dual-interview format is when the patient strongly requests it, such as in the case of someone whose severe anxiety or depression requires extra support.

TAKING NOTES

In most cases you will want to take notes. Few of us can remember even briefly all the material we hear, and you may not have the opportunity to write up your interview right away. So point out that you will be taking notes, and make sure that this is all right with the patient.

Nonetheless, you should try to keep note taking to a minimum. This will allow you to spend more time observing your patient's behavior and facial expressions for clues to feelings. You won't be able to get everything down on paper or to write complete sentences (other than the chief complaint, which we'll discuss in the next chapter). Instead, jot down key words that can indicate which issues to explore later or that can serve as reminders when you write up your report. Try to keep your pen in hand; this avoids the distraction of repeatedly picking it up. The only time you should lay it aside is when you discuss especially sensitive topics that the patient might not care to have recorded.

This brings up the "off the record" problem. Sometimes a patient will ask that you keep certain material in your head and out of the chart. When this request comes early in your relationship, it is usually better to comply, especially if it applies to a limited portion of the interview. If the patient seems extremely uncomfortable with any note taking, you can explain that you will need some notes for later review to help make sense of it all. In the rare event that the patient insists, give in, put down your pen, and later transcribe all that you can remember. What you want is to complete an informative interview, not to win a contest of wills. However, at some point—perhaps not right now when you are trying to complete the interview—you might raise the point again. Having a significant hole in the database could prove problematic, especially if this patient will be seen by other clinicians later on.

Reviewing a tape recording of a session can help you spot difficulties in your interview style. You can often uncover deficiencies that you would have missed with a less complete record of your conversation. As an everyday practice, however, it has drawbacks: Reviewing a tape takes a lot of time, and patients are far more likely to feel uncomfortable with tape recording than with note taking. If you do decide to make a tape recording, begin only after you have explained its educational purpose and obtained permission.

It may also be necessary to explain that state laws and professional ethics could require you to report certain information that has a bearing on the safety of others. This principle, formalized in 1974 by the *Tarasoff* decision in California, clearly states that health care personnel have a duty to protect identifiable persons against whom threats have been made. Although not all states have enacted such a statute, clinicians everywhere are advised to behave as if it has been enacted. Of course, if you are a student, you should never take such action on your own; discuss at once any threats or other concerns you have with a supervisor, who will then take the lead in discharging the duty to protect.

SAMPLE OPENINGS

Effective openings have many possible variations. Here is a good one.

> INTERVIEWER: Good morning, Mr. Dean. I'm Emily Watts, a third-year medical student. I'd like to talk with you for about an hour to learn as much as I can about people with problems like yours. Do you have the time to spend with me now?
>
> PATIENT: Yes, that will be fine.
>
> INTERVIEWER: Why don't you sit right here? *(Motions toward a chair.)* Do you mind if I take some notes?
>
> PATIENT: No, everyone else seems to.

This opening works because it quickly conveys information that is important to the patient: the interviewer's name and position, the purpose of the interview, and the time that will be required. The interviewer also manages the business of seating arrangements and obtaining permission for note taking. However, some patients may bridle at the notion of having a problem. Ms. Watts was interviewing an established patient, so her question went unchallenged. New patients might respond better to a simple "Please tell me why you are here."

Here's another useful opening:

> PATIENT: Are you the student they told me about?
>
> INTERVIEWER: No, I'm Dr. Holden, a psychology intern. I spoke with your therapist earlier this afternoon, and I'd like to spend some time with you to see what we can do to help you out. We can use this little room.
>
> PATIENT: *(Nods.)*
>
> INTERVIEWER: To help you best, I'm going to need all the information I can get. I'd like to jot down a few notes, if that's all right with you.
>
> PATIENT: No problem.

Sometimes the information-gathering phase takes more than a single interview. You might start the follow-up session by saying, "Have you thought of anything more to say from our previous discussion?" or "What did you say to your [wife, husband, daughter, etc.] about our last meeting?" Otherwise, just pick up where you left off last session when time ran out.

Chapter 2

Chief Complaint and Free Speech

The chief complaint states the patient's reasons for seeking care, whereas the free speech that immediately follows encourages the patient to talk about all these reasons. The words you use to prime the information pump can greatly affect its subsequent performance, and they fall into one of two principal interviewing styles: directive and nondirective.

DIRECTIVE VERSUS NONDIRECTIVE QUESTIONS

By asking many specific questions, a directive interviewer explicitly provides the structure that tells the patient what sort of information is wanted. The nondirective interviewer more passively absorbs whatever information the patient chooses to present. A nondirective style usually yields strong rapport and reliable facts. An exclusively nondirective style also produces less information, however. For example, without direction the patient may not realize that family history is important or could feel too embarrassed to volunteer highly personal information. A maximally effective initial interview will use both nondirective and directive questions.

Most of the early portion of your interview should be nondirective. This helps you establish your working relationship and learn what sort of problems and feelings are uppermost in your patient's mind. But your opening request for information should clearly state what you expect of your patient.

THE OPENING QUESTION

When you ask your first question, be specific. Let your patient know exactly what you want to hear about. If, like some nondirective interviewers, you leave matters completely up to the patient ("What would you like to talk about?"), you could end up with quite a lot of information about last Sunday's football game or the patient's new sports car. Eventually you would get the interview back on track, but at the cost of time and perhaps rapport with a patient who might wonder whether you knew what you really wanted.

You can avoid these difficulties by asking the right sort of question in the first place:

"Please tell me what problems made you come for treatment."

Notice that this request has two qualities that affect the type of information you will obtain:

- It tells the patient just what sort of information you seek.
- It is also open-ended. Open-ended inquiries are questions or statements that cannot readily be answered in a word or two. Because they invite patients to talk for a while about what seems important to them, they promote a relaxed interview style early in the interview that helps build rapport.

Open-ended questions and statements can serve two functions. Some simply request more information about a point:

"I'd like to hear some more about that."

"Could you expand on that?"

"What else happened?"

Others also move the story along toward the present:

"What happened after that?"

"And then what?"

"What did you do next?"

Open-ended requests broaden the scope of information that you might obtain; with more freedom to respond, patients tell you what is important to them. They let patients know that their stories are important to you. They also allow you to spend less time talking and more time observing. The importance of this will become more evident in Chapter 11 when we talk about the mental status examination.

Closed-ended questions more narrowly direct the sort of answer desired and can be answered in a few words. They can be "yes–no" or limited-choice questions ("Where were you born?" as opposed to "Tell me about your childhood"). They, too, are useful; they are sometimes necessary to obtain the most information in the least time. But in early parts of the interview, use open-ended questions that will encourage your patient to tell a story that touches on as many aspects of the case history as are relevant.

THE CHIEF COMPLAINT

The *chief complaint* is the patient's stated reason for seeking help. It is usually the first full sentence or two of the reply to your opening question:

"Tell me about the problem that brought you here."

Importance

The chief complaint is important for either of two reasons.

1. Because it is usually the problem uppermost in the patient's mind, it tells you what area you should explore first. Most patients have some sort of a specific problem or request. Here are some samples:

"I can't reach my goals."

"I have trouble forming relationships with women."

"I hear voices."

"I'm so depressed I feel that I can't go on."

Each of these typical examples expresses some discomfort, life problem, or fear that the patient wants help with.

2. By contrast, sometimes the chief complaint is a flat denial that anything is wrong. When this is the case, it tips you off about your patient's insight, intelligence, or cooperation. For example:

"There's nothing wrong with me. I'm only here because the judge ordered it."

"I don't remember anything about it."

"Absolute zero is coming, and when it gets here my brain is going to turn to bread."

Chief complaints like these three indicate serious pathology or resistance that requires special handling. Chapter 16 discusses patients who resist efforts at being interviewed.

Responding

Some chief complaints suggest that your patient doesn't quite understand the purpose of the interview. You will sometimes encounter this sort of vague or slightly quarrelsome chief complaint, so you should be prepared with some good responses.

INTERVIEWER: Why did you come here for treatment?

PATIENT: You can read all about it in my record.

INTERVIEWER: I could, but it would help me learn more about you if you'd tell me in your own words.

Here's how one interviewer reacted to a patient who, instead of a complaint, gave a prescription:

> PATIENT: I think I just need some vitamins.
>
> INTERVIEWER: Perhaps, but let's decide that after you tell me what's been bothering you.

Another patient made a plea for help in getting started:

> PATIENT: I really don't know where to begin.
>
> INTERVIEWER: Why don't you start with when your most recent trouble began?

Try to Learn the Real Reason for Coming

A patient's first words don't always express the real reason for seeking help. Some patients don't recognize the real reason, others may feel ashamed or fearful of what they'll be told. In either case, the stated chief complaint may be only a "ticket of admission" to the help a clinician can provide:

"I've been in such pain." (But the real pain is emotional.)

"I feel anxious nearly every moment I'm awake." (Heavy drinking isn't mentioned.)

"I'd like to discuss some of my relationships." (The patient is afraid to mention AIDS.)

"I want some advice about my mother. I wonder if she's becoming senile." (The patient really wonders, "Am I going crazy?")

Each of these initial complaints masks a deeper, less obvious reason for seeking help. Often you can ferret out the real problem later in the interview by asking:

"Is anything else bothering you?"

Sometimes you will be able to determine your patient's underlying motivation only after you have completed your initial evaluation.

Regardless of what chief complaint is presented, you should write it down in your patient's exact words. Later, you will want to contrast it with what you believe prompted the patient to seek help.

FREE SPEECH

During the few minutes following the chief complaint, your patient should have the chance to discuss freely the reasons for seeking treat-

ment. To encourage the widest possible range of information, allow the
story to emerge with little detailed probing or other interruption from
you. We may call this nondirected flow of information *free speech* to distinguish it from the relatively constrained question–answer format of
the later clinical interview.

What Is Free Speech?

Experienced interviewers recommend this period (as much as 8 or 10
minutes in an hour-long session) of free speech for several reasons.
Some of them are the reasons for asking any open-ended question:

- Free speech establishes you as someone who cares enough to listen to your patient's concerns.
- It provides the patient an opportunity to organize and explore
  the reasons for seeking treatment.
- You have the opportunity to learn what is uppermost in your patient's mind.
- It gives you the flavor of the patient's personality.
- Unhampered by any need to direct the conversation, you can
  start making observations about mood, behavior, and thought
  processes.
- Character traits may be more likely to emerge in a person who is
  speaking spontaneously than in one who is answering a stream
  of questions.
- When you share control during this portion of the conversation,
  you establish early the expectation that your patient will be an
  active partner throughout therapy.
- You can devote close attention to the content of your patient's
  speech. One study showed that as many as half the total symptoms reported by patients are mentioned in the first 3 minutes
  of an initial interview.
- It provides your patient an opportunity to bring up other concerns that weren't mentioned in the chief complaint.

Most patients will respond quickly and appropriately to your request that they talk about their problems. Getting them to tell you everything you need to know will take little redirection on your part.
Some have had so much experience telling their stories that they give
you complete, chronological accounts of their illnesses.

The opposite may be true of others. They have experienced too
many interviewers who want only specific answers to closed-ended
questions. You may have to teach these patients to give you an ex-

panded version of their feelings and experiences. If your patient persistently makes brief statements, then waits for more questions from you, you should explicitly state what you expect. For example:

"What I'd really like is for you to tell me in your own words about your problem. Later on I'll ask some specific questions that you can answer briefly."

In fact, few histories unfold like a textbook account of a classical mental health problem. Patients have their own ideas about what is important, and, regardless of the apparent value of their information, it is important that you let them make a stab at telling their stories. An occasional patient with mental retardation or severe psychosis might not be able to give you a satisfactory narration. Then you might have to fall back on a much more structured, question-and-answer strategy to obtain any history. But these patients will be infrequent, and every one who speaks at all will at least give you information in the form of the mental status observations you can make.

Allowing patients time to speak freely is at least as important now as it has ever been, but health care reimbursement models have put an ever-tightening squeeze on clinicians' time. It threatens to crowd out all but the most basic clinical interactions, tempting an interviewer to cut directly to the chase and focus too quickly on a patient's very first words. I know this because I've done it—and must occasionally remind myself of the importance of a prolonged period of free-running speech. If I do find that I've allowed too little time at the outset for free speech, I'll try to slip it in later on.

AREAS OF CLINICAL INTEREST

During free speech, your patient will probably mention one or more problems. These concerns can be emotional, physical, or social; most will fall into one of several major areas of clinical interest. When people become mental health patients, it is usually because of problems covered by these seven areas:

Difficulty thinking (cognitive disorders)
Substance use
Psychosis
Mood disturbance (depression or mania)
Anxiety, avoidance behavior, and arousal
Physical complaints
Social and personality problems

Each area of clinical interest comprises a number of diagnoses that have symptoms in common; of course, some of these diagnoses turn up in more than one area. Later, when you obtain the history of the present illness, you will systematically ask about the symptoms usually associated with whichever of these areas you have identified. This information will allow you to determine which of the associated diagnoses seems appropriate for your patient. But for now, during free speech, just make a note (mentally or on paper) about any subject that seems worth exploring later.

Signaling Areas of Clinical Interest

A number of symptoms and items of historical information specific to each area of clinical interest signal the need for further exploration. When you encounter one in your interview, consider an intensive review of that area (discussed in Chapter 13). These "red flag" symptoms are summarized in Table 2.

HOW MUCH TIME?

Unless your patient's speech is unusually vague or rambling, the chief complaint usually takes only a few seconds. However, the time you devote to free speech can vary tremendously. In the rare event that your patient is incoherent or nearly mute, you might decide within moments to adopt a more directive interview style. But with a patient who is well organized, experienced, and motivated to tell all, you could conceivably spend the entire interview in free speech, listening to a history that is presented just the way you would read it in a textbook.

Most patients will be neither of the above. Often you can listen without much interruption for the first 5 or 10 minutes. But don't try to stick to this recommendation too strictly—your allotment to free speech will depend on the total time you can spend interviewing and on what you already know about the history. As a rule, you should allow your patient to speak freely as long as the information you obtain seems important and relevant.

MOVING ON

The free-speech portion of the interview will draw to a close as you sense that you have obtained a broad outline of the problems that are uppermost in your patient's mind. Before proceeding to the next sec-

TABLE 2. Problems That Signal Areas of Clinical Interest

Difficulty thinking (cognitive disorders)
  Affect fluctuations
  Bizarre behavior
  Confusion
  Decreased judgment
  Delusions
  Hallucinations
  Memory defects
  Toxin ingestion
Substance misuse
  Alcohol use heavier than one or two
    drinks per day
  Arrests or other legal problems
  Financial: spending money needed
    for other items
  Health: blackouts, cirrhosis,
    abdominal pain, vomiting
  Illegal substance use
  Job loss, tardiness, demotions
  Memory impairment
  Social problems: fights, loss of
    friends
Psychosis
  Affect that is flat or inappropriate
  Bizarre behavior
  Confusion
  Delusions
  Fantasies or illogical ideas
  Hallucinations (of any of the senses)
  Insight or judgment that is disturbed
  Muteness
  Perceptual distortions (illusions,
    misinterpretations)
  Social withdrawal
  Speech that is hard to follow or
    incoherent
Mood disturbance: depression
  Activity level that is either markedly
    increased or decreased
  Anxiety symptoms
  Appetite changes
  Concentration poor
  Death wishes
  Feelings of worthlessness
  Interest decreased for usual activities
    (including sex)
  Sleeplessness or excessive sleepiness
  Substance misuse recently increased
  Suicidal ideas
  Tearfulness
  Weight loss or gain
Mood disturbance: mania
  Activity level increased
  Distractibility

Mood disturbance: mania (*cont.*)
  Grandiose sense of self-worth
  Judgment deteriorating
  Mood that is euphoric or irritable
  Planning many activities
  Sleep decreased (reduced need for
    sleep)
  Speech rapid, loud, hard to interrupt
  Substance misuse recently increased
  Thoughts moving rapidly from one
    idea to another
Anxiety disorders
  Anxiety
  Chest pain
  Compulsive behavior
  Dizziness
  Fear of going crazy
  Fear of dying or impending doom
  Fear of objects or situations
  Heaviness in the chest
  Irregular heartbeat
  Nervousness
  Obsessional ideas
  Palpitations
  Panic
  Shortness of breath
  Sweating
  Trauma: history of severe emotional
    or physical
  Trembling
  Worries
Physical complaints
  Appetite disturbance
  Convulsions
  Depression, chronic
  Headache
  History that is complicated
  Multiple complaints
  Neurological complaints
  Repeated treatment failures
  Sexual or physical abuse during
    childhood
  Substance misuse
  Vague history
  Weakness
  Weight changes (up or down)
Social and personality problems
  Anxiety
  Behaviors that seem odd or bizarre
  Dramatic presentation
  Drug or alcohol misuse
  Job loss, tardiness, demotions
  Legal difficulties
  Marital conflicts

tion of your interview, you should ask whether there are problems other than those already mentioned. This decreases the risk that you will overlook vital problem areas. (Even if you missed something big, it would probably show up later. Yet the whole point of the initial interview is to try to get *all* relevant information up front.)

This is also a good time to check on your understanding of all problems. Briefly summarize each, and invite your patient's assessment of your analysis.

> INTERVIEWER: Let's see if I have this right. You felt just fine until about 2 weeks ago, when you proposed to your girlfriend, and she accepted you. Since then you've had increasing attacks of anxiety, you've felt depressed, and you can't concentrate on your studies. Now you're afraid you might have heart disease because your pulse races. Is that about right?
>
> PATIENT: That's pretty much it.
>
> INTERVIEWER: I want to learn more about that, but first, is there anything else that's been bothering you?

Chapter 3

Developing Rapport

Rapport is the feeling of harmony and confidence that should exist between patient and clinician. As one of the goals of a good interview, good rapport has practical consequences. This point is especially relevant if you will be treating this patient in the future. The trust and confidence you begin to develop even in the opening minutes of the first session can greatly enhance your ability to manage a course of therapy. In fact, how well you convey your interest is the factor most likely to keep your patient in treatment.

But good rapport is also vital for obtaining information. During the evaluation phase of your relationship, positive rapport will help motivate your patient to talk spontaneously and to reveal important personal data.

The foundation for rapport is usually ready-made. Most patients come looking for help and expect that they will get it from a clinician You can build on this expectation by your words and body language, which should express real interest in the patient. Although it is possible that you might inadvertently say something upsetting, there is little you are likely to say or do that cannot be retrieved if you remain caring and sensitive to what your patient is experiencing.

THE BASIS OF RAPPORT

Right from the start, most patients will expect to like you. But real rapport between two individuals doesn't usually spring up overnight. It develops gradually, with long acquaintance, and requires the cooperation of both parties. Still, you can use certain behaviors to speed its growth.

Your demeanor is key. Remember that professionalism doesn't demand stiff formality. In fact, you should take care to avoid the image of the stone-faced therapist that has been popularized in the movies and in fiction. If you appear relaxed, interested, and sympathetic, your patient is more likely to feel safe and comfortable. Carefully monitor your facial expression: Don't frown, grimace, or show other signs that could be interpreted as disapproval. Although you should avoid fixed stares, which can make you appear cold and critical, be sure to make frequent eye contact, even if you are taking notes. Of course, you don't want to appear insincere, but appropriate smiles and nods will demonstrate that you are attentive and sympathetic. However, just at first I'd be a bit sparing in the use of praise. For one thing, praise used as a reinforcer can powerfully shape behavior. But early in any relationship, you don't know enough to be sure what behavior you will be reinforcing; you wouldn't want to praise apparent openness if your patient hasn't told you the whole truth, for instance.

The patient's own demeanor will probably shape your interaction more than any other factor. Body language—drooping shoulders, a clenched fist, restless feet, tears—often clearly indicates how your patient feels. Observe tone of voice for other clues to feelings. Suppose you have asked your patient, Mr. Kimble, how he and his wife get along, and he responds, "Just fine." If his tone is warm and light, the couple probably has relatively few interpersonal problems. If his "Just fine" is delivered between clenched teeth, in a dull monotone, or with a sigh, Mr. Kimble may be harboring feelings of hopelessness or anger that he can't put into words just yet.

Because you have arranged the furniture so you don't have a barrier between you, you can easily and naturally adjust even to minor shifts in your patient's affect, promoting rapport. If your patient is depressed, you will probably feel like drawing a little closer to show your concern. You can follow that natural inclination. If you sense hostility, you may feel like withdrawing physically, even if only a few inches. Doing so will help relax the tension by giving each of you more elbow room. Similarly, you may laugh when your patient makes a joke or display a worried frown of concern and support during a panic attack. By the time you have interviewed your first dozen patients, you will do these things automatically in response to the clues each patient unconsciously gives.

At the same time, you should carefully maintain a certain neutrality toward what you are told. If your patient criticizes relatives, you would be unlikely to defend them. But joining in the criticism risks offending someone whose feelings may be ambivalent. A safe response is an empathic comment that doesn't take sides.

PATIENT: My mother is a real bitch! She keeps trying to interfere between me and my husband.

INTERVIEWER: *(Leans slightly forward.)* That must be a real problem for you.

This interviewer's attitude—sympathetic, nonjudgmental, and respectful of patient and relatives alike—is likely to foster a good working relationship.

ASSESS YOUR OWN FEELINGS

How you feel about the patient can have important consequences. If your feelings are positive—here is the sort of person you would choose as a friend, for example—you will probably come across as warm and caring. Your attitude may serve as an encouragement to reveal additional sensitive information.

Heavily influenced by your own background and upbringing, your feelings could in turn affect your ability to make an accurate evaluation. Throughout the interview, you need to be aware of the nature and the sources of your feelings, especially when something about the patient distresses you. It could be a problem with personal hygiene, coarse language, or the expression of ethnic prejudice. Or this person may remind you of difficulties you had with one of your own relatives. In any case, you must carefully monitor how you respond. If you frown or otherwise appear uncomfortable, your patient may sense your disapproval and frustrate your efforts to gather accurate information.

Your goal is to express *empathy*, which means that on some level you can feel as your patient feels—that you can put yourself in the patient's place. Having empathy means understanding the motivation behind a patient's behavior, even though you may not agree that it was the right thing to do. (Surveys show that mental health clinicians score much higher than do other health care professionals in the ability to take another person's perspective.) You will probably convey your empathic feelings best if you keep in mind this thought: "What would it be like to stand in the shoes of this patient talking with me now?"

This job might seem daunting when your patient shows a lot of anger, anxiety, or even psychosis. Throughout your professional life, you will have to work with all sorts of people. Some of them will seem less agreeable than others, but you will find that there is something in nearly every patient to which you can relate. If you cannot respond pos-

itively to the content of what you are being told, perhaps you can sympathize with some of the feelings behind it. For example, a moderately
antisocial patient was speaking about his former therapist:

> PATIENT: I had no use for that guy. Once or twice I even thought
>   about blowing him away!
> INTERVIEWER: Sounds as if you were feeling really angry.

Trying to deal directly with the content of this patient's comment
would have forced the interviewer to choose whether to agree with or
to confront a potentially violent patient. By keying into the patient's anger, this interviewer said something that both parties could feel comfortable with.

All professionals have feelings, attitudes, and experiences that can
affect the image they project; we must all be constantly alert to prevent
these personal issues from impairing our effectiveness with patients.
Consider the effect of so ordinary an event as divorce:

> One clinician found that she was so upset during the time she was sep-
> arating from her husband that she could not effectively manage a pa-
> tient who was having similar problems.

> Another therapist, after a bruising telephone call from his ex-wife,
> postponed his next interview while he cooled off enough to focus on
> the patient's problems.

Many beginning interviewers have learned that they can alleviate pressure if they introduce themselves to patients as students. But regardless
of your stage of training or practice, your temperament and experience
will determine how you deal with your personal Achilles' heel. Whatever it is, your effectiveness with patients will increase if you remain
aware of your own limitations.

CONSIDER YOUR MANNER OF SPEAKING

For good rapport, the patient must know that you understand. It is
tempting to approach this directly by saying, "I know how you must feel
about . . . " Unhappily, this statement can ring hollow. By the time they
reach your office, many patients have heard it all too often from people
who don't really understand at all, or who may understand quite well
but do nothing to help. Some patients with severe problems, real or

perceived, feel that nobody could possibly appreciate what they are going through. You will probably be better off using some other response to suggest your compassion and interest:

"You must have felt terribly unhappy."

"I've never been in that position, so I can only imagine how you felt."

"That was a terrible experience. I can see that it upset you a great deal."

Sometimes you may find that you need to overemphasize your feelings a little. This suggestion might sound deceitful, but I don't mean it that way. Actors, for example, know that their recorded voices tend to flatten out and that they must overact to get across the feelings they intend to portray. In similar fashion, you may need to amplify your own emotional output to impress upon some patients how deeply you sympathize with them. You can accomplish this with your facial expressions, or with your voice by varying its volume, pitch, and emphasis. Even brief exclamations can do the job. An "Oh, wow!" that is suitably timed and intoned may convey understanding and compassion more effectively than a more elegant speech of condolence. Such emblems of your emotional involvement, which beginning interviewers often forget to use, can be vital to your patient and contribute to building rapport.

However, it's far too easy to go overboard. Consider the patient who comes to you with a story of betrayal by a spouse or lover, or injury in a military or civilian calamity. Of course, you will want to show your support, but if you express your own shock or horror too starkly, you risk reinforcing the traumatic effects you're there to dismantle. Sure, you can go ahead and express sympathy—you can even provide the support of a proffered tissue—but be careful not to portray your patient as a victim.

Consider the use of humor in your interactions with patients. Humor can be a great facilitator of communication: It helps people to relax and feel that they are among friends. But as a clinician, take care to judge your use of humor carefully. With any recent acquaintance, it is easy to misjudge and say something in jest that can be taken amiss; mental health patients are especially vulnerable to this sort of slip. Even a patient you know well could misinterpret an ill-considered remark. As always, put yourself in the patient's place: Consider how you'd feel if you thought your clinician was laughing at you.

In general, it is safe to laugh with, but never at, the patient. That means that you should generally let the patient start it. During your first few sessions, any use of humor should be gentle, and only when it is clear that the patient is in a frame of mind to appreciate it. Beware of making jokes (they might be misinterpreted as hostile or demeaning). Whenever the patient jests, be sure to evaluate whether this is a sub-conscious attempt to sidetrack both of you from a discussion of impor-tant material.

Experienced interviewers report that they sometimes seemingly undergo a personality change as they move from one patient to the next. They may adopt a formal tone with one, then settle into a folksy persona with the next patient. One interviewer persistently, and quite unconsciously, dropped his g's when talking with a patient from a rural background who spoke that way. Within limits these behaviors are probably acceptable, though you should be careful not to overdo them to the point of mimicry.

Regardless of your level of experience, at some point, with some patient, you will make an error. In the greater scheme of things, it will probably be of rather minor significance—you ask the same question twice, you forget the occupation of your patient's spouse, or you are suddenly aware that your mind has drifted and you can't recall the question your patient has just asked (or that you have!)—but both of you know that you've erred. You should take immediate steps to put it right. "Uh-oh, senior moment," I might say with a rueful smile. If you aren't so fortunate as to have old age for an excuse, you should admit that you focused for a moment on something else, and do whatever is necessary to correct your error (for example, ask the patient to restate the question). Almost always, the conversation will move safely for-ward.

TALK THE PATIENT'S LANGUAGE

Take pains to speak in terms your patient can understand. Your poorly educated patient may recognize "polite" terms for sexual or excretory functions, but the relationship you develop may be better if you use plain language. Listen to your patient's language and use it, as long as you feel comfortable doing so. Because teenagers and young adults of-ten distrust older people, they may respond more positively if you use language that is current for their generation. But be sure that your "cool" expression is still "in," or you risk being considered merely "square." (There is another point of view on this issue. Some adoles-cent patients may resent it enormously and become even more distrust-ful if you try to adopt their speech patterns.) How you speak to any pa-tient should be guided by the need for clarity and rapport, so monitor your patient's reactions and adjust your manner of speaking accord-ingly.

Certain terms may serve as red flags for many patients. These loaded words carry a message of illness, failure, or poor character, and you should generally avoid them. Here is a brief sample: *abortion, bad, brain damage, cancer, crazy, defective, fantasy, frigidity, hysterical, impotence, neurotic, obscene, perversion, victim*. You will encounter many more during your interviewing career. Be ready with neutral synonyms for such words, or, better, pick up on terms your patient already has used.

Avoid psychological jargon. Even simple terms like *psychosis* may be misunderstood, and your patient could think that you seem insensitive toward someone with less education than you. Also ensure that you understand your patient's own use of language; don't assume it is the same as yours. For example, to you "an occasional drink" may mean once a month, but to your patient it could mean "intermittently throughout the day." Does your teenaged patient drink *Coke* or snort coke? In the language of the street, "I was really paranoid" doesn't mean that the speaker felt psychotically persecuted, but merely frightened.

If your patient is foreign-born or was reared in another part of your own country, you may have trouble understanding one another. Don't let your manner imply that it is the patient who "talks funny." Rather, acknowledge that you have different accents and that at times you may have to ask one another for repetition. For a patient who hesitates or seems unsure of how to proceed, you can remove some of the pressure with the reassurance that it is "fine to take this at your own pace, so I can really understand what you're experiencing." On the flip side, to be sure you *do* understand, you may want to translate into simpler language the sometimes florid terms that patients use to express themselves perhaps to obfuscate, perhaps because they think a clinician wants to hear psychological terms.

PATIENT: I've always had a phobia about cats I've got four of 'em.

INTERVIEWER: So you're a real cat fancier!

Later on, perhaps, when you've gotten to know one another better, you can supply an accurate definition.

MAINTAIN BOUNDARIES

How clinicians should relate to their patients has been a moving target in recent years. The traditional image of an authoritarian lawgiver who decides *for* the patient has in many quarters been supplanted by that of a less formal collaborator who explores problems and their solutions *with* the patient. I strongly prefer the latter style. To me it feels more comfortable (it is less arrogant), and it encourages patients to participate in treatment decisions. In effect, it puts two minds to work, rather than loading all the responsibility on the clinician. When patients discuss and contribute to their own management plans, they are more likely to comply with treatment and less likely to complain about bumps in the road to improvement.

Yet even clinicians who encourage friendly collaboration need to maintain boundaries. When I practiced in California, it was customary to call patients by their first names. For adolescents this seemed just fine. But I heard even old men and women addressed in this overly familiar manner by mental health professionals young enough to be their grandchildren. It tends to infantilize patients, who, if they are hospital inpatients, have already lost considerable autonomy. It also increases the professional person's tendency to become *parentalistic*—that is, to make health care decisions that patients should be making for themselves.

However, before I make *too* big a deal of this, let me note that times have changed and that many therapists have maintained successful practices while they and their patients address one another in familiar terms. I still reject the idea of first names for hospitalized patients, and I continue to call my adult patients by last name and title (Miss, Ms., Mrs., or Mr. Green). This practice maximizes personal dignity and reinforces a sense of adulthood, even at a time when there may be loss of autonomy. It also encourages patients to keep a certain emotional distance by using my title and last name. This distance may sometimes help head off inappropriate attempts at amorous and other nonprofessional relationships.

If a patient appears offended when I don't agree to a first-name basis, I respond that it is my habit always to use last names and titles, and that it would be hard for me to change. (If you are still a student, your excuse might be that this is what your institution requires of trainees, if that's the case.) Rarely I have encountered patients who doggedly insist on using their first names. If I judge that sticking to my habit could harm our relationship, I will use *two* names—first and second or first and last—*plus* title. For example, when calling such a patient from the waiting room, I will announce, "Mrs. Joanne Cremier," and say it with a big, friendly smile. So far, this compromise has always proven satisfactory.

In general, it is a good idea not to reveal too much about yourself to your patients. This is especially true during the initial interview, when you really don't know one another very well.

A beginning psychiatry resident confided to his new patient that he was a reserve peace officer. He later learned to his chagrin that the patient had both a severe personality disorder and an abiding hatred of the police.

If you are having difficulty getting information from a patient, you might be able to encourage greater cooperation by identifying something that the two of you share. For example, you might remark that, just like the patient, you enjoy sailboating or were born in Indiana. Your status as fellow sailors or Hoosiers might nudge you a bit closer to the rapport you seek. This technique should be used sparingly—seldom more than once with a given patient—lest you begin to sound too familiar. You should also be careful not to let any resulting small talk distract you for long from the real purpose of your interview.

Why do patients ask personal questions? Some stem from simple curiosity; others may cloak concern about interviewers' professional backgrounds or ability to help. To provide reassurance about training and competence is one reason why clinicians in practice display a wall full of diplomas, licenses, and other certificates. Trainees often have the benefit of neither certificates nor wall. Still, to whatever degree possible, you should verbally provide this information when it is requested. Don't hesitate to invoke the names and positions of your supervisors if this is needed to reassure an especially anxious patient.

Some requests for personal information may be prompted by a largely unconscious desire to achieve a sense of equality between interviewer and patient. Others may cloak an attempt to avoid discussing sensitive material, and these should be handled firmly but with tact:

PATIENT: How old are you, anyway?

INTERVIEWER: Why do you want to know?

PATIENT: You seem so young to be doing this kind of work.

INTERVIEWER: Well, thank you for the compliment, but I don't think my age is especially relevant to our discussion; let's focus on you. Now, to get back to the question I asked . . .

In some circumstances, personal information may seem relevant to your interview. If you decide that this is the case, you should usually reveal something of yourself:

PATIENT: Were you raised in this city?

INTERVIEWER: What makes you ask that?

PATIENT: My mother told me to be sure to get a therapist who grew up here. She says no one else could really understand what it was like, growing up in a ghetto and all.

INTERVIEWER: I see. Actually, I didn't grow up here, but this is where I took most of my training. I've lived in town for nearly 8 years, so I think I have a pretty good idea of what some of your experiences must have been. But I have the feeling you'll be able to tell me a whole lot more.

Whenever it seems reasonable, I tend to answer questions frankly, because I believe it speeds the building of rapport.

SHOW YOUR EXPERTISE

You can pave yet another pathway to rapport by informing the patient that you know something about the presenting symptoms and what they could mean. This assessment will naturally come at the end of the initial interview, when you've obtained enough information to know what you're talking about. Then you'll probably say something like this:

"Your condition is actually pretty common—one of the most frequent problems patients bring to mental health clinicians. I've seen several similar cases just in the last few months. We have several good treatment approaches available, so we can look for a good outcome in your case."

Even if you are facing a rare condition, you can reassure the patient that you know where to turn for guidance:

"We can work through this problem together."

If you're a student, you probably won't have had much in the way of personal experience with your patient's condition—or any other. But you are connected with a training program that employs experienced teachers who have encountered many patients with similar conditions.

I would offer a few warnings about showing expertise. First, a natural consequence of empathy is respect, which implies that you should take pains to avoid sounding authoritarian. Sounding *authoritative* is fine, if it's accurate, but sounding *authoritarian* smacks of the old, parentalistic clinical style that seems disrespectful in the 21st century. It never did work all that well, anyway. Second, in your zeal to put your patient at ease, don't succumb to the patient's too-early request for information or advice. A part of being expert is waiting until you have the facts to justify offering support. Jumping in too soon with a diagnosis or with suggestions for treatment can sometimes lead to embarrassing backpedaling down the line. Finally, try to wear your erudition lightly. Preface your opinions with "I think" or "In my experience"— the patient will honor them just as well, and you'll avoid the need to live up to an aura of infallibility that no one can sustain.

Inevitably, you will encounter patients you just cannot work with. Sometimes this will be due to your own feelings—about unrepentant criminal behavior, perhaps, or about someone who reminds you far too strongly of your own former spouse. At other times you'll be tipped off by something the patient says, such as a statement of preference for "a Christian therapist" or some other therapeutic orientation that just plain doesn't fit.

Such patients will probably be few, but you have a duty to face them honestly. Of course, to be sure your first impressions are correct, you should complete the evaluation before deciding. Then you might say something like this:

"Quite frankly, I'm not sure I'm the right person to deal with your problem."

You'd go on to explain why you've come to this opinion (leaving out the unflattering bits) and where you would recommend the patient go next:

"Yours is the sort of problem that I haven't had much experience with. However, I know someone in this same building who has made a study of people with your kind of difficulty. If you'd like, I can write a note that describes my findings in your case."

Chapter 4

Managing the Early Patient Interview

A few minutes into most initial interview sessions, the patient should be relaxed and giving you the information you need; much of your task right now will be simply to keep your patient talking. Most patients feel highly motivated to talk, and you will usually need only to choose the device that will best encourage them to do so. (If this isn't the case with your interview, you can review the material in Chapters 16 and 17 for help.)

To keep speech flowing freely, intrude as little as you can. Anything you say—questions, comments, even clearing your throat—can prove distracting. As long as you are finding out why your patient came for treatment, you should keep out of the way. In practical terms, you will usually just listen for only the first couple of minutes or so. Then the flow of information will slow down or take a wrong turn, and you will have to intervene. Your choice of interventions can help determine the overall success of your interview.

NONVERBAL ENCOURAGEMENTS

Your most frequent challenge may be to deal with silence. Beginners often find silence hard to tolerate. They feel that every hole in the conversation, no matter how small, must be filled up with words. It is true that pauses greater than 10 or 15 seconds can make an interviewer seem cold, and this discourages some patients. Briefer pauses often mean only that your patient is trying to organize some thoughts for further discussion. Don't let anxiety cause you to derail a train of thought that has only paused to gather steam.

You must learn to walk the line between allowing brief pauses to let your patient think and long gaps that make you seem unfeeling or uninterested. A glance should tell you whether the narrative is still underway. Watch for the patient to draw another breath or to show other signs of activity, such as the moistening of lips.

You can encourage further speech by using nonverbal cues of your own. Be careful not to break eye contact; a smile or nod will say, "You're doing fine; just keep on going at your own pace." Another technique experienced interviewers sometimes use almost without thinking is to lean a little closer to show interest in what the patient is saying. Nonverbal cues of this sort are the simplest and often the most useful encouragements you can use. Without interrupting, they clearly signal that you are attentive and interested; they are part of a universal body language that asks the patient to continue. But don't overemphasize any of these gestures: A clinician who nods too vigorously or smiles too broadly may distract the patient, who wonders what these antics mean.

VERBAL ENCOURAGEMENTS

Body language helps, but you will also have to do some talking. Your choice of words is important: You want to facilitate, not distract. Therefore, speak as briefly as you can while still conveying your meaning.

A syllable or two is usually all it takes. "Yes" or "Mm-hmm" clearly indicates that the material is registering with you. Without being directive, brief interjections and phrases ask the patient to keep on talking. Use them frequently, perhaps interspersing them randomly with nonverbal encouragements. One such encouragement every minute or two should help keep your patient talking.

There are several other verbal techniques you can use to request additional information. These are more intrusive than those just mentioned, so you should use them sparingly. I will illustrate each—some of them have been termed "reflective listening"—with a brief example.

- Repeat your patient's own last word or two with a rising inflection in your voice to make a question of it.

  PATIENT: I was so upset that for hours I seemed to be hearing voices. *(Pauses.)*

  INTERVIEWER: "Voices"?

  PATIENT: In my head. I thought I heard the voice of my mother calling my name.

- Elaborate on a word the patient used earlier. This technique allows you to reach back to an idea that was *not* the last thought spoken.

PATIENT: I know I overreacted, but I was feeling desperate. I couldn't sleep or eat, and I screamed at my kids.

INTERVIEWER: You said you felt desperate. *(Pauses.)*

PATIENT: Yes, I even considered suicide.

- Directly request more information.

"Tell me more about that."
"How do you mean?"

- Re-request information when the patient seems to have misinterpreted your original question.

INTERVIEWER: What kind of work do you do?

PATIENT: It's at the foundry on Elm Street.

INTERVIEWER: And what kind of work do you do there?

- Offer brief summaries. These will often begin with "So you feel that . . . " or "Do you mean that . . . "

INTERVIEWER: So for about 6 months now you've been feeling depressed and anxious.

PATIENT: That's right. Lately I've even started to think terrible thoughts—thoughts about killing myself.

Sometimes you'll get information you don't really want. It isn't that descriptions of recent vacations, children's antics, and names of lovers are uninteresting, but they can take up time you could better spend pursuing other issues. Although you might be able to discourage this sort of verbal wild-goose chase by simply not reinforcing it, it is often better to be direct with your patient:

"That's interesting, and maybe we can get back to it later, but right now I'd like to know about . . . "

Or perhaps to be even more direct:

"No, let's keep our focus on information that can help me help you."

OFFERING REASSURANCE

Reassurance is anything you do to increase a patient's sense of confidence or well-being. Because it shows that you like or are interested in a person, it can also foster rapport. Used sparingly during the initial interview, supportive statements say, "I'm on your side. We'll get this job done."

Any interview can be therapeutic. Studies have shown that the mere act of sharing problems with another human being (even, in some cases, with a computer!) can help a person take a new view of old issues or put ideas together in novel ways. But with a new patient, you can't just jump in and start giving advice, making interpretations, or otherwise "doing therapy." Rather, the purpose of the initial interview is to obtain the information you need to plan treatment. On the other hand, you shouldn't pass up an opportunity to provide reassurance, as long as it doesn't interfere with the main goal of your interview. You might even raise the confidence of some patients enough that they will reveal especially sensitive material you would not otherwise have obtained.

Body language (smiles and nods) can be reassuring, but mostly you will reassure with speech. To be truly reassuring, what you say must be based in fact. You wouldn't get far saying, "You have a good head for finances," to a patient who in 45 years hasn't saved a nickel toward retirement. And choose your words carefully. Avoid clichés and other stereotyped expressions, which will make you sound as if you are responding only by rote, not from the heart.

Supportive reassurance must be factual, sincere, and specific to the situation. Here are two examples:

PATIENT: I did manage to get two promotions last year.

INTERVIEWER: So you've really done well with that job!

PATIENT: When he came at me with a knife, I jumped right through a second-story window onto a garage roof. It made me feel dumb. I thought I'd just saved him the work of cutting me to ribbons.

INTERVIEWER: It may have saved your life! Perhaps it was the only thing you could have done.

Avoid false generalizations that come too early in the interview or are based on too little fact. "I'm sure it will all work out," or "Those fears seem groundless," will probably ring hollow to most patients, especially those with paranoia or severe depression; they *know* things won't turn out well! Even those who are less severely ill might begin to question your knowledge if you leap in quickly with bland reassurances that cover too much ground to be believable.

Occasionally a patient will express concern based on a misconception about mental or physical phenomena. Then you can use your expertise to set the record straight without interfering with the history taking.

> PATIENT: I'd never even been to California before, but I suddenly thought, "I've been on this same San Francisco street before." I wondered if I was losing my mind.

> INTERVIEWER: That feeling is called *déjà vu*. It's very common, and doesn't mean anything at all is wrong. Now tell me what happened next.

Notice, however, that this interviewer did make the mistake of providing *unconditional* reassurance. Although *déjà vu* is nearly always a benign phenomenon, it is sometimes associated with neurological conditions such as temporal lobe epilepsy. But without more substantiating evidence, to suggest that there could be any pathological significance would also be a serious mistake. Here is a reasonable compromise: "It doesn't *usually* signify that anything is wrong."

Be careful to avoid offhand comments that may prove disquieting. One patient described a sexual encounter with her cousin, then said that she didn't know if that would be considered molestation. "It sure sounds like molestation to me," responded the young interviewer. This response had the potential for raising anxieties that the patient was not ready to deal with. ("How do you regard it?" would have been a safer response.)

Mostly, your efforts at reassurance and encouragement will meet with success. Nevertheless, any of these techniques can sometimes backfire. A patient with persecutory delusions might interpret even a friendly nod or smile as mockery. If you lean toward someone who is feeling angry, you might be rewarded not with more information, but with hostility or deepening silence. Judging when a patient will not be receptive can be tricky. Your best bet is to start slowly. Be friendly and pleasant, but not aggressively so.

Watch for cues. If you are being too aggressively forward, your patient may exhibit some of these behaviors:

> Loss of eye contact
> Frozen expression
> Decreased speech output
> Nervous shifting of position

If you spot any of these telltale signs, quickly change to a more reserved manner.

Chapter 5

History of the Present Illness

Once you feel that there are no additional major problem areas to discover, close the period of free speech and move smoothly into the history of the present illness. (However, throughout the balance of your history taking, listen carefully for other clues that might point the way for further explorations.) Now you will explore more thoroughly the problems that have brought the patient into treatment—the "meat" of the initial interview, including a description of symptoms, their timing, and possible stressors for each of the problems you've identified. To aid this process, you might consider the areas of clinical interest that you covered during free speech. These areas were first mentioned in Chapter 2; because they include material from the mental status examination, they will not be considered fully until Chapter 13.

Although some patients have no diagnosable disorder, it is a convention to label as "illness" whatever brings anyone in for evaluation. In this broad sense, then, marital disagreements and other problems of living—even the desire to understand oneself better—may constitute a present "illness" that no one, least of all the patient, would recognize as disease. But all of these problems do have precipitants, symptoms, course, and other features that will allow you to suggest an effective plan of action.

THE PRESENT EPISODE

Although you will eventually want to learn about any and all episodes, concentrate first on the current episode of illness. Your patient will be most concerned about it, and its details will be freshest in the minds of all your informants. Of course, you'll need a fund of basic information as to exactly what symptoms you can expect to find in an episode of illness. For that, you'll need to refer to textbooks and other resources that cover this material (I've written one or two of these myself). Appendix D in this book presents a semistructured interview that covers the symptoms typically found in the more common mental disorders. If your early interviewing experiences are anything like mine (see the very beginning of the Introduction to this book), you'll benefit by returning to your patient to ask the questions you've forgotten the first—or second—time around.

DESCRIBING SYMPTOMS

Learn as much as you can about each symptom your patient reports. (Remember that a *symptom* is any subjective sensation that makes the patient think that something is wrong. A symptom could be a pain, a hallucination, a feeling of anxiety, or any of many other thoughts, feelings, or behaviors.) Clarify any descriptive terms that are used: For example, what does *nervous* mean to the patient?

Characterize each symptom as fully as you can. Is it always present, or does it come and go (episodic)? If episodic, as is the case with anxiety attacks and many depressions, how often does it occur? How intense is it? Is it always the same, or does it vary? Remember that symptoms can wax and wane with time or with changes in the environment. Has the patient noticed any factors (such as activity or time of day) that seem to be associated with the symptom? Has the intensity or frequency of the symptom been increasing, staying the same, or decreasing? When your patient has the symptom, how long does it last? In what context does it occur? (Only at night? Only when alone? Or at any time at all?)

How does the patient describe the symptom? Pain can feel cutting, burning, crushing, sharp, or dull. Auditory hallucinations can be described as to their content (noises, mumbles, isolated words, complete sentences), location (inside the patient's head, in the air, out in the hall), and intensity (ranging from loud screams to faraway whispers). Other sorts of hallucination—of vision, touch, smell, or taste—can be described similarly. I'll have more to say about this in Chapter 12.

VEGETATIVE SYMPTOMS

Many patients with serious problems such as anxiety attacks, depressions, and psychoses have experienced *vegetative symptoms.* This old term refers to body functions that are concerned with maintaining health and vigor. Vegetative symptoms include problems with sleep, appetite, weight change, energy level, and sexual interest.

Not every patient will spontaneously report these symptoms, but they are found in so many of the more serious mental disorders that they serve as a useful screening tool. You should ask about them routinely. Look especially for evidence of *change* from previous normal functioning. You may find one or more of the following responses:

• *Sleep.* Your patient may complain of either excessive sleepiness (hypersomnia) or inability to sleep (insomnia). If the latter, find out what portion of the normal sleep period is affected—early (initial insomnia), middle (interval insomnia), or late (terminal insomnia). Terminal insomnia is usually associated with more severe mental problems, such as depression with melancholia. Initial insomnia is much more common; many normal adults experience this from time to time when they have problems of living. Interval insomnia, in the form of awakening with nightmares, may be found in patients who drink alcohol heavily or who have posttraumatic stress disorder (PTSD). Here is how you might inquire about problems with sleep:

INTERVIEWER: Have you had any problems with your sleeping?

PATIENT: Yeah, it's been murder.

INTERVIEWER: What sort of trouble have you had?

PATIENT: What do you mean?

INTERVIEWER: Well, what part of the night do you not sleep well?

PATIENT: Oh. Mostly, it's trouble getting to sleep.

INTERVIEWER: Do you ever wake up early in the morning, before it's time to get up, and then you can't get back to sleep?

PATIENT: Yeah, that too. I do that a lot.

INTERVIEWER: How long do you usually sleep?

PATIENT: Lately, I guess . . . probably only 4 or 5 hours.

INTERVIEWER: And do you feel rested when you wake up?

PATIENT: Yeah, rested like I've been hauling bricks all night!

INTERVIEWER: How much of a change is this for you?

• *Appetite and weight.* These, too, may increase or decrease with an episode of illness. You should also learn how significant the change has been (how much weight has the patient gained or lost, and over what period of time?) Also ask whether this weight change was intentional. Some patients will tell you that they have not weighed themselves recently; asking whether clothing has become too loose or too tight may help you judge.

• *Energy level.* Does the patient complain of feeling constantly tired? Is this a change from what's usual for this person? Has it interfered in some way with performance at work or school, or with getting jobs done around the house? You may also hear complaints of change in other body functions, such as bowel habits. For example, some severely depressed patients experience constipation.

• *Diurnal variation of mood.* This phrase refers to the tendency of some patients to feel better during a certain part of the day. Patients with severe depression often feel worse upon arising and better as the day goes on. By bedtime they may feel nearly normal. Those who are less depressed are more likely to report feeling better early in the day, but depressed, sluggish, and weary by nightfall.

• *Sexual interest and performance.* Sexual functioning usually depends strongly upon the individual's sense of well-being. Therefore, loss of interest in sex is often an early casualty of mental distress. Also learn how these aspects of the patient's sex life have changed: frequency, ability, and enjoyment. The direction of change could be either up or down, depending on the specific mental health problem. Number and choice of partners can also be affected if judgment is impaired. A more detailed description of sexual symptoms and patterns will be given in Chapter 9.

CONSEQUENCES OF ILLNESS

Mental disorder can interfere with the entire range of human interaction. For several reasons, it is important to learn how your patient's illness has affected functioning and relationships in all of life's areas, including social, educational/occupational, and familial.

1. It may provide your most reliable index of severity. So far, most of the history you have heard is highly subjective: You depend on your patient's ability to sort out facts from opinions. Partly because it can be verified by talking with informants, the fact that a patient has not gone to work for a week may be subject to less distortion than, say, how much vodka this same patient has consumed.

2. The diagnosis of some disorders depends heavily on social consequences: What have been the effects on the patient? On others? Substance use disorders and antisocial personality disorder are examples of conditions that can entail legal, financial, health, and interpersonal problems.

3. You may learn that relatives blame the patient for being fired, getting divorced, or separating from family members. Yet these and

various other ruptured human relationships are really *effects* of mental disorder. This view may prove useful to patient and relatives alike: Teaching family and friends about the consequences of illness can help get your patient off the hook.

To learn what social problems your patient's illness has caused, start with an open-ended question that doesn't limit the information you might obtain. If your patient asks what your question means, respond with some examples of the sort of facts that would interest you.

INTERVIEWER: What sort of difficulties has this problem caused you?

PATIENT: What do you mean, difficulties?

INTERVIEWER: For example, it would help to know whether your problem has changed the way you get along with your family, your friends, the job, hobbies—that sort of thing.

Be sure to obtain details about any positive answers. Areas to explore include the following:

• *Marital/couple.* Patients who are even moderately ill commonly experience discord in their marriages and other love relationships. All too often, mental disorder can lead to divorce or breakup.

• *Interpersonal.* Has your patient felt estranged from relatives or shunned by friends? Can you tell whether this is only a perceived problem, or has behavior been problematic long enough that others really do avoid the patient?

• *Legal.* Have there been legal difficulties? They are especially likely when the history is complicated by alcohol or other substance use. Ask:

"Have you ever had any police or legal difficulties?"

"Have you ever been arrested? How many times?"

"Have you been in jail? For a total of how long?"

"Have you ever been committed to an institution or placed under the control of a conservator, guardian, or fiduciary?"

These serious legal steps are usually taken only after a long siege of severe mental illness. Be sure to obtain details: events leading up to the legal action; duration; name and responsibilities of the legally responsible person; and the effect the action has had upon the course of the disorder.

• *Occupational/educational.* As a result of emotional problems, has the patient ever missed work, quit work, or been fired? How often has this happened? Difficulties with job performance are sometimes noted by supervisors or coworkers even before family members take much notice of the patient's difficulties. For younger patients, the questions to consider would be about school attendance and performance.

• *Disability payments.* Have benefits been awarded from the Department of Veterans Affairs (VA), the Social Security Administration, a state compensation board, or private insurance? For what disorder? What is the dollar amount? How long will the payments last?

• *Interests.* Has interest in hobbies, reading, or watching TV changed? What about chores at home? Has interest in sex either increased or decreased? What about sexual performance? Have there been complaints of impotence, painful intercourse, or inability to have climax? There's more about this in Chapter 9.

• *Symptoms.* How much discomfort do the symptoms cause? What fears does your patient have about the meanings of the symptoms? Do they seem to imply death or permanent disability? Insanity? This information will also help you evaluate depth of insight and soundness of judgment, which we'll discuss in Chapter 12.

ONSET AND SEQUENCE OF SYMPTOMS

In addition to a complete and accurate description of the symptoms, you should establish their timing and sequence. When did these problems begin? Sometimes the onset may be reported quite precisely: "I started drinking again last New Year's Eve," or "I woke up feeling depressed a week ago Thursday." But more often the answer will be less exact, either because the patient is vague or because that episode began so gradually that you cannot pinpoint the onset.

Try to encourage precision about the onset of especially noticeable symptoms. (Sometimes details are especially important, as in the case of the first episode of panic or the horrific event precipitating PTSD.) Patients can often remember the first time they experienced such important problems as death wishes or loss of interest in sex. You might be able to relate onset to noteworthy dates or events.

INTERVIEWER: Had you started to feel depressed by the Fourth of July last year?

PATIENT: No, I don't think so.

INTERVIEWER: What about in the fall, around the time of your birthday?

No matter how much you prompt, some patients simply can't give a date or even an approximation: "I only know it's been a long time. A very long time." Pressing further for a precise answer will probably only frustrate both of you. Try focusing instead on something the patient may have thought about many times:

"When did you last feel well?"

If even this effort fails, at least try to learn which of your patient's several problems started first. It is often important for diagnosis and treatment to know, for example, whether an episode of depression or a bout of drinking began earlier. So ask:

"Which symptoms did you notice first, the drinking or the depression?"

"How long did it take before the other symptom developed?"

If symptoms fluctuate:

"Do they do so together?"

STRESSORS

Of course, having mental symptoms is enormously stressful itself, but here we will consider stress in a different sense. A *stressor* is any condition or event that seems to cause, precipitate, or worsen a patient's mental health problems.

"My husband ran off with his secretary."

"I didn't want to be dependent on medicine any longer, so I stopped taking it."

"My cat died."

The variety of possible stressors is vast, and what might be mildly stressful for one person could seem catastrophic to another. For years the diagnostic manuals have listed nine groups of potential psychosocial and environmental problems, comprising many individual stressors. In Table 3, I have paraphrased many of these stressors. They should have occurred within the year prior to your evaluation. If they took place earlier, they must be a focus of treatment or have contributed to the development of the mental disorder to count as a current stressor. When stating them on Axis IV, be as specific as possible.

Patients often mention stressors during free speech, or even when stating the chief complaint. If they don't, you will have to ask. A good time to do so is right after you have pinned down the approximate onset of the episode of illness. If you find a stressor, try to learn how it affected the course of your patient's difficulty. Ask:

"Was anything happening then that might have started your symptoms?"

TABLE 3. Psychosocial and Environmental Problems

These stressors may have been caused by an Axis I or Axis II disorder, or they may be independent events.

Access to health care services: inadequate insurance or health care services; lack of transportation to health care services

Economic: marked poverty; inadequate finances or welfare support

Educational: academic problems; arguments with classmates or teachers; illiteracy; inadequate school environment

Housing: homelessness; inadequate housing; dangerous neighborhood; arguments with landlord or neighbors

Legal system/crime: arrest; incarceration; litigation; being the victim of crime

Occupational: stressful work conditions or schedule; job change or dissatisfaction; arguments with supervisor or coworkers; retirement; unemployment; threatened job loss

Social environment: death or loss of friend; difficulty with acculturation; discrimination; living alone; social isolation

Support group: death or illness of relative; family disruption by divorce or separation; parent's remarriage; physical or sexual abuse; discord with relative

Other: arguments with nonfamily caregivers (counselor, social workers, physician); unavailable social service agencies; exposure to disasters, war, or other hostilities

---

"How did it affect you?"

If your patient can think of no possible stressor, you should run through a list of possibilities, pausing briefly to allow thinking time:

"Could there have been anything that happened at home? At work? With friends? Any legal problems? Sickness? Problems with the kids? With your spouse?"

For some episodes of illness you'll find no stressors at all, but to a patient almost anything can seem a possible cause of emotional disorder. Therefore, events reported as stressors may include births, deaths, marriages, divorces, job loss, broken love affairs, health problems, and virtually any other emotional trauma you can think of, as well as many life experiences that might seem routine.

But just because your patient identifies something as a stressor, this doesn't mean that it actually caused the disorder to happen. Often two events simply occur by coincidence, but we humans tend to blame any problem on whatever happened before it. For example, if you carefully checked the time course of Mrs. Albertson's depression, you might find that she had some symptoms—perhaps insomnia and some crying spells—even before her husband left her.

Another patient's "stressor" may seem an unlikely cause of illness—

as in the case of the woman whose overwhelming depression started, she said, when she learned her niece was pregnant. Whether or not the stressor seems related to the disorder, note it down. You can evaluate it later in the light of everything else you learn about your patient.

Even though you might find nothing that has precipitated the episode of mental illness, try to answer this question: Why does your patient appear for evaluation now? In some cases, it will not have been the patient's choice, but someone else who perceived the need for help in a suicide attempt, the purchase of a gun, or acute intoxication. If the answer isn't so obvious, the best approach is to ask:

"This problem has been bothering you for a long time. What made you seek help now?"

When the patient has come voluntarily for evaluation, you are likely to hear about the urging of concerned relatives, fear of losing a valued job, or the patient's own anxiety about worsening symptoms.

PREVIOUS EPISODES

Knowing about previous episodes of the same or a similar mental condition can help you determine diagnosis and prognosis for the future. By this time you may already have heard details about any prior episodes. If not, ask:

"When was the first time you felt like this?"

"Did you first seek treatment then or later?"

"Why did you delay?"

"What was the diagnosis?" (There may have been more than one.)

Since that first attack, has there ever been complete recovery, or has the patient continued to have some residual symptoms or a change of personality? This issue of complete recovery can be critically important. For example, it can help differentiate schizophrenia (from which most patients never totally recover) from mood disorder with psychosis (which usually resolves completely).

How has your patient reacted to previous symptoms or prior episodes of illness? Some patients may have simply ignored them; others might have tried to escape by quitting work, running away from home, attempting suicide, or abusing alcohol or other drugs. People who experience auditory hallucinations sometimes play the radio loudly to drown out the sound. A few will have talked with a friend or a religious counselor. Whatever coping behavior was used, this information may help you evaluate the severity of the present episode by comparing it with earlier episodes. It could also help you predict how your patient would behave if the illness continued untreated.

PREVIOUS TREATMENT

Has your patient received treatment before? If so, who provided it? Try to learn the name, and certainly the profession, of the therapist. How long did treatment last?

You should also try to evaluate how well the patient complied with treatment. If you ask a straight question about this, pride or guilt may cause some patients to have trouble answering the question fairly. Try instead:

"Were you usually able to follow your therapist's directions?"
If the answer to that question is "No," ask:

"What sort of trouble did you have?"

Were drugs prescribed? If so, which ones and at what doses? Were there any side effects to drug therapy? If your patient doesn't know the names of previous medications, a physical description of the tablets or capsules may give you or a pharmacist consultant some clues. A list of side effects may also help you with drug identification. Find out whether injectable medications were ever used, especially the long-acting injectable antipsychotics such as the decanoate form of flu-phenazine (Prolixin) and haloperidol (Haldol).

What have been the effects of previous treatment—has anything helped? If so, try to get an opinion as to which treatment helped most (talking with a therapist? behavior therapy? electroconvulsive therapy? medications?). You could be surprised. Even though an antipsychotic might be the current medication, your patient might answer that lithium helped most, and ask for it again.

Was the patient ever hospitalized? If so, how many times? Where, and for how long? If time is short and your patient is both knowledge-able and cooperative, you might instead ask for a written summary of previous hospitalizations and treatment to be given to you at your next interview.

Chapter 6

Getting the Facts about the Present Illness

Of all portions of the initial mental health interview, the history of the present illness is probably the most important. (It is also frequently neglected.) Here is where you will develop most of the information and test the hypotheses that provide the basis for your diagnosis. This process requires that you obtain highly valid information; that is, it should reflect as closely as possible the true facts of your patient's history. You can take several steps to increase the validity of the information you record in your history of the present illness.

BE CLEAR ABOUT THE GOALS OF YOUR INTERVIEW

Ideally, your patient will understand your expectations for accuracy from the very beginning of your interview. Still, in the middle of the interview, your apparently truthful patient may appear to be holding back on you. Something in that patient's manner may tell you—a hesitation of speech or an unwillingness to look you in the eye. Of course, your first task should be to try to understand any such behavior; we'll cover in detail the reasons for patient resistance in Chapter 16. For minor evasions and omissions, it may be enough simply to restate the goal of your interview:

"I know some of these topics are hard to talk about, but to help you most, I need every scrap of information I can get."

If you are a student, you will have less authority to require cooperation, so you might try something like this:

"I'm sorry to be causing you distress with this line of questioning, but you've really been helping me with my studies. I know it's painful to talk about, but maybe getting in touch with some of these memories and feelings could even help you understand your problems."

It can be especially hard to obtain good-quality facts from teenagers. Some teens worry a lot about what you might tell their parents; others may mistrust everyone more than 5 years older than they are. Whatever the cause, some teenagers have trouble telling the truth. It sometimes helps to repeat your reassurances about confidentiality. I say something like this:

"As you'd expect, after we're finished I will have to talk with your parents. But anything I might tell them I will first discuss with you. And as long as I think you're safe, if you tell me anything that you don't want me to repeat, I'll respect that confidence."

In some states you can counsel or treat teenagers for certain indications such as venereal disease and birth control, even without informing their parents. By assuring confidentiality when teens might be afraid to tell their parents, these states have enacted laws in the hopes of encouraging young people to consult appropriate caregivers about important health conditions. In such a case you might work with your patient to determine the best way of informing the parent, but you shouldn't take it upon yourself to volunteer this information. If a teenager is brought in by a parent, then you would usually consult the parent—after informing your patient what you plan to say.

Information that isn't valid can be confusing, especially in the initial interview, so some clinicians begin interviews with teenagers by indicating that they prefer silence to misinformation. Here's how they might put it:

"A lot of the questions I am going to ask you are personal. Some of them may be pretty embarrassing or even frightening. But if I'm to help you, it's important that I not get confused by something that isn't the truth. So if you can't bear to discuss what I'm asking about, please don't make up an answer. Just say that you don't want to talk about that now, and we'll go on to something else."

TRACK YOUR DISTRACTIONS

Hardly any interviewer proceeds smoothly and logically, covering one topic completely before moving on to another. In fact, experienced interviewers expect to be distracted from time to time by—well, the unexpected. When new material interrupts the flow of your interview, you can either pursue it immediately or, if you feel the first topic is more important, make a note to come back to it later. If you choose the latter course, you should acknowledge that your patient has said something important and promise that you will return to it shortly.

PATIENT: Yesterday I felt so disgusted with myself that I got out my suitcase, just to see how it felt in my hand.

INTERVIEWER: You must have been feeling pretty bad, to think about running away. I'll ask you more about those thoughts in a few minutes, after we've finished talking about your drinking.

In clinical interviewing, you must constantly reconcile two opposing principles: getting all the necessary information while avoiding the bog of excessive detail. For example, you'd certainly want to know about the family uproar that occurred last month when your patient was becoming severely depressed, but not at the expense of uncovering enough symptoms of depression to make a solid diagnosis. Resolving this dilemma often means putting off until later questions that, however much you'd like their answers, must take a back seat to other, more burning issues. It's an ideal time to make some notes for future reference.

USE OPEN-ENDED QUESTIONS

Above all else, you want information that is valid. Studies have shown that patients give the most valid information when they are allowed to answer freely, in their own words, and as completely as they wish. So, whenever possible, phrase your question in an open-ended way that allows the widest possible scope of response. Here are some examples:

Instead of "Did you have insomnia when you were most depressed?" try "How was your sleep then?" (Your patient might have been sleeping too much, rather than too little.)

Instead of "How many times have you been hospitalized?" try "Tell me about your previous hospitalizations." (The details could reveal suicide attempts or bouts of drinking.)

Instead of "Did you lose your appetite?" try "To what extent did your appetite change?" (The phrase "to what extent" can change nearly any closed-ended question into an open-ended one.)

TALK THE PATIENT'S LANGUAGE

Even the most experienced interviewers must guard against using technical words that patients might not understand.

"Has your libido remained healthy?" asked one professor of psychiatry during ward rounds. The patient, a burly high school dropout, looked perplexed.

If you use an unfamiliar word and are asked to define it, you won't lose anything but a little time.

Some patients think they understand when they don't. If they answer the question they *thought* you asked, the information you get might not be accurate. Others are reluctant to admit their ignorance and so say nothing. You will improve validity if you pitch your questions at a level the patient can understand. At the same time, be careful not to talk down to your patient.

> An interviewer asked one patient, a man with a master's degree in psychology, "How's your thinker?" The patient at first did not understand. When the clinician's meaning was finally explained, the patient felt so insulted that he left the room without finishing the interview.

Although most patients will not react so extremely, remember to approach all adults (and children, for that matter) with full regard for their intelligence and feelings.

In polite society, everyone uses circumlocutions at one time or another. For example, "sleeping with" is commonly used to mean "having sexual relations with"—sleep may have nothing to do with it. You should try to preserve amenities, of course, but your first obligation should be to communicate accurately. Asking whether your patient had "sex before getting married" is discreet, but inaccurate; nearly everybody has, even if it is only masturbation. If you really need to know about a history of sexual intercourse, ask that question in so many words. In Chapter 9 we'll take up some methods to help you approach the sensitive subjects of sex, suicide, and substance use.

You should work hard to be sure that you understand what your patient is trying to say. For example, what does "I was off the wall" mean? To find out, you could do one of two things:

1. State your understanding of the expression: "You mean, you felt very upset?"
2. Simply ask what was meant: "I don't understand how your statement relates to what we were talking about."

Ensuring good communication requires your constant vigilance. It is all too easy to assume that you know what your patient means, when in fact the two of you are speaking in different idioms.

In the same vein, be careful not to judge other people's behavior by your own. A common example is duration of sleep. You might suppose that your patient, who sleeps only 6 hours each night, suffers from insomnia, but for some people that's plenty (Thomas Edison slept only

4). Keep in mind the almost endless variety of human preferences and habits, and guard against the temptation to impose your standards on others.

CHOOSE THE RIGHT PROBING QUESTIONS

When you want to know about something, just ask. A simple request for information will often produce what you need with a minimum of effort. Your patient will probably appreciate your directness; if you use an open-ended question, you'll probably get the details.

When it comes time to delve more deeply into your patient's presenting problems, choose your probing questions with two principles in mind:

1. Select probes that will resolve unanswered questions. It's more efficient to concentrate your efforts on areas your patient has not already covered.
2. If your questions show that you know a lot about the illness, you will be perceived as knowledgeable. The resulting dividend of rapport and trust should lead to increased sharing of information.

At this point in your interview, you are interested in the facts, so questions that begin with "Why . . . " are often better avoided. This is especially true if the questions refer to the patient's opinions or to other people's behavior. Besides, "Why . . . " questions can prove frustrating to a patient who lacks insight, and this frustration can inhibit the formation of rapport.

"Why do you think you're having these symptoms now?"
"Why did your boss say that?"
"Why did your son leave home?"

Each of these questions invites speculation rather than facts. Later you may want to hear about possible interpretations, but at first you should try to avoid the opinions and concentrate on the data that will allow you to form your own conclusions. Try asking instead for more details or for some typical examples. (Fair warning: later on, I'll break my own rule and mention a couple of specific situations where you might use "Why . . . " questions to good effect.)

Getting a good history depends in part on knowing what questions will help you better understand the facts about your patient's symptoms or problems. Each symptom has its unique set of details that must be explored, but for a full, rich exploration of any behavior or event, certain items of information are always necessary. They include accurate details about these aspects of your patient's symptoms:

Type
Severity
Frequency
Duration
Context in which they occur

Because you will now be looking for specific details, you will be using more closed-ended questions—those that can be answered in a few words and *don't* invite further comment from your patient. You should still include some open-ended questions, which will stimulate your patient to relate additional material that you may not have thought to ask about. In the following example, the clinician uses a mixture of closed- and open-ended questions to explore a patient's anxiety attacks:

INTERVIEWER: When did you first notice these episodes of anxiety? [Closed-ended]

PATIENT: I guess it must have been about 2 months ago—I had just started my new job with the county.

INTERVIEWER: Would you describe an episode for me? [Open-ended]

PATIENT: It's pretty much the same every time. For no reason I start to feel nervous, and then I'm afraid I won't be able to breathe. It's awfully scary.

INTERVIEWER: How often have they occurred? [Closed-ended]

PATIENT: It's been getting more frequent. I'm not sure I can say.

INTERVIEWER: Well, has it been several times a day, once a day, once a week? [Closed-ended, multiple-choice]

PATIENT: About once or twice a day now, I'd say.

INTERVIEWER: What do you do about it? [Open-ended]

PATIENT: Usually I just sit down. I'm usually too shaky to stand, anyway. After about 15 minutes, it starts to go away.

INTERVIEWER: What sort of help have you sought before? [Open-ended]

Some rules of interviewing seem obvious, but they should be mentioned for the sake of completeness.

- *Don't phrase questions in the negative.* ("You haven't been drinking heavily, have you?") The effect is to telegraph an expected answer, which in this case would be "Heck, no."
- *Don't ask double questions.* ("Have you had trouble with your sleep or appetite?") Double questions may seem efficient, but they are often confusing. The patient may respond to one part of the question and ignore the other, without your realizing it.
- *Avoid leading questions.* ("Has your drinking ever caused you a really serious problem, such as missing work?") A leading question is one that (often broadly) hints at the answer expected; judges on TV crime shows overrule leading questions, and so should you. They represent the opposite of your quest for honest, open-ended inquiry: "Have you ever missed work because of drinking?"
- *Encourage precision.* Where appropriate, ask for dates, times, and numbers.
- *Keep questions brief.* Long questions with much explanatory detail can confuse the patient; they also occupy time you could be using to obtain information.
- *Keep on the lookout for new leads.* Even when you are hot on the trail of vital information, be alert for hints of other directions to explore later.

> PATIENT: . . . That's about the story of my first suicide attempt. It really upset my mother, so bad she had a nervous breakdown. Now did you want to hear about the other attempt?
>
> INTERVIEWER: (*Noting on pad, "Mother's breakdown."*) Yes, please.

CONFRONTATIONS

Of course, *confrontation* does not mean showing anger, much less coming to blows. In the context of a mental health interview, it simply means pointing out something that requires clarification. It could be an inconsistency between two points of the history, or between the story and how the patient appears to feel about it. The purpose of the confrontation is to help you and the patient communicate better.

> INTERVIEWER: I've noticed that whenever I ask about your father, you glance away. Did you realize that?
>
> PATIENT: No, I didn't.
>
> INTERVIEWER: What do you suppose it means?

In the usual initial interview, you should try to avoid any confrontation more than the mild sort just mentioned. In the first visit or two, you don't know one another well at all; your patient could feel tricked or trapped by a relative stranger who points out inconsistencies. That could lead in turn to decreased cooperation with the history taking, or, in extreme cases, to a breakdown in communications. But if you seem to be getting contradictory information on an important point, try to enhance validity by asking for clarification.

When you do ask, be gentle. The experience of being interrogated is an unpleasant one; it makes the subject feel attacked and defensive. If instead you make your confrontations in a warm, empathic way, they are less likely to be rejected. If the patient sees you as interested and concerned, the confrontation should lead to an increase in self-exploration.

You can also make the confrontation seem less like a challenge by choosing your phrases carefully. You might express puzzlement and ask for help:

"Here's something I don't understand. You just said that your husband drove you to the hospital, but I thought that earlier you told me he had run off with his secretary."

Notice the "I thought." It implies that the interviewer might have been mistaken. The overall effect of the confrontation just quoted is to make interviewer and patient collaborators in the search for truth. In another example, to a patient who has made what seems to you an illogical (perhaps delusional) connection, you might simply probe, "I don't think I quite follow that."

Suppose you observe that your patient's appearance and thought content do not jibe. A confrontation asks for clarification:

"What you told me about your mother-in-law is sad, but you seem to be smiling. There must be something else to this story."

Whatever the issue, try to restrict your confrontations to one or two essential issues. Otherwise, you do put your rapport with your new patient at risk. To be sure that you reserve this treatment for only the most important issues, it may be better to save confrontation until close to the end of the interview. Your relationship should be stronger by then (risk will be lessened), and you will have already obtained most of your information (less to lose). Any risk you do take will be in the service of resolving important issues.

Chapter 7

Interviewing about Feelings

Dates, events, and other facts provide only the bare bones of your patient's problems; they must be fleshed out with feelings and reactions to give the problems substance. Whatever the nature of the presenting problems—even in patients with psychoses—feelings about the illness, and indeed about the interview itself, will probably be among the most important information you obtain during the entire interview. Yet studies have shown that of all the topics that must be covered in an initial mental health interview, the one most often ignored by beginning interviewers is feelings.

NEGATIVE AND POSITIVE FEELINGS

People can experience an impressive range of feelings. In listing a few of them (Table 4), I have tried to be comprehensive. Some are major moods or affects; others are variants or combinations. All are represented by commonly used words. Although in nearly every case a noun form exists, I have listed the adjective forms (with occasional synonyms), because that is how people use these words in reference to themselves. For example, a patient would be more likely to say, "I feel anxious," than "I have anxiety."

In most cases I have paired feelings with their opposites. Note that the negative feelings considerably outnumber the positive ones. I have omitted most of the obvious antonyms (*un-* and *in-* words) and have not included some words that are too vague to be useful as descriptors, such as *bad*, *good*, *nervous*, and *uncomfortable*. Because I wanted to include only those terms that are used to describe how people feel, in some cases I have listed no antonym. Thus *innocent* isn't given as an antonym for *guilty*, because people don't usually state that they *feel* innocent—"I *am* innocent" proclaims conviction, not emotion.

TABLE 4. Negative and Positive Feelings

Negative feelings	Positive feelings
Afraid, fearful, apprehensive	Confident
Angry	
Anxious	Contented, calm, peaceful
Apathetic, indifferent	Eager, enthusiastic, interested
Ashamed	Proud
Confused, perplexed, puzzled	Certain, sure
Desiring	
Disappointed	Fulfilled
Disgusted	Delighted
Dissatisfied	Satisfied
Embarrassed	
Envious	
Foolish	
Frustrated	Encouraged
Guilty	
Hateful	Affectionate, loving
Helpless, dependent	Independent
Hopeless, trapped	Hopeful
Humiliated	
Impatient	Patient
Indignant	Pleased
Inferior	Important
Jealous	
Lonely	Sociable
Pessimistic	Optimistic
Regretful	
Rejected	Accepted
Resentful	
Sad, unhappy, depressed	Cheerful, happy, euphoric
Shy, timid	Confident
Surprised, astonished, amazed	Prepared
Suspicious	Trustful
Tense	Relaxed
Uncertain	Determined
Useless, worthless	Useful, worthwhile
Vulnerable	Secure
Wary	
Worried	Carefree
	Appreciative, grateful
	Sympathetic

You can obtain information about feelings from most normally expressive people just by careful watching and listening. But some patients are reluctant to share their feelings; even when they are willing to talk, they hide their emotions deeply. Then you will have to go prospecting to elicit feelings.

ELICITING FEELINGS

Many patients—perhaps most—will express their feelings adequately if you just ask. Patients don't seem to mind this method. In fact, studies show that this direct approach is preferred by most patients and informants, as long as the interviewer has a warm and caring manner and is attentive, courteous, and responsive to cues.

Successful examiners effectively use two techniques that are especially good at eliciting emotions. These are the already-mentioned direct requests and open-ended questions.

Direct Requests for Feelings

Watch for the opportunity to ask about the feelings associated with any of the facts you have been discussing. Simply asking is probably the most effective method of eliciting emotions, but be careful to use the word *feelings* or a synonym. If you slip and say, for example, "What do you *think?*" you risk harvesting a lot of factual and cognitive material, especially if your patient is highly educated or otherwise tends to intellectualize. Here are a couple of examples of useful requests for feelings:

"How did you feel when you found out that you would have to move?"

"What was your state of mind when you were served with that subpoena?"

Patients are used to answering questions and will usually give you information about nearly any emotional state that you seem interested enough to ask about.

Open-Ended Questions

Without specifically asking how the patient feels, open-ended questions encourage the free expression of emotions. This method works because its relative freedom encourages patients to speak at length. The more people talk, the more likely they are to reveal emotion-laden information.

This technique, which is really just an extension of free speech, suggests that you care about how the patient perceives the situation as a whole. On the other hand, closed-ended, short-answer questions may suggest that you have already decided what is significant. This could reduce your patient's motivation to tell the entire story. Furthermore, it seems obvious that the less time you spend asking questions, the more time your patient will have to reveal feelings.

Open-ended questions can also help patients who have trouble sorting out or accepting emotions that conflict with one another—as in the old joke about watching your mother-in-law drive over a cliff in your new car. To describe conflicting emotions, we often use the term *ambivalence*; most people find it hard to express ambivalent feelings in just a few words. But a comparatively long run of uninterrupted talk may provide the time necessary for the patient to think about and express such feelings. Here's an example of an open-ended question that revealed decidedly mixed feelings:

> INTERVIEWER: A few minutes ago, you said that your wife was talking about divorce. Could you tell me more about that?
>
> PATIENT: It's been an awful time for me . . . I know that . . . well, I've always felt that if you've failed in your marriage, you've failed in life. At least, that's what my mother always said.
>
> INTERVIEWER: *(Nods encouragement.)*
>
> PATIENT: But when I think about it . . . you know, there's so much trouble we've had getting along, almost since . . . well, since the kids were born. Maybe we haven't really had much of a marriage at all. Maybe there are some things worse than divorce.

OTHER TECHNIQUES

Several situations can make it hard to elicit emotions from patients. Here are a few of them:

• From childhood, some people are discouraged from revealing their feelings or displaying emotions. When they are grown up, this "macho" view of appropriate behavior can lead them to deny their feelings. The most obvious example is when the childhood admonition "Boys don't cry" becomes "Men should show that they don't care." The same fate can befall women, too.

• Some patients don't recognize their own feelings or have difficulty connecting their feelings to their experiences. Perhaps this, too, develops from childhood experiences. In extreme cases, people grow up unable to recognize or describe how they feel—a condition called *alexithymia*.

• Still others may be reluctant to express themselves, especially to someone they don't know well, because it makes them feel vulnerable. "If you show a hard exterior, no one can hurt you" is how they might put it. In contrast to those with alexithymia, these people know how they feel and could put their emotions into words, but the need for self-protection wins out.

To elicit feelings in one of these situations may require you to use such techniques as expressions of concern, reflection of feelings, picking up on emotional cues, and interpretation.

Expressions of Concern or Sympathy

Controlled studies have shown that any expression of concern or sympathy by a clinician may encourage a patient to share feelings. This is especially likely to work if your patient has already begun to share some feelings. The sympathetic expression you use can be either verbal or behavioral, such as facial expressions or other body language.

> PATIENT: I've worked for that company for 15 years, but when a supervisory position opens up, the boss passes me over for his own nephew. It really burns me!
>
> INTERVIEWER: *(Frowns sympathetically.)* It makes me feel unhappy just hearing about it! I think that anyone in that situation would feel hurt and angry.
>
> PATIENT: I was beyond that—I was totally blown away. I wanted to flush myself out of existence! I still feel that way, sometimes.

Reflection of Feelings

Reflection of feelings means explicitly stating the emotion you think the patient might have felt in a given situation.

> PATIENT: My daughter has always been a little wild, but last night she didn't come home until nearly daybreak.
>
> INTERVIEWER: I'll bet you were nearly frantic.

Of course, this technique runs the risk that your interpretation could be wrong. But if it is, and your patient says so, you have at least accomplished your goal of promoting a discussion of feelings.

Picking Up on Emotional Cues

Picking up on emotional cues means being constantly alert for indications of high emotional concern. Often these will be nonverbal cues: a slight frown, moistening of the eyes, or any other idiom of body language. Your response might be verbal:

"I thought you looked a little sad when you were talking about your mother. What were you feeling?"

You might also indicate your interest and support with some quiet action of your own, such as passing a box of facial tissues to someone who has begun to cry.

Interpretation

In interpretation, you draw parallels between the emotional content of current and past situations.

> PATIENT: My husband never listens to my opinion on things.
>
> INTERVIEWER: From what you told me before, it sounds like the way your father treated you when you were a teenager.

The technique of interpretation can be tricky to use. The patient must be receptive, looking for explanations of behavior; ideally, the patient should be the one who suggests the connection. If not, offer the interpretation tentatively: It might be briskly rejected. Generally, I'd tend to stay away from interpretations during the initial interview; they are a device best used in later therapy by experienced clinicians.

Studies show that each of the techniques above can encourage a reticent patient or informant to offer up more emotions and to examine them at greater depth. However, none of them will discourage a normally expressive person from revealing emotions. They also require less in the way of detailed, extensive probing than do techniques that are less responsive to the needs of patients.

Analogy

Finally, for the patient who absolutely cannot identify the feelings that accompany a given situation, you could ask about times when similar feelings might have been experienced.

"Did you feel anything like this when your mother died?"

"Did you feel this way that time your boss used you as a bad example in front of the entire staff?"

FOLLOWING UP FOR DETAILS

Once you have uncovered some feelings, increase the depth of the interview by asking for more. Probe to elicit examples and to evaluate details.

> INTERVIEWER: I'd like to hear some more about those rage attacks. When do you feel that way?
>
> PATIENT: For one thing, it's whenever we go to visit my father-in-law.
>
> INTERVIEWER: Have you had some previous unpleasant experiences with him?
>
> PATIENT: I'll say! He almost ruined my marriage with some of his sly cracks.
>
> INTERVIEWER: I'd like to hear an example of how you felt then.

Be sure to ask follow-up probing questions when your patient gives you the opportunity. Beginners sometimes uncover evidence of significant events or pathology, only to ignore it in the subsequent dialogue. Here is an unfortunate example:

> INTERVIEWER: Were you ever approached for sex in any way when you were a child?
>
> PATIENT: Well, yes, I was.
>
> INTERVIEWER: *(Writes down "Yes.")* Where are you employed now?

Perhaps this interviewer felt uncomfortable at pressing ahead for the details, but the patient was left to deal with the frustration of pent-up information. Positive information should be followed up until you have learned who, what, when, where, why, and how.

DEFENSE MECHANISMS

When following up, you should also learn what your patient does to cope with feelings. These strategies for dealing with emotions and behaviors are called *defense mechanisms*. They may seem almost endless in their number and variety—consult standard texts for a more exhaustive listing. Following are a few of the more common ones. Rather than just stating definitions, I will try to clarify what is meant with examples of defense mechanisms that might be used by an aspiring politician who feels anxiety and anger about losing a city council election.

Potentially Harmful Defense Mechanisms

In the potentially harmful group, I've included those mechanisms that generally allow a person to avoid confronting the effects of feelings or emotions. When stressed, most of us occasionally resort to such measures to shore up our egos.

> *Acting out.* [The politician smashes the camera of a news photographer who is trying to take a picture.]
>
> *Denial.* "The recount will show that I really won."
>
> *Devaluation.* "It's a lousy job anyway—the hours are murder, and nothing but complaints from the taxpayers."
>
> *Displacement.* [The politician goes home and kicks the cat.]
>
> *Dissociation.* [The politician awakens one morning in strange surroundings, unable to recall any of the events of the past 3 days.]
>
> *Fantasy.* "Next year I'll run for Congress—and win!"
>
> *Intellectualization.* "I look at this defeat only as an example of 'democracy in action.'"
>
> *Projection.* [Unconscious thought: "I'd like to kill him."] "He's plotting to kill me."
>
> *Repression.* [The politician "forgets" to attend a banquet in honor of the victor.]
>
> *Splitting.* "Some politicians are good, some bad; my opponent's one of the bad ones."
>
> *Reaction formation.* [Thought: "He's a miserable low-life."] "I'm proud to support the honorable council member."
>
> *Somatization.* [The candidate develops persistent chest pain of unexplained origin . . .] " . . . so I couldn't have served anyway."

Effective Defense Mechanisms

Better-integrated adults rely principally on some of the more mature defense mechanisms.

> *Altruism.* "I'll support him; he has better qualifications than I do."
>
> *Humor.* "In the campaign I said he was honorable; he said I was a jerk. Perhaps we were both wrong."
>
> *Sublimation.* "I'll write a book about the campaign."
>
> *Suppression.* "I'll put it to the back of my mind, and concentrate on the business at hand."

HANDLING EXCESSIVELY EMOTIONAL PATIENTS

Although you usually want to encourage the expression of emotions, some patients are so emotional that it impedes their communication with other people, including therapists. People can experience excessive emotionality for a variety of reasons.

- They may be people who are angry, sometimes without knowing why.
- Others, such as those with somatization disorder or antisocial personality disorder, have learned that high-volume emotions help them get their way. Drama has therefore become a way of life.
- Even some people who don't have such severe underlying psychopathology use high emotional output to control their families or friends.
- Some people have been reared in families where feelings are expressed loudly and often. By their imitation of others, this behavior becomes habitual.
- Anxiety causes some to behave this way.
- A few cannot stand the loneliness of silence.
- Perhaps your patient, recalling experiences with other clinicians, fears that you won't be interested or that there won't be enough time to tell the whole story.

Whatever the cause, excessive emotionality can focus too much of your attention on feelings, leaving insufficient time for gathering facts. In such a situation, try to adopt a brisk, controlling manner in which you firmly direct the course of the interview. Several techniques can help you accomplish this objective.

1. Acknowledge the emotion. You may be able to turn down the heat by just putting a label on the emotion. Then the patient sees that you recognize the feeling and no longer needs to attract your attention to it.

> PATIENT: *(Shouting)* She's not going to jerk me around that way, not ever again!
>
> INTERVIEWER: You really feel angry. Frustrated and angry.
>
> PATIENT: *(More quietly)* Well, sure. Who wouldn't be? Wait'll you hear what she did last week.

This technique shows that you understand and accept how your patient feels, so it is probably the best one to use. Try it first.

2. Talk quietly. If your patient shouts, try *lowering* your own voice. It will be hard for most people to maintain high-volume output when you are speaking so softly that you can barely be heard.

3. Explain again what information you are trying to get:

"What I really want at this point is to learn about your family history. Perhaps later we can talk some more about your husband's girlfriend."

4. Redirect any of the patient's questions or comments that change the topic.

INTERVIEWER: Now I'd like to hear about your son. You said that he was living with his mother?

PATIENT: That's right, and she hasn't let me even talk to him on the phone for the past 3 months. Don't you think I should get a court order?

INTERVIEWER: We might be able to talk about that later. Right now I really need to know about your relationship with your son. Have you been close?

5. Switch to a closed-ended style. The opposite of open-ended requests, this style indicates what sort of specific answer you would like to hear. It also tends to discourage further comment by the patient.

INTERVIEWER: Could you tell me about your first marriage?

PATIENT: It was a disaster! I've never forgiven that man! He was a complete brute! One time I cried for a month without stopping. Why, I couldn't even—

INTERVIEWER: *(Interrupts, recognizing that open-ended questions aren't useful.)* Was he a drinker?

PATIENT: Oh gosh, yes, he drank like a camel. He—

INTERVIEWER: *(Interrupts.)* How long did the marriage last?

PATIENT: Until I was 26, about 4 years. He was never—

INTERVIEWER: Was the divorce your idea, or his?

This interviewer was prepared to go on interrupting until the patient learned to stick to the main topic.

6. If you are still having trouble, check to be sure that the patient understands what you want. Here is how you might phrase this confrontation:

"We seem to be having some trouble here with our communication. Have I made it clear what I need to know?"

The aim of each these techniques is to reduce the patient's scope for excessive verbal and behavioral output. They should help you obtain the diagnostic information you need without sacrificing rapport.

Occasionally, even these techniques are insufficient. If an outpouring of tears or other feelings prevents you from obtaining the information you need from a hospitalized patient, you may have to break off the interview long enough for the patient to get a better grip. Say something like this:

"I can see you're too upset to continue today. Let's take a rest for now. I'll stop back and see you again in the morning, when you've had some sleep."

Chapter 8

Personal and Social History

Health care professionals don't treat illnesses; they treat people. You therefore need to know the context in which your patient's complaints have occurred. This requires learning all you can about family background and other biographical data. The process not only will help you get to know your patient, but may reveal material that illuminates and extends your knowledge of the cause and context of mental disorder. Some of it may have a direct bearing on the cause of an illness or on its treatment. Your patient has spent a lifetime accumulating these experiences, so there is almost no limit to the amount and variety of the information you can find. What you learn will be determined by the purpose of your present interview and the time you can devote to it.

While you are gathering biographical information, maintain a healthy skepticism about its validity. Human memory is fallible, especially when the human has an intense personal interest in what is being remembered. Accurate recall is more likely for major historical events such as births, deaths, and marriages, and for recent events that constitute the history of the present illness.

Some material is especially subject to distortion: early childhood events, everything reported secondhand, interpersonal disputes, and any other item that requires interpretation. You should be constantly evaluating the validity of all interview data against your own internal standards ("Does this story seem likely? Does it even seem possible?"). But you should also use external checks on accuracy, such as previous medical records and interviews with relatives and friends (see Chapter 15).

In this and subsequent chapters, I will use *italics* to point out some of the possible interpretations of the material as we discuss it.

CHILDHOOD AND ADOLESCENCE

Childhood Nuclear Family

A logical starting place is with your patient's birth. In what city/state/country did it occur? Was the patient an only child? If there were brothers and sisters, how many were there of each? What was your patient's position in the sibship (first, second, middle, youngest, or only child)? How well did your patient get along with siblings? Was one sibling favored over the others? *Older children in a sibship tend to receive more atten-tion when they are young, whereas middle children may be relatively neglected; youngest children may be babied or spoiled. Genetic disorders that are obvious at birth (such as Down syndrome) tend to occur late in a sibship.*

If your patient was one of twins, were they identical (one-egg) or fraternal (two-egg) twins? *Identical twins have inherited the same genetic material; fraternal twins are no more genetically alike than ordinary siblings. Some mental disorders, including schizophrenia and bipolar disorders, are much more likely if your patient is the identical twin of someone who has such a disorder.*

Did your patient feel wanted as a child? How close was the relation-ship with the parents? Did this change with adolescence? Was the pa-tient reared by both parents? If not, was this due to death? Divorce? Military service? *Absence of a parent (especially the father) has been associ-ated with antisocial personality disorder. In some studies, early death of a par-ent has been associated with adult-onset depression.*

Occasionally a patient will tell you, "I never knew my father." You should gently try to learn whether the parents were ever married. (Using "Is it possible that . . . " can soften this question considerably.) *Even in our modern era, being born "illegitimate" is a lifelong source of dis-comfort and embarrassment for some people.*

Whatever the exact nature of your patient's nuclear family, you should try to learn something about how the parents (or surrogates) re-lated to one another. Did they communicate well with one another? Show affection? Did they quarrel often? Fight? Did one physically abuse the other? How did their relationship affect the emotional cli-mate in the home while your patient was growing up? *People often model their adult relationships with others on what they observed as the "norm" dur-ing childhood. On the other hand, some people go to extremes to be different from a parent whose behavior was perceived as undesirable or unattractive.*

If your patient was adopted, at what age did this take place? Can you learn anything about the biological parents or about the circum-stances leading to adoption? Was the adoption intrafamilial (this is, were the adoptive parents blood relatives of the patient) or extrafamilial? *Many adopted people, especially adolescents and young adults, feel incomplete because they don't know their biological parents. This can result in a quest for roots that drives some to extraordinary lengths to discover (and in some cases become acquainted with) the birth parents who gave them up.*

Growing Up

What was the age of each parent when your patient was born? Were they mature enough to provide responsible care? Did both work regularly? What were their jobs? Were they good providers? Did they have enough time left over to spend with children? What sort of disciplinary techniques were used? Were these harsh, firm, relaxed, or inconsistent?

If either parent was gone from home for an extended period of time, find out why. (Illness? A job far from home? Jail? Was your patient a "military brat"?) Did the family live in one place, or were there frequent moves? Did the family ever really put down roots somewhere?

Were there other losses, such as the death of a sibling, grandparent, or other close relative?

Find out about hobbies, clubs, and other extracurricular interests. Was your patient sociable? A loner? *Many people with schizophrenia have been isolated or loners for most of their lives.*

Try to obtain a general picture of the childhood environment and your patient's place in it. Here are some questions that might help you with this broad task:

"Could you tell me something about your childhood?"
"What was life like for you then?"
"How do you feel about your sibling(s)?"
"Who were your childhood friends?"
"Did you feel different from other kids?"
"How did you spend your free time?"
"Did you belong to organizations such as the Scouts or the Y?"
"Did you participate in organized sports?"
"Where did your family go on vacations?"
"Did your family have pets?"
"What chores or other responsibilities did you have?"
"What summer or after-school jobs did you have?"
"What did you want to be when you grew up?"
"With whom did you identify?"
"Was sex discussed in the home?"
"What were your parents' attitudes toward sex?"
"When did you first become interested in having a romantic relationship?"

Asking about Abuse

Many patients were physically abused as children—an experience that can significantly affect adult personality. This information can be difficult to obtain; sometimes these patients do not themselves realize the extent to which they were abused as children. You should nonetheless make an effort to learn whether your patient's childhood involved such experiences. You can lead into these sensitive topics gradually:

"How well do you feel your parents provided for you?"

"What methods of discipline did your parents use?"

"Did you ever feel that you were mistreated as a child?"

Positive replies to questions about abuse must be pursued thoroughly, if carefully. You will need to develop the following areas of information:

How often did this abuse occur?

Who administered it? Did both parents participate?

If one of them tried to shield the child, who was it?

What form did the abuse take? (Beatings? If so, what with?)

How often did it occur?

What was the provocation, if any?

At the time, did the patient feel that this abuse was deserved? What about now?

What effect did these experiences have on the patient as a child?

As an adult, how does the patient feel about these experiences now?

You'll need to ask about sexual abuse, too; we'll cover this issue in Chapter 9.

Childhood Health

Early developmental milestones (such as the ages at which a child learns to sit, stand, walk, speak words, and speak sentences) are usually not worth pursuing. Most of what your patient knows about milestones has probably been passed along as family mythology, which is highly subject to distortion. (Who remembers being breast-fed or toilet-trained?) But if you suspect mental retardation or developmental difficulties such as a specific learning disorder, these milestones may be important enough to ask informants about them.

Try to learn something about overall childhood health. Were there frequent visits to doctors, hospitalizations, operations, or long absences from school for health reasons? How did the family deal with illness? (Overprotection? Rejection?) If your patient was a sickly child, did the parents and other relatives "reward" illness behavior with a great deal of attention? *Overprotection or rewards for illness may precede some somatoform disorders.*

What was your patient's temperament and activity level, especially around ages 5 to 10? Was this child quiet and withdrawn or outgoing and friendly? *Temperament characteristics appear in the first few months of life and tend to persist throughout childhood, even into the adult years. They may correlate with adult mental disorders.*

Does your patient report any of these relatively common childhood problems?

Bedwetting
Tics
Stuttering
Obesity
Nightmares
Phobias

If so, what treatment (if any) was attempted? Did it help? How did these problems affect relations with siblings or schoolmates? *Any of these conditions suggests that the patient was under stress as a child. Due to its increased frequency, obesity may in recent years have become somewhat more accepted, but it retains a serious potential source of childhood hazing.*

Were there any concerns about masturbation? At what age did puberty begin? If female, was your patient prepared for the onset of menses? If so, who told her? At what age did they begin? Was she concerned or teased about breast development? *Teens of either sex can be exquisitely sensitive about being noticed. Developmental delay (or acceleration) may have caused your patient some degree of embarrassment.*

When did dating begin? What feelings were associated with this? Sexual history will be covered in Chapter 9.

Education

How well did your patient do academically, and what was the last grade completed? Did your patient like school? If there were academic problems, what subjects caused the most trouble? Were there any specific problems with reading (dyslexia)? Were there behavior problems in school? Truancy? What were the consequences? (Sent to principal? Paddling? Suspension or expulsion?)

Did your patient repeat grades or have difficulty concentrating on schoolwork? *Short attention span and low school performance suggest attention-deficit/hyperactivity disorder. Some of these patients (little boys, espe-cially) were markedly hyperactive as children, and may even have learned to walk early.*

Did your patient ever miss school for long periods of time? If so, why? Was there any history of school refusal? How old was your patient when it occurred? *School refusal (once known as "school phobia") is fairly common in young children and does not necessarily predict later pathology.*

If your patient quit before graduating from high school, what was the reason? What did your patient do then? Work? Join the military? You should also learn whether a GED was attempted or attained (the initials stand for General Equivalency Diploma or tests of General Edu-cational Development).

Finally, at what age did your patient make the transition from a life of dependency on parents or others to one of self-sufficiency?

LIFE AS AN ADULT

Work History

Employment history can help you judge both your patient's underlying potential and the effect of recent illness on performance. This informa-tion is also relatively objective: Work history seems to be distorted less than more personal, perhaps more embarrassing portions of the social history. You should therefore spend some time inquiring into the de-tails of your patient's job history.

What is your patient's current occupation? Is it stimulating, satisfy-ing? How does it match earlier ambitions? How long has your patient worked for the current employer? If the patient was ever unemployed, why and for how long? If employed only briefly, how many jobs have there been in the last 5 years? Has each job change been for a better one? How much time is spent working? Investigate any gap, change of direction, or lack of promotion.

If your patient was ever fired from a job, what were the circum-stances? If the patient is unemployed now, why? When did your patient last work regularly? If currently unemployed, what is the means of sup-port? *Multiple jobs of brief duration are often found in antisocial personality disorder. No job at all, or none for many years, is commonplace among patients with chronic schizophrenia.*

While you are about it, find out about adult leisure activities. Does your patient have any hobbies? Belong to any clubs or other organiza-tions? Have there been efforts at continuing education as an adult? What about talents? To find out more, you can ask:

"What do you think you're good at?"

Military History

Has your patient served in the armed forces? (Don't omit this topic for female patients.) If the answer is "Yes," ask:

"What branch?"

"Was this a volunteer enlistment, or were you drafted?"

"How long did you serve?"

"What was your job in the military?"

"What was the highest rank you attained?"

"Did you have any disciplinary problems?" (These include courts-martial, Articles 15, captain's masts, and lower-grade punishments.)

"What kind of discharge did you receive?" (Honorable? General? Dishonorable? Medical?)

"Did you see combat? If so, for how long? What was your role?"

"Were you ever wounded?"

"Do you have a service-connected disability?" (This could be due either to wounds or to a non-combat-related accident or illness.)

"Were you a prisoner of war?"

"As a result of your experiences, have you persistently relived your experiences or had bad dreams or anniversary reactions?" *Symptoms that persist after any severe trauma can indicate PTSD. This condition has been reported in 10% or more of Vietnam-era combat veterans, and it is also turning up in large numbers among Iraq War returnees. It may also occur after civilian calamities, such as car wrecks and natural disasters.*

Legal History

Ask about any legal problems. These might include lawsuits over insurance or disability (especially likely in the case of a chronic illness, injury, or pain), evictions, and feuds with neighbors. In these litigious times, nearly any sort of dispute seems possible. *Legal history can serve as a clue to personality disorders, as well as illnesses such as bipolar disorders and substance misuse.*

Has your patient ever been arrested? If so, at what age? What were the circumstances? How many times did this occur? What was the outcome? (Probation? Time in prison?) Was this in local confinement or in a penitentiary? What was the total duration of time served?

Has there been a continuing pattern of illegal behavior from adolescence throughout adult life? If so, have these criminal activities always taken place in the context of substance use, or have they also occurred when the patient was clean and sober? Have there been other illegal activities for which your patient has never been caught? It might be worthwhile to ask specifically about shoplifting, which is a relatively common behavior, especially in children and young adults. *In antisocial* personality disorder, there is a continuing pattern of illegal acts from at least age 15 (and often much earlier). Partly because it carries such a poor prognosis, antisocial personality disorder is a diagnosis you should not make in any patient whose illegal behavior has occurred entirely under the influence of drugs or alcohol.

Religion

To what religion does your patient belong (if any)? Is this different from any religious affiliation of childhood? How often does your patient attend services? How does religion inform your patient's life? *Religion is useful to know about for several reasons. It can provide clues to possible sources of support and comfort, and may reveal something of your patient's values and system of ethics. It may also suggest to what degree there has been a break with parents. Increasingly, authorities advocate exploration of the patient's spirituality and belief in God.*

Current Living Situation

Where does your patient live now? (House? Apartment? Mobile home? Rented room? Board and care facility? On the street?) What is the neighborhood like?

Does your patient live alone or with someone? With whom? How well does your patient provide self-care? If there has been wandering, you might not learn this from the patient; this is material for which you may have to depend on informants. *Wandering is commonly found in patients with cognitive disorders.*

From what your patient says, can you characterize the quality of the home? Is there privacy for each person who lives there? Are there pets? Are there sufficient means of communication, including telephone, postal service, e-mail? What means of transportation does your patient use—car? bus? train?

Has your patient ever been homeless? If so, for how long? What were the circumstances?

What is your patient's financial situation? What is the source of income? Is it steady? Be sure to include jobs, disability compensation, Social Security, annuities, alimony, and investments. Ask:

"Has money been a problem for you?"

Social Network

You can begin to assess the quality of social relationships by asking:

"To whom do you feel close in your family?"

"What about among your friends?"

"How often do you see these people?"

If responsible for providing care for another adult, such as a parent, other relative, or friend, how does your patient feel about these duties? Can you tell how well this function is carried out?

How much of a social support network does your patient have? Try to find out about the quality of relationships with family, friends, and coworkers. Are there memberships in any clubs or support groups? Have any government or private agencies helped out? What about home food services like Meals on Wheels? If there are grown children, how close is their relationship with the patient?

Does the patient pursue leisure interests alone or with other people?

Marital Status

It has become commonplace for couples to live together without being married. I will use the terms *spouse* and *partner* to include any intimate relationship between two people, without regard to legal status or gender.

You might start by asking:

"Tell me about your spouse." (How does what you hear from the patient square with what you observe?)

"What do you see as the strong points of your relationship?" (Like all open-ended questions, this one gives enough scope to discuss whatever seems important. The report, favorable or not, could indicate the overall state of the relationship.)

Here are some specific items of information you should learn about:

Is the patient currently married?
Have there been any common-law marriages or long-term relationships?
Are the patient and spouse currently living together?
What are the relative ages of spouse and patient?
How long have they been together?
If they are married, how long did they know one another before the ceremony?
How many marriages have there been for each partner?
If there have been prior marriages, how old was the patient each time?
Why did prior marriages or other long-term relationships end?
How have emotional problems affected the patient's current relationship?

How well does the partner support the patient during periods of illness or disability?

If the patient is divorced, what were the circumstances of the separation? Who initiated it? Why? Do the former spouses still maintain a relationship? If so, how amicable is it?

Certain issues, including money, sex, children, and relatives, commonly provide fodder for disputes in contemporary marriages. They can develop into mammoth feuds between patients and their families as the burden of mental disorder produces an uncommon number and variety of arguments, fights, affairs, separations, and divorces. Expect to invest considerable time in—and gain extensive information from—inquiries into the quality of your patient's marriage or other love relationship. Following are some of the questions you can ask to elicit routine problems that can produce friction in any relationship:

"How well do you and your spouse communicate?" (Some couples almost never have a serious discussion; successful couples take the time to air their grievances, preferences, and points of view.)

"Does each of you consider the other a best friend?"

"How do you argue?" (Are old issues constantly brought up, or do they get laid to rest? Do the partners commonly say things they later regret?)

"What do you argue about?"

If there are children, you should find out:

How many are there from each marriage?

Are there stepchildren?

What ages and genders are all the children?

Were there ever any children conceived outside marriage?

What is the patient's relationship with each of the children?

Do patient and spouse agree about sharing responsibility for child care?

Questions about sexual adjustment and preference logically belong here. These can be difficult to discuss, so I'll address them in a separate chapter on sensitive subjects (Chapter 9).

Avocations and Interests

OK, so it isn't going to make or break the diagnosis of schizophrenia or a bipolar disorder; still, you want to know something of how your patient spends leisure time, or would like to if any became available. What can you infer from hobbies (e.g., primarily solitary pastimes such as stamp collecting or photography, outdoor activities such as bird watching) and interests (TV, movies, reading, shopping)? *About 5% of adults identify themselves as compulsive shoppers; such a history could tip you off to other pathology, such as depression, gambling, or binge eating.* Are sporting activities participatory, such as dancing, tennis, or golf, or mainly ones viewed from the grandstand (or home theater couch)? Have there been any recent changes in the type or intensity of leisure interests, or in the patient's ability to focus attention while pursuing these interests? If so, can you tell why?

MEDICAL HISTORY

Even if you are not a physician, don't pass medical history by. It is vital for every practitioner to know about this topic and the next one, the review of systems—both of which have practical implications for diagnosis, treatment, and prognosis. For example, in 2007 a report pointed out that mentally ill patients die, on average, 25 years earlier than do people in the general population—not only because of suicide (though that is a major cause), but from conditions such as heart and lung disease, diabetes, and infectious diseases that include HIV/AIDS. All of these are treatable, but you have to identify them first. Furthermore, some patients with symptoms of mental illness actually turn out to have treatable medical conditions as everyday as thyroid problems and Lyme disease. I can assure you that the issues to be covered in these two sections are no more difficult than any of the other areas we have already discussed.

Has your patient had any previous major illnesses? If so, what were they? Did they result in hospitalization? Have there been any operations? If so, what were they? When did they occur? Did the patient ever receive a blood transfusion? If so, is this patient at risk for AIDS? If serious medical illness or operations occurred during childhood, how did the patient perceive them at the time? What about allergies to pollen, dust, or animals?

While you are taking this history, you might try to ascertain how well your patient has complied with recommendations made by physicians and other therapists. Many people, especially those who don't know you very well, may have trouble admitting to poor compliance. Try asking:

"Has it always been easy for you to follow your doctor's advice?"
"When have you had difficulty?"

You will find more advice on dealing with difficult patient behaviors in Chapters 16 and 17.

Ask about any obvious physical problems. Don't be shy about bringing up stuttering, an eye patch, a missing limb, or a severe limp. Any of these could have a bearing on the present problem. They may also have prompted teasing during childhood. Even if physical defects are not causing emotional problems now, they may well have done so at some time in the past. You might say:

"I noticed that you stammered once or twice while we were talking. I wonder what sort of problems that might have caused when you were a child."

"Children can be pretty cruel about birthmarks. Could you tell me about yours?"

Medications

In the history of the present illness, you have already learned about the medicines prescribed for emotional disorders. Now ask whether your patient regularly takes any other medications. This information is especially important when the presenting problems include depression, psychosis, or anxiety. Any of these can be caused or made worse by commonly prescribed medications. Pay special attention to birth control pills, other hormones (such as thyroid hormones or steroids), pain pills, and drugs for blood pressure. For each medicine, try to learn dose, frequency, and how long your patient has been taking it. Has the patient recently stopped taking any other medications? *Of course, you are looking for the possibility that side effects could explain some of the symptoms you are investigating. Keep reading.*

Side Effects

Have there been side effects (unwanted effects) or drug reactions? This topic is often ignored by beginning interviewers, but it can influence the choice of therapies. Try to get a description of the side effect or drug reaction:

What happened?
How long after the first dose did it occur?
Was treatment needed?

If the patient ever tried the drug again, did it produce the same reaction? *Often patients assume that a drug has caused physical or mental symptoms when the two events were only coincidental. The question of cause and effect is sometimes settled when the drug is started again, and the symptoms either reappear or do not.*

You are most likely to hear complaints about rashes developing from sulfa or penicillin, but it is more important to learn about untoward reactions to psychotropic medications. True allergies to these drugs are rare, but side effects are not. Here are some of the more common ones:

Antidepressants: drowsiness, dry mouth, skin rash, dizziness, nausea, weight gain, blurred vision, constipation
Antianxiety agents: drowsiness, forgetfulness or confusion, dizziness
Lithium: skin rash, tremor, excessive urination, thirst
Antipsychotics: low blood pressure, extrapyramidal side effects

Extrapyramidal side effects are neurological symptoms that can be caused by taking antipsychotic medication. The four types are common enough that every mental health professional can expect to encounter each of them from time to time. The first three occur soon after starting medication and can be treated with antiparkinsonian drugs such as trihexyphenidyl (Artane) or diphenhydramine (Benadryl).

1. *Acute dystonia* develops within a few hours of the first dose of an antipsychotic drug. It is characterized by a sharp, cramping pain of the neck that may cause the head to turn to the side. Sometimes the gaze rolls upward. This side effect can be painful and frightening and can constitute a real emergency.

2. *Akathisia* usually begins within a few days of starting antipsychotics. Patients experience it as a profound restlessness, often with an inability to sit still that results in pacing.

3. *Pseudoparkinsonism* also occurs soon after starting medication. The patient experiences a decreased mobility of facial expression (masked facies); a tendency to walk with short, shuffling steps; and a back-and-forth tremor of the hands when they are relaxed, as when resting on a table. This tremor resembles the motion that old-time druggists would use to form drugs into pills; hence the term *pill-rolling tremor.*

4. *Tardive dyskinesia* usually does not begin until the patient has been using antipsychotics for months or years. Someone with tardive dyskinesia typically has uncontrollable motions of the tongue, jaw, and lips that result in persistent pursing, chewing, or licking movements. Patients themselves are often almost entirely unaware that they are doing this; it is not a debilitating disorder, but it is unsightly. *Tardive dyskinesia is all the more important because it has no specific treatment. Unless the antipsychotic drug is discontinued quickly, tardive dyskine*

sia can become permanent, persisting even after the medication is eventually stopped.

REVIEW OF SYSTEMS

In the review of systems, you ask patients to identify any symptoms they have had from a list that you recite. That list comprises symptoms from all the different organ systems of the body. The rationale for using it is that patients will recognize more symptoms by passive identification than if you depend upon their spontaneous, active recall.

A complete medical review of systems is long and not especially relevant to the initial mental health examination. However, you should ask about the following:

Disturbance of appetite *(found in severe depression, anorexia nervosa, and bulimia nervosa; over- or undereating may begin as early as childhood).*

Head injury *(characteristic of cognitive disorders, though in 2007 researchers reported social awkwardness and a change in the response to moral dilemmas in patients who had had brain tumors or strokes that affected the ventromedial area of the brain's prefrontal cortex).*

History of unconsciousness, dizziness, or fainting spells *(suggests cognitive disorders, somatization disorder).*

Convulsions (seizures). These may be either biological or psychogenic in nature. Ask about these symptoms: loss of conscious ness, loss of control of bowels or bladder, tongue biting, and auras (any premonition or sensation warning the patient that a seizure is about to begin).

Symptoms of premenstrual dysphoric disorder. Before menses there may be persistent anger, labile mood, trouble with sleep, fatigue, tension, trouble concentrating, and physical symptoms such as weight gain. *Premenstrual dysphoric disorder is easy to ignore, especially if you are a male interviewer. But it is fairly common among women of childbearing age and can cause symptoms of depression.*

Somatization Disorder

In addition to these general-purpose questions, there is a specialized review of systems you can use to diagnose somatization disorder—a chronic illness that usually begins in the teens or early 20s and is seen in perhaps 8% of female mental health patients. Although this review is somewhat cumbersome to use, it remains the only reliable way to diagnose somatization disorder. The patient must respond positively to at least eight symptoms from the list in Appendix B. To count as significant,

1. any symptom must not be fully explained by a general medical condition or substance use, *or*
2. if a medical condition does seem to be related, the symptoms or impairments must exceed what you'd expect, based on the findings.

FAMILY HISTORY

With the family history, you have the opportunity to accomplish three tasks: (1) develop a brief biographical sketch of parents, siblings, spouse (or significant other), and children; (2) learn about the relationships between patient and relatives, both current and during childhood; and (3) learn whether mental disorders run in your patient's family, including distant relatives. (Remember that the transmission of a familial disorder could be either genetic or environmental.)

You might start with an open-ended request for information about your patient's current family at home:

"Tell me how you get along with your [spouse, children]."

"What sort of people are [were] your parents?"

A few additional probing questions along these lines should help you answer the first two questions about family history. Keep in mind that you should obtain your patient's assessment of both the childhood and adult families.

By this time you have probably already learned such basics as parents' occupations and ages of siblings, but you might not know how much contact your patient has had with them as an adult. If there has been a rupture of these relationships, find out why. The answer could tell you something about the personalities of the relatives, and also of your patient.

To learn what sort of mental disorders may run in your patient's family, you'll need to be explicit. Naturally, you want to know whether any blood relatives had symptoms similar to the patient's, but to be clear that you are looking for even more, carefully define the disorders and the relatives you are inquiring about:

"I'd like to know whether any of your blood relatives ever had any nervous or mental disorders. By 'blood relatives' I mean your parents, brothers, sisters, children, grandparents, uncles, aunts, cousins, nieces, and nephews. Has any of these people ever had nervousness, nervous breakdown, psychosis or schizophrenia, depression, problems from drug or alcohol dependence, suicide or suicide attempts, delinquency, hypochondriasis [define this term if you think the patient won't understand], mental hospitalization, or arrests or incarcerations? Any relatives who were considered odd or eccentric, or who had difficult personalities?"

This is a long speech, but it tells the patient exactly what you want to know and which relatives to consider.

Move through the list of disorders slowly enough to give your patient time to think, and probe for details of any positive answers. Just because someone (even a mental health professional) diagnosed Cousin Louise as having schizophrenia, this doesn't guarantee that she did have it. The relative could have misunderstood the diagnosis, or the clinician could have been wrong. Try to learn Louise's age when she fell ill and what her symptoms were. What sort of treatment did she receive? How did she respond? What was the ultimate outcome—chronic illness or complete recovery? Did she ever have another episode?

PERSONALITY TRAITS AND DISORDERS

We can define *personality* as the combination of all the mental, emotional, behavioral, and social aspects that make us individual human beings. The term *character* is often used synonymously with *personality*. How individuals perceive, think about, and relate to the environment and to themselves form patterns of behavior called *personality traits* that persist for long periods of time, often throughout life. Personality (or character) traits can be detected as early as the first few months of life; they shape behavior forever after and may become even more pronounced with advancing age. These patterns govern relationships with friends, lovers, bosses, and colleagues, as well as with more casual social contacts.

Much of one's personality is under the surface, not readily apparent to others or even to the individual. Psychological testing can help reveal aspects of your patient's personality, but you probably won't have this sort of material available during an initial interview. Your own impression will often depend upon several sources of information:

Your patient's self-assessment
Interviews with people who know the patient well (covered in
    Chapter 15)

Information about relationships, attitudes, and behaviors with
other people

Behaviors you observe during your interview session

The Patient's Self-Assessment

Try to learn what characterized your patient's personality prior to the
first episode of mental disorder; this is often referred to as the
premorbid personality. Some of the following open-ended questions may
help you evaluate premorbid personality:

"Describe yourself for me." This is intended as an invitation. If the
response is "What do you mean?" you could prompt with some of the
following questions:

"What sort of a person are you normally?" (Watch especially for
answers indicating self-esteem that is either low or inflated, or for responses that contradict facts you already know.)

"What do you like best about yourself?"

"What is your mood normally?"

"What were you like as a teenager?"

Be especially alert for evidence of lifelong behavior patterns. Your
patient may use certain phrases that will tip you off:

"For as long as I can remember, I've made friends easily."

"All my life I've been an 'up' sort of person—until my illness."

The two examples just given suggest behaviors and attitudes that
generally work well for people. Indeed, in assessing personality it is
important not to focus solely on weaknesses, but on strengths as well.
For example, how would you describe your patient's intelligence? Previous successes? Coping skills? Support system? Don't let your quest for
psychopathology blind you to the predictive power of a normal premorbid personality. A preponderance of positive character traits suggests that your patient will be less inconvenienced by the current illness, will enjoy better social support while ill, and, once the current
siege has lifted, will have a better chance for eventually returning to
complete mental health.

Following is a list of personality characteristics that are generally
considered positive:

Agreeable	Forgiving
Charming	Independent
Cheerful	Inquisitive
Confident	Open
Conscientious	Optimistic
Dependable	Outgoing

Punctual	Steady
Relaxed	Trusting

In the initial mental health interview, you'll often encounter life-long patterns of maladjustment or interpersonal conflicts. Here are some typical self-evaluations from patients:

"I've always been an anxious, tense person. Kinda depressed."

"I've been a loner all my life."

"People are no damn good. I don't like them, they don't like me."

"I've never felt comfortable around people—not unless I was drinking."

"I've never been successful the way I'd hoped."

"As long as I can remember I have avoided conflict, whatever the cost."

A list of some of these negative personality traits would include the following:

Aggressive	Passive
Anxious	Perfectionistic
Changeable	Quarrelsome
Compulsive	Resentful
Controlling	Rigid
Fussy	Self-centered
Gloomy	Suspicious
Histrionic	Shy
Introverted	Tense
Irritable	Volatile
Jealous	Worrisome
Neurotic	

A few other traits could be read as positive, negative, or neither:

Demonstrative	Sensitive
Meticulous	Serious
Reserved	

Relationships with Others

During a single interview with any patient, you may have trouble assessing personality. Some mental health patients give distorted assessments: The picture you obtain may be either too gloomy or overly optimistic. Still, you might obtain valuable information by trying to learn how others view your patient—from the patient's own perspective:

"What sorts of situations do people think you have trouble handling?"

"How well do you control your temper?"

"Does anyone in your family think you have a problem with [alcohol, drugs, your temper]?"

What can you learn about your patient's prejudices and regard for other people? Ask:

"How do you feel about your boss?"

"Is your spouse always as supportive as you'd like?"

"Is there anyone—any type of person—you can't stand?"

Although I ordinarily try to avoid them, questions beginning with "Why . . . " may help sort out your patient's motivations and style of relating to other people:

"Why do you think your brother wants your mother to move in with him?"

"You said you can't work well with one of your partners. Why is that?"

A more objective indicator of personality traits is the history, as it is related by the patient and especially by informants. For example, from the employment history, you could learn something about your patient's adherence to the work ethic: Consider the age of first employment, number of jobs, unbroken pattern of employment, and history of moonlighting. From the marital history, you can learn about your patient's fidelity and capacity for forming relationships. Throughout the history, you will have examples of how your patient has responded to various stressors.

Rather than taking what you see or hear at face value, try to evaluate all of this information against behavior you already know about. For example, suppose you have already heard that a sibling was favored by their father, and that ethnicity gives a coworker the inside track to promotion. How do these opinions square with your patient's claim to being an open and trusting person?

Observed Behaviors

Some of the behaviors you observe during the interview may reveal important character traits. Watch for actions or comments that seem to go beyond what you would expect during an interview situation. For example, your patient:

Yawns, slouches, gazes about the room, and otherwise appears uninterested

Invades your personal space by picking things up from your desk

Asks for time out to smoke a cigarette

Questions your credentials as a therapist

Criticizes your clothing or hairstyle

Uses strong words to express prejudice against some ethnic or religious group

Tries to argue about something you have said

Brags about qualities that others might seek to conceal, such as sexual liaisons, physical aggression, illegal activities, or substance use

Recognizing Personality Disorder

By itself, none of the behaviors I've mentioned above means that there is actual character pathology. In aggregate, however, or combined with your historical information, they may suggest one or more of the *personality disorders*. These diagnoses are made only when character traits are so inflexible and poorly adapted to the requirements of life that they cause considerable distress or impair the person's functioning in the realms of social, work, or other areas.

A personality disorder isn't so much an illness as a way of life. It implies long-standing behavior that causes problems for the patient. It often has its roots in childhood and may stem either from environmental influences or from the patient's inherited genetic material. Sometimes both causes are implicated.

A personality disorder should be diagnosed on the basis of behaviors, sustained through a lifetime, that suggest interpersonal conflict or maladjustment and problems with cognition (how people perceive and interpret themselves, others, and all that happens around them), affectivity (how they respond emotionally, including its type and how intense, labile, and appropriate it is), and impulse control.

To give the flavor of personality disorders, here are some that have been defined across the decades. The five that are asterisked are generally considered to have better validity than the rest; I've described them more completely in Appendix B.

*Antisocial.** The irresponsible, often criminal behavior of these people begins in childhood or early adolescence. Pathological childhood behavior includes truancy, running away, cruelty, fighting, destructiveness, lying, stealing, and robbery. As adults they may also default on debts, fail to care for dependents, fail to maintain monogamous relationships, and show no remorse for their behavior. This is perhaps the personality disorder diagnosis made with greatest validity, principally because so much depends on verifiable historical data.

Avoidant. These timid people are so easily wounded by criticism that they hesitate to become involved with others. They may fear the embarrassment of showing emotion or of saying things that seem foolish. They may have no close friends, and they exaggerate the risks of undertaking pursuits outside their usual routines.

*Borderline.** These impulsive people make recurrent suicide threats or attempts. Affectively unstable, they often show intense, inappropriate anger. They feel empty or bored, and they frantically try to avoid abandonment. They are uncertain about who they are and unable to maintain stable interpersonal relationships.

Dependent. These people have trouble starting projects or making independent decisions, even to the extent of agreeing with others who may be wrong. Often preoccupied with fears of abandonment, they feel helpless when alone and miserable when relationships end. They are easily hurt by criticism and will volunteer for unpleasant tasks to gain people's favor.

Histrionic. Overly emotional, vague, and attention-seeking, these patients need constant reassurance about their attractiveness. They may be self-centered and sexually seductive.

Narcissistic. Narcissistic people are self-important and often preoccupied with envy, fantasies of success, or ruminations about the uniqueness of their own problems. Their sense of entitlement and lack of empathy may cause them to take advantage of others. They vigorously reject criticism, and need constant attention and admiration.

*Obsessive–compulsive.** Perfectionism and rigidity characterize these people. Often workaholics, they tend to be indecisive, excessively scrupulous, and preoccupied with detail. They insist that others do things their way. They have trouble expressing affection, tend to lack generosity, and may even resist throwing away worthless objects they no longer need.

Paranoid. These people expect to be threatened or humiliated; other people's behavior seems to confirm these expectations. They can be quick to take offense and slow to forgive; often they have few confidants, question the loyalty of others, and read hidden meaning into innocent remarks.

*Schizoid.** These patients care little for social relationships, have a restricted emotional range, and seem indifferent to criticism or praise. Tending to be solitary, they avoid close (including sexual) relationships.

*Schizotypal.** Such patients have so much difficulty with interpersonal relationships that they appear peculiar or strange to others. Lacking close friends, they are uncomfortable in social situations. They may show suspiciousness, unusual perceptions or thinking, an eccentric manner of speaking, and inappropriate affect.

In considering these descriptions, we need to keep a couple of points in mind. First, many people, perhaps the majority of our patients, have distressing social problems that are *not* caused by personality disorder. A tyrannical boss can create dissension at work; a psychotic spouse can wreak havoc with a marriage. Chronic psychosis can alienate patients from their families. Every day, kids use drugs and the stock market swallows someone's savings. We also need to make sure that the pattern of behavior hasn't been caused by, say, a depression, substance misuse, or a medical condition. We protect against this sort of error by making sure that we have covered all possibilities during the information-gathering phase of evaluation.

The second point to remember has to do with the limitations inherent in a single interview, no matter how careful and extensive. Especially with personality disorder, the material you need for diagnosis may be revealed only as time deepens your experience with this patient.

Chapter 9

Sensitive Subjects

Getting up the courage to cover certain subjects can be a challenge. Though the material itself is pretty straightforward, our society largely regards these sensitive topics—which include sex, substance use, and suicidal behavior—as deeply private. Consequently, the patient may feel guilt or shame, whereas the interviewer must cast aside a lifetime of teaching, personal doubts, and perhaps prejudice. But because their exploration is critically important to your interview, if your patient does not mention them spontaneously, you must at some point bring them up yourself. You may delay until the latter portions of the interview, after you know the patient a little better, but don't wait until the very end: You could run out of time and still have important material yet to cover. Any interviewer who ignores these topics risks committing serious errors of diagnosis and treatment.

SUICIDAL BEHAVIOR

Delving into suicidal behavior is an absolute must. This rule holds even if there has been no hint of death wishes or suicidal ideas at any time during the interview. To violate the rule risks ignoring potentially life-threatening ideas and behaviors in a patient who may be too ashamed or too embarrassed to mention them spontaneously. Although the vast majority of mental health patients do not kill themselves, nearly every mental health diagnosis confers some degree of suicide risk beyond that found in the general population.

When asking about suicidal behavior, you may feel some discomfort of your own. Beginning interviewers sometimes worry that mentioning this topic could plant the idea in a patient's mind. The truth is that any patient at serious risk for suicide will have considered it long before anyone thinks to ask. The real risk is not asking soon enough.

Then you might learn only too late how gravely ill your patient really was.

If your patient is the one who raises the topic, you can pursue it with a degree of comfort. Absent such an opening, it is vitally important that you raise the question yourself. Unless your patient seems unusually uncomfortable, you don't need to precede these questions with apologies or explanations. Most patients will feel about as comfortable as you appear to feel.

In the context of the mental health interview, it is perfectly all right simply to ask:

"Have you ever had any thoughts of hurting or killing yourself?" If the answer is "No," and this seems to jibe with the patient's mood and recent behavior, you can accept it as simple fact and move on to another topic. If the response is equivocal or delivered with telltale body language, such as a hesitating manner or suddenly downcast gaze, you must pursue the matter with further questioning.

Of course, you must also be careful not to damage rapport. Should your questioning seem to cause increasing discomfort (hesitation, tears), you may need to comment on the distress:

"You look so sad that I hate to pursue this subject, but I really feel that I must."

To someone who has attempted suicide or has been otherwise violent, you might say:

"Your recent experience makes me worry that you might try it again. Has anything changed that might influence you one way or another?"

Some clinicians believe that patients may respond more truthfully if you avoid the "S-word," *suicide*. If you wish, you can gradually work toward your goal with a series of increasingly explicit questions:

1. "Have you been having any disturbing or gloomy thoughts?"
2. "Have any of these thoughts been desperate ones?"
3. "Have you ever wished you were dead?"
4. "Have you thought about harming yourself?"
5. "Have you made any plans to take your own life?"
6. "Have you ever made any actual attempts?"

It is important to expand upon a "Yes" answer to any of the questions above by asking a suitable, open-ended follow-up question:

"Could you tell me some more about that?"

"What happened then?"

If the actual attempts occurred prior to this episode—sometimes in the distant past—memories may be dim. But you should learn as much as you can about previous attempts. The information will help you (1) predict what your patient might do next, and (2) assess what actions you should take. So get answers to these questions:

- How many previous attempts have there been?
- When did they occur?
- Where was the patient at the time?
- What was the patient's mood at the time?
- What methods were used for the attempts?
- Was the attempt made under the influence of drugs or alcohol? (If so, had there been other attempts when the patient was straight and sober?)
- Did the patient have other mental disorders at the time? (In addition to substance use, you especially should learn about depression and psychosis.)
- What were the stressors that preceded the suicidal behavior? (Look for such losses as separation or divorce, death of a loved one, job loss, or retirement. However, any upsetting event in the life of the patient or of a friend or relative could serve as a precipitant.)
- How serious were the attempts?

Physical and Psychological Seriousness

We can judge the seriousness of a suicide attempt in two ways: (1) How physically harmful was the attempt? (2) How strong was the patient's intent to die? An attempt that is serious either physically or psychologically increases the likelihood that this patient will commit suicide in the future. When you are assessing your new patient for suicide potential, you should have these guidelines in mind.

A suicide attempt is physically serious when it results (or could result) in significant bodily harm. By this standard, a severed jugular vein, a deep coma, or a gunshot wound to the chest would be a physically serious attempt. So would be the ingestion of 100 tricyclic antidepressant tablets, even if the patient's stomach is pumped before coma sets in. Without prompt medical attention, fewer than half that number of antidepressants could be fatal.

At the other extreme are those attempts that are highly unlikely to cause any serious harm, let alone death. They include such acts as lightly scratching the wrist and swallowing four or five aspirin tablets. Such behaviors, which are sometimes called "gestures," suggest that the patient had in mind some purpose other than dying. In making this judgment, you set aside the physical implications and consider the psychological seriousness of the attempt, to learn what intention lay behind it. Was there a genuine wish to die, or was it a cry for help? Here are some of the possible motives for attempted suicide:

A genuine wish to die
The desire to attract help
Escape from some intolerable situation
Relief from mental distress
An attempt to influence someone

Many patients who have made psychologically serious attempts can clearly state their feelings:

"I'm sorry I didn't succeed."

"I'll try it again."

Others may be less clear, or perhaps ambivalent. For them you must ask:

"What did you think would be the outcome of your overdose [or other attempt]?"

For some, your best course could be to infer intention from behavior. The patient who attempts suicide alone in a hotel room under an assumed name is clearly more bent on self-destruction than is one whose attempt occurs at home just before the expected return of a spouse.

Here are some other questions that can help you judge the psychological seriousness of intent:

"Did you impulsively decide to make the attempt, or had you been planning it for a while?" *Planning and preparation are usually associated with more serious attempts.*

"Before the attempt, had you written or revised a will, given away property, or taken out life insurance?" *Any of these behaviors suggests planning.*

"Did you write a suicide note?" *More evidence of planning.*

"Was someone with you when you made the attempt?" *A "yes" answer suggests that the patient had arranged a means of rescue.*

"What did you do after you made the attempt?" (Lie down to wait for the end? Call for help? Phone a suicide hotline?) *Inaction should ring an alarm.*

"How did you feel when you were rescued?" *"Anger" sounds more serious than "relief."*

You must correlate whatever you learn about these previous suicide ideas and attempts with your patient's current thinking on the subject. It is vital to learn whether your patient has ideas or plans that could prove lethal, especially within the next few hours or days. Ask:

"Have you felt suicidal recently?"

"What have been your thoughts about it?"

"Have you made any plans?"

(If so:) "What are they?"

"Do you think you are likely to carry them out?"

"What has stopped you in the past?"

"When is it likely to happen?"

"What effect do you think it would have on others?"

"Do you feel you have any reason to live?"

"Could anything make suicide seem less a possibility?"

As a general rule, I avoid using the term *manipulative* in describing a suicide attempt. For one thing, most patients who attempt (or complete) suicide are somewhat ambivalent about their actions, so most attempts are manipulative to a degree. More important, this term tends to cause clinicians and families alike to relax their vigilance at a time when they may need it most.

Any current ideas or plans that could prove harmful require rapid action. If you are a student, this means contacting the treating clinician at once, to be certain that the patient's thoughts and plans are fully known. This action on your part is essential, even if it means violating a confidence or promise of confidentiality you have made previously. *Preventing suicide and other harm to patients is an absolute duty of every health care professional. To carry out this duty effectively, all clinicians must feel confident that everyone who has contact with the patient will share vital information. If you must break a confidence to ensure the safety of a patient, be assured that the vast majority of patients will not blame you for your action. In fact, most patients later feel intensely grateful for such a life-saving "betrayal."*

VIOLENCE AND ITS PREVENTION

A history of violent behavior is relatively uncommon, but it is at least as important to learn about as suicide. It can have serious implications for patients as well as for intended victims.

If your patient admits to legal difficulties such as arrests or time in confinement, you will have a natural lead-in to questions about violence. Much violence is domestic, so another good time to inquire is when you learn that the patient has been divorced or has been a partner in a troubled marriage. (Don't neglect to learn about beatings or other mistreatment that the patient might have received *from* a domestic partner.)

If no natural lead-in occurs, you will have to ask. As with self-harm, you can work up to the subject gradually:

1. "Have you ever had feelings of uncontrollable rage?"
2. "Have you had any thoughts about harming others?"
3. "Have you ever had trouble controlling your impulses?"
4. "As an adult, have you been involved in fights?"
5. "Were you ever arrested for fighting or for other violent behavior?"

Positive answers must be explored:

"What were the circumstances of the violent acts?"
"When did they occur?"
"Who was involved?"
"How did you feel about this?"
"Did the behavior involve substance use?"
"What was the effect on the victim?"
"What happened to you as a result?"
"Were you arrested?"
"Were you convicted?"
"How much time did you serve?"

Throughout, try to understand what lies behind your patient's violent ideas or behavior, and what might be causing these feelings. You might find, for example:

Anger at a motorist who has damaged the patient's car
Depression that results from genetic inheritance plus heavy drinking
Envy of a coworker who has won a coveted promotion to vice-president
Frustration that the Internal Revenue Service continues to send dunning notices for an assessment the patient has already paid
Greed when confronted with the possibility of inheriting a large estate
Hatred for an ex-spouse
Revenge for a sister's death at the hands of a mugger

A temptation for anyone, including a highly experienced clinician, who interviews a patient with the potential to be violent is to become immersed in obtaining the relevant information, to the exclusion of all other considerations. The principal one of these should be personal safety. I don't mean to alarm anyone; your risk from any individual patient is small. Yet one survey found that over half of mental health professionals had been threatened or assaulted by a patient within the previous year. Years ago, I was the target of a battering patient, and it is something I'll go a long way to prevent happening again. In a nutshell, here's how to go about it.

1. Ensure that you have an unimpeded exit route from the room where you are working. This means that there should be nothing and no one between you and your escape.

2. Make sure that someone is within earshot or can instantly answer a warning buzzer or other alarm.

3. Be especially alert when your patient has a prior history of violence; the recidivism rate for assault is sky-high. The danger is especially high for a patient who should be taking antipsychotic drugs, but isn't.

4. Keep alert to the nuances of voice (rising pitch or tempo), words (threats and insults), and body language (a clenched fist, narrowed gaze, or agitated pacing) that can indicate a need for action.

5. As soon as you sense danger, act. You'll need to put aside your usual instincts about soothing the patient (no leaning close to provide comfort, no touching for reassurance). Instead, announce calmly what you're about to do—"Mr. Smyth, I'm about to stand up and walk to the door"—a verbal warning to avert sudden alarm in a startled patient. Then do just as you've promised.

6. Once you are out of the room, get help from anyone who is available: other staff, building security, or police.

As for your office, every inpatient or outpatient facility should have a set of emergency procedures that serve as the basis for drills. The details will involve deciding who calls 911, who shows up at the door to answer any sort of alarm, and how to present a show of force in a manner that is as casual and nonthreatening as possible under the circumstances.

SUBSTANCE MISUSE

At least 1 of every 13 adult Americans has a problem with substance misuse. The figure is even higher among mental health patients, of whom perhaps 25% misuse substances. Some experience with substances that can be misused has become almost a rite of passage for American teenagers. It is so common—and its effects upon patient and environment can be so far-reaching—that substance use must be covered in the initial interview of every mental health patient, regardless of sex, age, or presenting complaint.

Alcohol

Despite the educational efforts of mental health professionals and Twelve-Step organizations like Alcoholics Anonymous, many people still view substance misuse as a disorder of morals. As a result, patients and interviewers alike find this issue difficult to discuss. Perhaps you can find a natural lead-in. Some family history might tip you off.

> PATIENT: So you can see, my childhood was nearly ruined by Mom's drinking.
>
> INTERVIEWER: Sounds pretty difficult, all right. And what about you—do you do any drinking yourself?

Just at that moment it might be inconvenient to change course, as this interviewer did, and pursue a new subject. You might instead decide to keep on eliciting childhood history and later refer back to what the patient said about family history:

> INTERVIEWER: A few minutes ago you mentioned your mother's drinking. It made me wonder—have you ever been a heavy drinker yourself?

If your patient doesn't raise the subject of drug and alcohol use, you will have to create your own opportunity. Alcohol is more socially acceptable, so you can ask about it with less risk of embarrassment. Assume that your patient, like most adults, is no teetotaler. You will be right more often than not, and the assumption of some drinking may ease the stigma if your patient's drinking has been excessive. Find out how often and how much your patient drinks:

"Now I'd like to know about some of your habits. First, in an average month, on how many days do you have at least one drink of alcohol?"

Note how the form of this question requests a precise answer, framed in terms of days per month. This discourages vague or evasive answers such as "Not very much" or "Only on social occasions." (You can count the following drinks as having roughly the same alcohol content: a 12-ounce beer, a 6-ounce glass of wine, and a 1-ounce shot of 80-proof hard liquor.)

Next you might ask:

"On the average day that you have at least one drink, how many drinks do you usually have?"

These two numbers—drinks per day and days per month—allow

you to calculate your patient's average number of drinks per month. As you do more interviews, you will develop a feel for what is usual and what is excessive. More than 60 drinks per month (2 per day, on average) is worrisome; more than 100 per month is far above the norm. But even a number below 60 can suggest a drinking problem if many of the drinks are consumed over just a few individual days: Binge drinking is one of the possible patterns of abusive drinking.

Even if the patient denies current heavy drinking, learn how much drinking there has been in the past. Has the patient been a lifelong teetotaler, or is this a recent change? ("I don't touch alcohol" may mean "I haven't had a drink since Sunday. For breakfast.") Ask:

"Was there ever a time in your life when you used alcohol more heavily than you do now?"
Obtain follow-up information about days per month, drinks per day, and the reasons for stopping.

Alcoholism (now more accurately called *alcohol dependence*) is a disorder that is defined by its consequences. The amount a person consumes is an important clue, but the diagnosis itself is based on the effects drinking has on the individual and on the environment. Therefore, unless your patient denies ever having a problem with drinking, you will need to ask questions about several categories of consequences.

For medical problems, ask:

"Has drinking caused you to have liver trouble, vomiting spells, or other medical problems?"

"Were you ever told to quit drinking because of your health? And did you?"

"Have you ever suffered from blackouts? That means that the morning after drinking, you can't remember what happened the night before." (As demonstrated in this question, be sure to define what you mean by *blackout*—some patients won't know the term.)

One of the criteria for alcohol (or any substance) dependence is using more than the patient intends. This is sometimes difficult to ascertain—especially with teenagers, who aren't known for setting limits, but rather drink for the effect it provides. Instead, try to ascertain loss of control:

"Have you ever tried to quit drinking?"

"Have you ever set rules about drinking, such as 'Never drink before four in the afternoon?' "

"Do you ever gulp drinks?"

"Once you take your first drink, do you have trouble stopping?"
For personal and interpersonal problems, ask:

"Do you sometimes feel guilty about how much you drink?"

"Have you ever gotten into fights when drinking?"

"Has drinking ever caused a divorce or other serious domestic problems?"

"Has it lost you friends?"

For job problems, ask:

"Has drinking ever caused you to be absent from work? Late to work?"

"Have you ever been fired from a job because of drinking?"

For legal problems, ask:

"Have you ever been arrested for alcohol-related behavior?"

"Have you had any arrests for driving while intoxicated?" (If so, find out what happened in court.)

"Have you ever caused an accident while driving under the influence?"

For financial problems, ask:

"Have you ever spent money on alcohol that should have gone for necessities like food?"

"Have you had any other financial difficulties because of drinking?"

If any of these questions yields a positive response, ask:

"Have you ever been concerned about your drinking?"

"Have you ever thought that you were alcoholic?"

"What has been your longest period of sobriety?"

"How did you achieve that?"

"Were you ever treated for the use of alcohol?"

"What happened as a result of treatment?"

Street Drugs

With street drugs, the procedure is similar. Your questions about alcohol use will lead naturally into this subject. Ask:

"Have you ever used street drugs of any sort?"

As with alcohol use, you will want to learn when drug use began and when it ended. Define the type of drug; the frequency of use; and the effects of use on the patient, friends, and relatives.

One problem you may encounter is not knowing the slang terminology for drugs commonly misused. If you don't understand a term, just ask; patients love to teach their care providers. I've listed a few of the terms you might hear used, but there are hundreds more. You can find many of them on the Web (www.pride.org/slangdrugterms.htm).

Hypnotics: downers, ludes, yellow jackets, tranks, reds, rainbows, Christmas trees

Cocaine: snow, coke, rock, crack

Hallucinogens: LSD, acid, PCP, mescaline, peyote, STP

Narcotics: H, horse, smack, junk (heroin); schoolboy (codeine); little D (dilaudid); Miss Emma (morphine)
Marijuana: pot, grass, tea, hash, joint, reefer, Mary Jane
Central nervous system stimulants: uppers, bennies, black beauties, crank, speed

In addition, special names may be used by various ethnic groups or in diverse parts of the country, and the terminology is fluid, changing as new cohorts of users come of age.

Prescribed or Over-the-Counter Medications

Don't forget to inquire into overuse of medicines:
"Have you ever taken more of a prescription medication than your doctor prescribed?"
"Do you ever overuse over-the-counter drugs?"
Again you need to know when, what, how much and what the effects were.
And, for any substance, you'd like to know the answer to this question: "What does it do for you that causes you to keep using it?"

SEXUAL LIFE

Patients often expect questions about sex. For most, it's an accepted part of consulting a mental health professional. However, this line of questioning makes some people feel uncomfortable, so you could be better off delaying it until later in the interview. By then you will be better acquainted with the patient, who may view these sensitive issues in the context of other necessary psychological, medical, and social information.

To learn about this important area in the life of nearly everyone, you must be able to discuss it openly, without showing disapproval or censure. Clinicians in training often have difficulty questioning patients about their sex lives. Sometimes this is due to an unfamiliarity with the questions that should be asked, but it may relate to personal standards of sexual conduct—which in turn are the results of upbringing and culture. Here it is vital to recognize your own standards and acknowledge that your patient has the right to a different set. And because a frank discussion of sex can be titillating to both parties, the sexual history is an area where, more than ever, you need a firm grip on your professional boundaries.

During the present illness or the personal and social history, you may have already learned something about the relationship between patient and partner that provides a natural introduction to the subject of sex. If this has not happened, or if the patient has no current partner, a straightforward request for information is in order. An open-ended question will provide both comfort for you and scope for the patient to respond:

"Now I would like you to tell me about your sexual functioning." The form of this question assumes that most people have sex, and that this is acceptable and normal.

If the first response is a question of the patient's own ("How do you mean?"), you might elaborate as follows:

"I'm trying to learn two things. First, how is your sexual functioning usually? And second, how has it been affected by the problem that brought you into treatment?" (Note that this speech, which deliberately breaks the rule about not asking two questions at once, tells the patient the scope of what you are trying to learn.)

The ensuing discussion should give you the following sorts of information:

> At what age did the patient first learn about sex?
> What was the nature of early sexual experiences?
> At what age did they occur?
> How did the patient react to them?

Sexual Preference

Some mental health clinicians prefer to start their inquiries about sex with a straightforward question:

"What is your sexual preference?"

This approach has the virtue of (usually) eliciting a clear answer early, therefore avoiding the possibility of embarrassing misunderstandings later. Be careful not to assume that a married patient has no history of homosexuality.

For anyone with such a history, you should try to learn:

> Is the patient bisexual or exclusively homosexual?
> If the latter, about what percentage of sexual encounters are heterosexual?
> Does the patient find this sexual orientation comfortable (ego-syntonic) or uncomfortable (ego-dystonic)?
> How well has the patient integrated sexual orientation with lifestyle?
> Has the patient wanted or attempted to change?

Although dreams and fantasies are not often productive in an initial interview, the presence of homosexual fantasies may help in the evaluation of patients who seem unclear as to their basic orientation.

Sexual Practices

When there is a history of sexual difficulty, a great many questions should be asked that you wouldn't delve into routinely. When these questions must be broached, they are often better left until a subsequent interview. Use your common sense. Once you have assured yourself that the patient and partner are happy together and function well sexually, you can probably employ a general question:

"Have there been any issues of a sexual nature that we haven't yet talked about?"

In the event of sexual dysfunction, however, some of the following issues will be appropriate for discussion:

- Has the sexual problem been lifelong, or was it recently acquired?
- What are the current sleeping arrangements?
- Have there been problems with intercourse? (Do they necessitate abstinence?)
- Is sex pleasurable for the patient?
- What about for the partner? (Until sex preference and practices are known, it is safer to use *partner* than a gender-specific noun.) *Women are much more likely than men to report lack of sexual pleasure.*
- If the patient is married or in a long-term relationship, have there been outside affairs? If so, how many? How often? How recent?
- Does the couple communicate clearly about sex?
- What is the frequency of sexual relations? Has this changed recently, or with age?
- Who usually initiates sex?
- Are the partners hesitant to approach one another for sex, perhaps due to other interpersonal problems?
- Does the couple use foreplay? How long does it last? What constitutes foreplay? (Talking? Kissing? Genital touching?) *Because many men do not realize that arousal takes longer for a woman than for a man, their female partners may report that foreplay is too brief and that intercourse itself is unsatisfying.*
- If oral sex is practiced, are both partners enthusiastic about it?
- How often does the patient achieve climax? *Anorgasmia (lack of*

climax) *is fairly common among women, who may nonetheless experience strong sex desire. Some can achieve climax only under certain circumstances, such as with masturbation. Ability to achieve climax, like
sexual interest, may be decreased by illness (physical or mental) and
anxiety.*

- How often does the patient masturbate? Does this represent a
  problem for either the patient or the partner?
- What method of birth control (if any) does the couple use? Do
  the partners agree about the timing or prevention of concep-
  tion?
- Have there been sex partners outside the current relationship?
- Has either partner had any history of sexually transmitted disease?

Common Sexual Issues

Sexual functioning comprises the areas of desire, arousal, and orgasm.
Even if desire seems to have waned, does the patient still have sexual
thoughts or fantasies? Be alert for several relatively common sexual
problems:

Impotence (inability to achieve or maintain erection). How long ago
did it start? Is it total or partial? Does it occur only with specific partners? Has it been medically investigated? Treated?
Note that impotence is quite different from lack of sexual desire.

Dyspareunia (pain with intercourse). Common in women, this condition has rarely been reported in men, too. Its cause can be
biological or emotional. Is it severe enough to interfere with
sexual functioning or pleasure?

Premature ejaculation. When a man too quickly reaches the stage of
ejaculatory inevitability (to use the Masters and Johnson
term), both partners can experience frustration and lack of
pleasure.

Retarded ejaculation. This can be the result of emotional factors,
such as guilt, or of certain medications. The classic one is
thioridazine (Mellaril), which has even been used to treat premature ejaculation.

Concerns about possible homosexuality or bisexuality. Whereas such behavior may be important for the patient, and so constitute le-
gitimate grounds for investigation by a mental health clinician, it is important to make patients aware that it is not

considered an illness, rather a form of normal sexual preference.

When you are learning about the patient's sexual life, ask for specific instances in which the problem arose. If technique seems to be the
issue, ask for a description in behavioral terms: "First I . . . then she
does . . . but that usually doesn't work, so we . . . " As for any nonsexual
problem, find out when it began, how often and under what circumstances it occurs, how severe it is (is it getting worse?), what has been
done about it, and what seems to help.

Paraphilias

Relatively uncommon are the paraphilias, which comprise a number of
disorders in which the patient is aroused by a stimulus other than a
consenting adult human, or by the humiliation or suffering of the patient or sexual partner. The diagnosis is made only when the desire has
occurred repeatedly for least 6 months and when the patient has acted
on the urge or has been markedly distressed by it. Almost all such patients are men, and they often experience as many as three or more
types of these urges, which can interfere with the ability to enjoy normal sexual and love relationships. The specific paraphilias are as follows:

> *Exhibitionism.* These patients have fantasies and urges that involve
>   the sudden exposure of their genitals to a stranger, usually a
>   female. Patients who act upon these fantasies usually don't at-
>   tempt physical contact with the victim and usually pose no
>   physical danger.
> *Fetishism.* Fetishists are sexually aroused by inanimate objects—of-
>   ten shoes or women's underwear, which are used by the pa-
>   tients themselves or are worn by a partner for sexual activity.
> *Frotteurism.* Frotteurs are aroused by touching or rubbing against a
>   nonconsenting person. Frottage usually takes place in a crowd
>   and may involve contact through clothing with hands or geni-
>   tals.
> *Pedophilia.* These patients have sexual fantasies and urges about
>   young children (usually age 13 or under). Most pedophiles
>   prefer girls, but some are aroused by boys or by children of ei-
>   ther gender. The disorder is usually chronic and may involve
>   various sexual activities, including looking, undressing, and
>   physical contact.
> *Sexual masochism.* The sexual fantasies and behaviors of these pa-

tients involve being beaten, bound, or otherwise humiliated or made to suffer. In extreme cases, death from suffocation can result.

Sexual sadism. These patients are sexually aroused by inflicting physical or psychological pain on partners, who may be either consenting or nonconsenting. Such behavior may increase over time, sometimes to the point that these patients cause severe injury and even death.

Transvestic fetishism. Occurring only in heterosexual males, this disorder involves sexual arousal from dressing in women's clothing.

Voyeurism. Voyeurs ("peeping Toms") are aroused by watching an unsuspecting person who is nude, in the act of disrobing, or having sex.

Other paraphilias. Other paraphilias include sexual arousal from animals, body excretions, cadavers, and "talking dirty" on the telephone.

Sexually Transmitted Diseases

For all patients, be alert for a history of sexually transmitted diseases, including herpes, syphilis, and gonorrhea. Especially ask about risk factors for AIDS: multiple sex partners, sex with drug users, or homosexual relationships. If any answer is "Yes," you'll need to ask whether condoms are used. If so, what percentage of the time? Has the patient ever been tested for HIV? If so, how recently? What were the results?

SEXUAL ABUSE

Childhood Molestation

A history of childhood sexual experience is distressingly common, especially among mental health patients. Yet this area is often left unexplored, even by experienced clinicians. *Childhood sexual experiences have been linked to many adult disorders, including borderline personality disorder, eating disorders, dissociative identity disorder, and somatization disorder.*

Even if none of these conditions is present, memories of early sexual behavior may present concerns that require discussion and reassurance. Therefore, you must ask. But ask in a way that avoids the loaded term *molestation:*

"When you were a child, were you ever approached for sex by another child or by an adult?"

Any positive answer should be explored thoroughly. In particular, obtain the following details:

> What actually happened?
> Was there physical contact?
> How old was the patient then?
> How many times did the incidents occur?
> Who was the perpetrator?
> Was there a blood relationship between perpetrator and patient?
> How did the patient react to the incident(s)?
> Were the parents told?
> What were their reactions?
> How have these incidents affected the patient, either during childhood or as an adult?

An occasional patient will give equivocal answers such as "I'm not sure," or "I really can't remember much about my childhood." Such a response should alert you that somewhere in your patient's background may lie experiences too distressing to be tolerated as conscious memory. Further probing at this time probably won't uncover much additional information, but do try to identify as exactly as possible the interval that has been forgotten ("ages 6 through 12" or "throughout junior high"). It may help later with the memory recovery process.

This is one time when you should probably not alert your patient that you will return to the subject later. A promise to pursue long-buried traumatic memories may seem threatening and could interfere with the rapport you are trying to build. Instead, say:

"It sounds as if you have some doubt about this area. That's all right—nobody remembers everything from childhood. But if anything about early sexual experiences comes back to you, I'd like to hear about it later. It could be important."

Do make a careful note to return to the subject in a later interview, when your relationship is on solid ground.

Rape and Spouse Abuse

For decades (at least), the crime of rape has been seriously underreported. This fact is probably explained by victims' feelings of shame and embarrassment and their fear of notoriety. With the publicity of "celebrity rape" trials and our enhanced understanding of victim psychology, these attitudes may have lessened somewhat in recent years. Nonetheless, it remains all too common that patients (nearly all of them female) have as adults suffered rape or other forms of sexual abuse. (The U.S. military reported that sexual assault increased by 24% in 2006 over the previous year.) Mental health interviewers must be able to draw forth the information needed to determine the best course of action for these patients, many of whom have been severely traumatized by their experiences.

Usually the preferred first approach is a sympathetic, unstructured invitation to describe the events and their consequences:

"Please tell me about these experiences."

With gentle, probing questions, you should then try to obtain the following information:

> What were the circumstances? (Surroundings? Patient's age?)
> Who was the perpetrator? (Relative? Acquaintance? Stranger? Gang?)
> How many times did it occur?
> Did the patient know the perpetrator?
> Were they related?
> Was the use of alcohol or drugs involved? If so, by whom?
> What feelings did the patient have at the time?
> Who has been told?
> Has the story been heard sympathetically?
> Has legal action been taken? If not, why not?
> What have been the lingering effects of the experiences? (Look for fear, anger, shame, anxiety, depression, and symptoms of posttraumatic stress.)

Similar multiple emotions can be evoked by sexual and physical abuse from spouses. Victims may also be reluctant to report this crime for fear of reprisals, such as further abuse or abandonment.

Chapter 10

Control of the Later Interview

During most of the early interview, you have encouraged your patient to discuss problems freely. By the time you move on to the personal and social history, you will need to exercise more control over the form of your interview. This will enable you to use your time efficiently to cover all the material and probe the important remaining areas. A number of verbal and nonverbal techniques can help direct the patient's responses and maximize the amount of material obtained.

TAKE CHARGE

Some patients take direction so well that you can exercise control just by gently interjecting an occasional guiding question. Patients who are circumstantial or perhaps just plain talkative will need more active measures of control. Those with manic pressure of speech or psychotic suspiciousness may require almost constant redirection.

Of course, you will have to temper your own verbal output. Novice interviewers must be especially wary: Anxiety sometimes causes them to speak too often or at excessive length. Remember that the main purpose of your questions and interventions is to facilitate the flow of information from the patient. In order to occupy as little time as possible with explanations, state your questions clearly and succinctly.

With the need to cover so much ground, you may not be able to respond as completely as you would like to issues your patient raises. For example, on hearing that your patient was teased as a child, your natural impulse may be to sympathize and ask for examples, effects, and the patient's reactions. But perhaps it is late in the session, and you still must uncover any history of sexual abuse. You may have to defer some of these natural responses until another session. For now, you could briefly sympathize and then indicate your interest by asking about other childhood traumas you want to know about anyway.

> PATIENT: . . . so I felt that I was the butt of every schoolyard joke and prank.

> INTERVIEWER: That sort of experience can really make a kid miserable. Did you have other sorts of distressing problems as a child? For example, did any one ever approach you about sex?

You should try to avoid abrupt transitions, which can impair rapport. Instead, try one of these techniques:

- You can change the subject with more grace if you first make an empathic comment, as did the interviewer in the example above.
- Stop taking notes, and put down your pen. If you continue to write, your patient may feel encouraged to continue talking about the same subject.
- If you must interrupt, try raising your forefinger (raising an entire hand seems peremptory) and taking a breath to signal that you need a turn to speak.
- Try moving quickly to get in a word between two of your patient's sentences. Although this requires vigilance and can sometimes be a real struggle, it usually works well, especially if you manage to intervene at the end of a thought.
- If your patient brings up something that you already have covered sufficiently, indicate the need for a change of direction:

"I'd like to hear more about that later, if we have time. For now, let's talk instead about . . . "

"I think I understand about your insomnia. But has your appetite changed any?" (Notice that asking a "yes–no" question suggests that now you'd like a short answer.)

"I need to interrupt here to ask about something else that's important . . . "

- Nod or smile when you do get the sort of brief answer you want. This reinforcement will encourage further brevity.

But some patients simply don't respond well to hints. For someone who continues to ramble, you may have to be more direct. A good approach is to state clearly your needs and your proposed solution:

"For me to help you best, it's important that we cover a lot of ground. That means we'll have to move on now to another area."

"Our time is getting a little short . . ."

"Let's stick with the main topic . . ."

You may have to indicate the new direction more than once before an especially talkative patient gets the message. But keep at it—you must obtain all of your diagnostic material.

CLOSED-ENDED QUESTIONS

In the earlier portions of the interview, open-ended questions are recommended, because they help patients communicate with greater clarity and scope. Later in the interview, when you know what sort of specific information may be relevant to diagnosis and therapy, closed-ended questions work especially well.

Closed-ended questions are those that can be answered "Yes" or "No," or that request a specific answer (such as, the patient's place of birth or duration of marriage). They allow you to pin down diagnostic criteria and clarify previous responses, so you obtain a more complete picture of your patient's problems. They are also less likely to promote evasiveness on the part of a patient who would like to hold back certain types of information. In addition, they will help you ascertain significant negatives, such as the *absence* of sexual problems or psychosis; from open-ended questions alone, you might not learn that your patient doesn't have these symptoms.

Another closed-ended technique is to substitute a multiple-choice request when your patient can't answer a question that is less well defined:

INTERVIEWER: For about how long have you been using cocaine?

PATIENT: Well, I . . . that is . . . uh, I don't know exactly.

INTERVIEWER: Well, has it been a week or 2, or more like 6 months, or perhaps a year or more?

PATIENT: Oh, it's been over a year. Maybe 3 years, anyway.

You should also be aware of the potential drawbacks of closed-ended questions. Patients who are more verbal may resent closed-ended questions if they think you care more about the process of getting the information than you do about the person who is supplying it. Also, the "yes–no" format denies patients the chance to give a gradient of response. The answer you get could mislead rather than educate you. Here is an unfortunate example:

> INTERVIEWER: Did you have problems relating to your father when you were a child?
>
> PATIENT: (*Thinking*, "Let's see, I couldn't stand the Old Man, so I never paid any attention to what he said. I guess the answer I can give is ... ") No.

Closed-ended questions can be valuable, but you should avoid suggesting how you would like your patient to answer. Such *leading questions* broadly hint that there are certain standards or behaviors you approve of. A leading question severely limits the scope and validity of the information you will obtain. For example, don't indicate your idea of "average":

> INTERVIEWER: How much alcohol do you drink?
>
> PATIENT: Oh, I'd say it's about average.
>
> INTERVIEWER: Two or three times a week?
>
> PATIENT: Well, sure.

A better response for this interviewer would have been "What is 'average' for you?" In fact, beware of any leading formulation that suggests what you regard as normal. Instead of "Is your relationship with your father a good one?" try the open-ended "How do you get along with your father?"

Closed-ended questions may actually inhibit some patients from responding fully. This is why they should only be used later in the interview, after you have built rapport and your patient has developed the habit of giving full responses. Because you must do a larger share of the talking, closed-ended questions occupy more of your time and give the patient the chance to screen out possible replies that are embarrassing or that seem "irrelevant." In consequence, the information you gather could prove false or incomplete.

Nevertheless, this highly structured style of requesting information may be appropriate for patients who are not used to the interview process or for those whose verbal skills have never been well developed. This will apply especially to patients with severe mental illness such as untreated schizophrenia; to some with mental retardation; and to those who, for a variety of reasons, are reluctant to be interviewed in the first place. Such patients may require extensive use of "yes–no" questions.

Regardless of how far you have progressed in the interview, you will probably succeed best if you continue to use a mixture of open- and closed-ended questions. For example, after you have obtained a string of rapid-fire answers that confirm a diagnosis of alcoholism, you might relieve the monotony (and tension) by asking something open-ended:

"That was a lot of questions. Now perhaps you could tell me how you plan to deal with your drinking in the future."

By combining styles, you can obtain detailed, structured information as well as encourage your patient to generate important new material; the combination of styles should help you obtain material that has maximum validity.

SENSITIVITY TRAINING

It is important to remember that highly structured questioning needn't (and shouldn't) be abrasive or otherwise unpleasant. You can soften any question with a sympathetic facial expression or tone of voice. But you should also phrase your requests to help your patient talk about a variety of sensitive issues:

• "I know that your wife's death makes it hard for you to talk about her." This comment acknowledges that the topic is important enough to pursue, despite the patient's obvious distress.

• "How do you think other people would deal with a daughter who's gotten into trouble with the law?" By asking how others might react or feel, you may be able to reduce your patient's sense of personal involvement and responsibility. This particular expression also suggests that the patient is not alone in suffering from this sort of experience. The result could be information that you would otherwise miss.

• "What if the police picked you up for drinking—how would you feel?" Using supposition, you help your patient achieve some distance from an emotionally charged situation.

• "Have you ever had the opportunity to tell your wife you were sorry for hitting her?" Here you soften the question by suggesting that chance might have prevented some praiseworthy action that your patient should have taken, but didn't.

TRANSITIONS

Effective interviewing isn't just asking one question after another. You must also pay attention to the overall coherence of what you and the patient are saying. The sentence or phrase you use to get from one topic to the next is called a *transition*. Because it points the way to where you are going, a careful transition keeps the patient from feeling blindly herded. Transitions also help you tie the entire story together.

The best transitions are couched in language that flows naturally, as in a conversation. Try to let each question take off from a portion of the previous answer. Whenever possible, use the patient's own words as a vehicle for exploration:

> PATIENT: . . . so our finances really changed for the better when my wife got a full-time job.
>
> INTERVIEWER: And what about your relationship—did it change after your wife got a full-time job?

Interviews can't always proceed in a linear fashion. If you are discussing important topic *A* when *B* is mentioned, your interview could become scattered unless you get closure on *A* before moving on. Later, if you reintroduce *B* by referring to your patient's earlier statement, you will have made a smooth transition. For example:

"A few minutes ago you mentioned that the depression seems to get better when you drink alcohol. Could you tell me some more about the drinking?"

You can use any common factor—time, place, family relationships, a job—to smooth the flow of the conversation:

> PATIENT: . . . so it was just after my brother left for Iraq that my mother died.
>
> INTERVIEWER: And what were you doing at that time?

No one likes to be given the third degree; patients are no exception. You should therefore try to make your interview feel like a conversation, not an interrogation. Smooth transitions help to create that feeling. But when you have to make an abrupt transition, flag it so the patient realizes that you are changing gears intentionally:

"I think I've got a good picture of your drinking. Now I'd like to move on to something different. Could you tell me whether you've ever had problems with other substances, such as marijuana or cocaine?"

Once you and your patient have become accustomed to one another, you will probably find that a single word, appropriately emphasized, can signal a change of topics:

"*Now* please tell me what happened when you and your husband were cooking and selling methamphetamine."

The one time you may feel tempted to make a fairly abrupt transition is if your patient becomes hostile or anxious. Even then, you should attempt to smooth the transition by acknowledging the shift—and the patient's right to whatever upset feelings you may have inadvertently elicited. For example:

"I can see that it's pretty upsetting to talk about how your wife ran off with her lover. I don't blame you. It's an area we can easily skip for now. Instead, let me ask you some more about your new girlfriend."

If it is your patient who abruptly changes the subject, you should try to learn why.

Chapter 11

Mental Status Exam I: Behavioral Aspects

WHAT IS THE MENTAL STATUS EXAM?

The *mental status exam* is simply your evaluation of the patient's current mental functioning. Originally a part of the traditional neurological exam, now it is a staple of the initial mental health examination. This and the following chapter discuss the complete mental status exam. The amount and type of material presented here may seem daunting at first, but once learned, it becomes automatic and easy to cover in a few minutes.

The mental status exam is usually divided into several parts. They can be arranged many different ways. Arrange your mental status exam any way you wish, as long as you cover all the parts. Your best bet is to choose a format, memorize it, and perform your mental status exam the same way every time until it has become second nature.

The following format has worked well for many professionals. It divides the mental status exam into two large areas: behavioral and cognitive.

Behavioral Aspects

To obtain the behavioral material, you don't have to ask special questions or perform tests. Mostly you just observe speech and behavior while you are talking to your patient (although in the area of mood, there are some questions to ask). The behavioral aspects are as follows:

1. General appearance and behavior
2. Mood
3. Flow of thought

Cognitive Aspects

The cognitive portions of the mental status exam are concerned with what your patient is thinking (talking) about. Their evaluation demands more activity on your part. They include the following:

1. Content of thought
2. Perception
3. Cognition
4. Insight and judgment

The cognitive aspects will be described in Chapter 12.

I will define and explain the standard terms you need to know. Italics will indicate some of the *possible* interpretations you might put on this information. Remember, though, that many more interpretations may be possible, and that isolated bits of even quite unusual behavior may be completely normal. Throughout your interview, you should be constantly evaluating what you observe of your patient's present behavior against what the history would lead you to expect.

GENERAL APPEARANCE AND BEHAVIOR

You can learn a great deal about a patient just by looking. Most of the following are characteristics that you should begin to notice first thing in your interview, even before anyone says a word.

Physical Characteristics

What is your patient's ethnicity? *Various studies suggest that Hispanic patients report symptoms differently from Anglos. Some diagnoses are more common among, for example, Native Americans. Any patient may have difficulty relating to a clinician of a different ethnicity.*

How old would you say this person is? Do apparent age and stated age jibe? *Age can suggest certain diagnoses. Personality disorder and schizophrenia are more likely in a young patient (late teens to mid-30s), whereas symptoms of melancholia or Alzheimer's dementia are more common in older patients.*

Notice your patient's body build. Is it slender? Stocky? Muscular? What about posture? (Erect? Slumped?) Are walking and other movements graceful or jerky? Is there a limp? Are there unusual physical characteristics, such as scars, tattoos, or missing limbs? How would you assess the patient's general nutrition? (Obese? Slender? Wasted?) *Ab-*

normal thinness suggests anorexia nervosa. Poor nutrition is most often unre-
lated to mental disorder, but it can indicate a chronic debilitating physical dis-
ease, depression, substance misuse, or homelessness.

When you shake hands during your introductions, notice whether
the patient's palms are dry or damp. Is the grip firm and hearty, or
limp and halfhearted?

Alertness

Your patient's alertness can be graded along a continuum.

- *Full or normal alertness* implies awareness of the environment
  and the ability to respond quickly to a variety of sensory stimuli.
- *Drowsiness* and *clouding of consciousness* refer somewhat impre-
  cisely to someone who is awake but less than fully alert. Drowsiness suggests that the patient can be stimulated to full wakefulness. Clouding of consciousness may be less transient, as in a
  person who has taken a drug overdose; it implies greater pathology.
- *Stupor* is a state of unconsciousness. The stuporous patient will
  respond with partial arousal to vigorous, repeated physical stimuli such as shaking or pinching.
- *Coma* is a condition from which the patient cannot be aroused at
  all, even by stimuli such as deep pain or noxious odors.

It isn't uncommon to encounter fluctuating consciousness during
a single interview session. *Carefully note any alterations in level of con-*
sciousness; they can affect your interpretation of the formal tests, as well as your
informal observations of the patient's behavior.

Some patients will appear to be more alert than is usually considered normal. These people may rapidly and repeatedly glance about
the room, as if suspiciously scanning the environment for danger. *Such*
hypervigilance or hyperalertness is found in paranoid disorders and PTSD.

Clothing and Hygiene

Is your patient's clothing clean and well cared for or dirty and tattered?
Is it casual or formal? Contemporary or out of date? Is it appropriate to
the climate and to the circumstances of your meeting? Notice any jewelry. *Bright colors may suggest mania; something as ordinary as a mis-*
buttoned shirt or coat could indicate dementia. Bizarre dress, such as an adult
wearing a Boy Scout uniform, suggests psychosis.

What is your patient's hairstyle and hair color? Is there any facial hair? What about personal hygiene? *If the patient is disheveled or malodorous, suspect serious illness such as schizophrenia or substance dependence.*

Motor Activity

Try to assess dominant body attitude: Is it one of apparent relaxation, or does the patient sit tensely on the edge of the chair?

Notice the amount of motor activity. As you talk, does your patient sit quietly? Does this seem to approach immobility at times? *True immobility is rare and can be due to catatonia. Classically described as a feature of schizophrenia, immobility is actually encountered in a variety of other psychiatric conditions and in frontal lobe brain dysfunction with various physical causes.*

Much more common in mental health patients is excessive motion. Does your patient fidget, jiggle a leg up and down, or frequently arise from the chair to pace? *These behaviors may be due to* akathisia, *a side effect of the older type of antipsychotic drugs, which may still be used to control psychosis. Sometimes akathisia can become so severe that a patient literally cannot sit still and spends much time pacing restlessly around the room. Occasional uneasy shifting of position is more likely to be the consequence of simple anxiety.*

Mostly, a patient's gestures will just express spoken feelings or emphasize verbalized statements ("talking with the hands"). Some gestures, however, convey unvoiced ideas—such as the circled OK of thumb and forefinger or the not-so-OK raised middle finger. Observe your patient's hands. Are they folded at rest, or are fists kept tightly clenched? Are fingernails dirty, bitten, stained, or carefully manicured? Is there a tremor? *This could be due to anxiety, but tremor of a pill-rolling type is often seen in Parkinson's disease and in pseudoparkinsonism (a frequent side effect of older antipsychotic drugs).*

Notice any behavior such as inappropriate scratching, touching, or rubbing in public. Does this person pick at skin or clothing? *One possible explanation is delirium, which can have a variety of physical or chemical causes. One type is delirium tremens (DTs), found in severe alcohol dependence.*

It is extremely important, especially in chronically ill mental patients, to look for the involuntary movements of face and limbs associated with tardive dyskinesia. Are there any twisting or writhing movements of the extremities? What about, chewing, facial grimacing, puckering of lips, or protrusions of the tongue? These movements may be gross and unmistakable, but more often they will be mild and may be hard to identify. If in doubt, ask to see your patient's tongue; wormlike fasciculations may be the only early sign of tardive dyskinesia.

You may notice other unusual behaviors. Look for any *manner-isms*—unnecessary behaviors that are part of a goal-directed activity. (An example would be the flourish that some people make with a pen before writing something.) *Mannerisms are common and normal; to some degree, we all have them.* On the other hand, *stereotypies* are behaviors that are not goal-directed. An example would be a patient who repeatedly pauses to make the peace sign to no apparent purpose. *Posturing* is when a patient strikes and holds a pose (such as a hand tucked inside a shirt front, like Napoleon) that appears to have no purpose. Purpose-less *negativism* may be shown by persistent silence or by turning away from the examiner. In *waxy flexibility*, the patient's rigidly held limbs can be moved only slowly and with pressure from you, as if you were bending a rod of soft wax. Patients with *catalepsy* will maintain any odd or unusual posture you place them in, despite the fact that you urge them to relax. *Stereotypies, posturing, waxy flexibility, negativism, and cata-lepsy are infrequently encountered today, and then only in the most seriously ill of hospitalized patients. They usually signify psychosis—most often schizophre-nia.*

Facial Expression

Does the patient smile and generally show normal mobility of facial ex-pression? *A fixed, motionless expression could indicate senility, the rigidity common in Parkinson's disease, or pseudoparkinsonism from antipsychotic drugs.* How well does this patient make eye contact with you? *A psychotic patient may stare fixedly at you; in depression, the gaze may seem riveted to the floor.* As you converse, does your patient repeatedly glance around the room, as if noticing something you cannot see or attending to voices no one else can hear? *These behaviors of responding to an internal stimulus may be encountered in patients who have psychoses of various types.* Are there any tics of eyes, mouth, or other body parts?

You should watch for any other behaviors that contradict the infor-mation your patient is giving you verbally:

> You notice the motor restlessness of akathisia, when your patient denies taking antipsychotics.
> Your patient has a sad face and appears to be about to cry, but claims to feel cheerful.

Voice

As you talk, notice the volume, pitch, and clarity of your patient's voice. Does it have a normal lilt (called *prosody*), or is it monotonous and dull? From the use of grammar, can you tell anything about education or family background? Does an accent identify the country or region in which the patient was reared? Does the patient stutter, lisp, mumble, or demonstrate some other speech impediment? Are there mannerisms of speech, such as words or phrases used habitually? How would you characterize the tone of voice: friendly, angry, or sad?

Attitude toward Examiner

There are several continuums along which you could describe your patient's apparent relationship to you:

    Cooperative → obstructionistic
    Friendly → hostile
    Open → secretive
    Involved → apathetic

How far to the left your patient scores on each of these factors will help determine the amount of information you can expect to obtain, as well as the strength of your rapport. In addition, note any evidence of seductiveness or evasiveness.

MOOD

The terms *mood* and *affect* have been variously defined. Nowadays, some clinicians use them interchangeably. I will use *mood* to mean the way a person claims to be feeling, and *affect* to mean how the person appears to be feeling. Therefore, the term *affect* signifies not only stated mood, but facial expression, posture, eye contact (or its lack), and tearfulness as well.

Mood (or affect) is described in several dimensions: type, lability, appropriateness, and (by some observers) intensity.

Type

What is the patient's *type* of mood? This means simply the basic quality of mood. In Chapter 7 I have presented some 60 expressions of feeling (see Table 4), but they can be boiled down to just a few basic moods. Trouble is, there isn't a lot of agreement as to exactly what's basic. Here's my take on the best consensus judgment of a dozen or more experts on basic emotions:

Anger	Joy
Anxiety	Love
Contempt	Sadness
Disgust	Shame
Fear	Surprise
Guilt	

One mood will usually predominate. When it does not, "normal" or "about medium" serves as an adequate description.

Your patient's mood will probably be obvious from what you have already observed. If not, ask:

"How are you feeling now?"

"What is your mood at this time?"

If you detect sadness, you might inquire:

"Do you feel like crying?"

An occasional patient will burst into tears—a response that can be distressing for a beginning interviewer, but is sometimes therapeutic for the patient. Have some facial tissues available for this situation, and try to learn what feelings lie behind the cloudburst.

You can also infer a good deal from your patient's body language. Here are a few nonverbal cues to feelings:

Anger: clenched jaw, knotted fists, flushing of face or neck, drumming fingers, extended neck veins, fixed stare

Anxiety: jiggling foot, twisting fingers, affected casualness (such as toothpicking)

Sadness: moistening of eyes, drooping shoulders, slowed movements

Shame: poor eye contact, blushing, shrugging

Some patients have difficulty describing, or even recognizing, how they feel. A few cannot seem to do it at all. I'll mention again the term *alexithymia*, which is sometimes used to describe the inability to recognize or describe one's feelings.

Lability

Even normal people will sometimes show two or more moods within a brief time span. For example, at a funny yet tender moment in a movie or play, anyone might laugh and weep almost at the same time. But wide swings of mood are often abnormal and should be watched for in a mental health interview. Such mood swings are termed *increased lability* of mood. *Patients with somatization disorder may show dramatic swings of mood from ecstasy to tears, all in a matter of minutes. A patient with manic euphoria may suddenly burst into bitter tears, then rapidly return to bubbling good nature (the term* microdepression *is sometimes used to described this phenomenon). In the dementias, rapid mood swings can be so severe as to deserve the term* affective incontinence.

The opposite picture occurs when the patient shows reduced variation of mood. This lack of response to environmental stimuli is called *flattening* of mood. The term *blunting* has been used as a synonym, although some writers use *flattening* to mean a compressed range of mood and reserve *blunting* for a lack of emotional sensitivity. *However the terms are defined, these patients, classically identified as having schizophrenia, seem unable to relate to other people's emotions. Relative immobility of mood is also found in severe depression and in Parkinson's disease and other neurological conditions.* Blandness *of affect, in which nothing much ever seems to ruffle the patient, classically occurs in the dementias.*

Appropriateness

Appropriateness of mood is your estimate of how well the patient's mood matches the situation and the content of thought. Your judgment will be affected by two cultures: your own and the patient's. Although most people show inappropriate emotional reactions from time to time, a pronounced inappropriateness is common in certain diagnostic groups. *Someone who giggles or laughs while, for example, describing something sad (such as the death of a close relative) may be suffering from schizophrenia, disorganized type. Pathological affect (either inappropriate laughing or weeping) may be encountered in pseudobulbar palsy, which can have a variety of causes, including multiple sclerosis and strokes. Patients with somatization disorder will sometimes talk about their physical incapacities (paralysis, blindness) with a nonchalance more appropriate to a weather report. This special type of inappropriate mood is called* la belle indifférence *(French for "lofty indifference").*

Although you should be continually alert for these and other signs of otherwise unexpressed feeling, it is important not to overinterpret. Try instead to relate what you observe to what you hear and to what you yourself might feel under similar circumstances. Are tears warranted by the topic being discussed, or does your patient appear to be unnaturally sad? Does the smile seem genuine, or is it forced, perhaps hiding true feelings?

Intensity

Although the designation is subjective and therefore somewhat arbitrary, you can grade *intensity* of mood as mild, moderate, or severe (think of the progression from dysthymia through major depression without and with psychosis). You might also want to note the *reactivity* of a mood: Is it fleeting, prolonged, or somewhere in between?

FLOW OF THOUGHT

The term *flow of thought* is a slight misnomer. What we are interested in *is* the thought, but what we actually perceive is the flow of speech. We assume that the speech we hear reflects the patient's thoughts.

Most of the problems described here are usually apparent only during the acute phase of illness. They can be grouped into two overall categories: (1) defects of *association* (the way words are joined together to make phrases and sentences), and (2) abnormal *rate and rhythm*.

Unhappily, mental health clinicians don't always agree about these definitions, so I've tried to adopt a consensus view. However, you will be safest if you record in quotes actual examples of your patient's speech. This will remind you later exactly what the patient said, will help anyone who reads your write-up to understand what you mean by the terms you use, and will provide a recorded basis for judging future change in thought patterns that may occur with treatment.

Be careful not to attribute undue pathological significance to your patient's manner of speaking. Speech patterns different from yours can be shaped by neurological or other medical disorders, by cultural influences, or by growing up speaking a different primary language.

Association

First, notice whether speech is *spontaneous* or occurs only in response to questions. If the latter, you should take some pains to induce the patient to talk spontaneously:

"I'm grateful for all the answers you've given me. But now I think it would help if you'll just talk for a while about your problems. That way, I'll get a better feeling for what is bothering you."

If you don't succeed with this, the amount of information you can obtain about speech patterns will obviously be somewhat limited. Record examples of what speech there is, and note the attempts you made to obtain more.

Derailment. Sometimes called *loose associations*, derailment is a breakdown of thought association in which one idea seems to run into another. The two ideas may be related or unrelated. You can understand the sequence of words, but their general direction seems to be governed not by logic but by rhymes, puns, or other rules that might not be apparent to an observer. What comes out is speech that seems to mean something to the patient but not to you:

"She tells me something in one morning and out the other."

"Half a loaf is better than the whole enchilada."

"I'll never go back to that store again. I don't have enough sand for my shoes."

A special type of derailment is *flight of ideas*, in which a word or phrase from one thought stimulates the patient to take off on another. The thoughts do not appear to be related by logic. The patient will usually completely lose the thread of the original question.

INTERVIEWER: When did you enter the hospital?

PATIENT: I came in on a Monday. Monday is wash day. That's what I'm gonna do—wash that man right outta my hair. He's the tortoise and I'm the hare.

Patients with mania often have flight of ideas associated with push of speech (described later in this chapter).

Tangentiality (tangential speech). These terms describe an answer that seems irrelevant to the question asked. If there is some relationship between question and answer, it is hard to discern.

INTERVIEWER: How long did you live in Wichita?

PATIENT: Even anteaters like to French-kiss.

Derailments and tangentiality are classically encountered in psychosis, often schizophrenia, but patients with mania can also exhibit these symptoms.

Poverty of speech. This is a marked reduction from normal in the amount of spontaneous speech. The patient answers briefly when you expect elaboration, and, unless prompted, may say nothing for long periods. When this behavior is carried to the extreme of muteness, there is little or no speech at all. *Patients with depression may show poverty of speech. Muteness is more characteristic of schizophrenia, but it is sometimes found in somatization disorder. It must be distinguished from aphonia of neurological origin.*

The following terms designate speech pathology that is seldom encountered in clinical interviews. I will define them briefly, but unless you work on the back ward of a large psychiatric hospital, you are unlikely to encounter any of these behaviors more than once every few years. Most occur classically in schizophrenia, but any may be found in psychoses of cognitive origin. When you do encounter an example, be sure to record it and try to learn why the patient has responded that way.

Thought blocking. The train of thought stops suddenly, before it arrives at the station. The patient can usually give no explanation more adequate than that the thought has been "forgotten."

Alliteration. A phrase or sentence intentionally contains multiple repetitions of the same or similar sounds: "I ran the risk, Doctor dear, of recognizing revolting rabbits racing in the roadster."

Clang associations. The choice of individual words is governed by rhyming or other similarity of sound, not by the requirements of communication.

> INTERVIEWER: Who brought you to the hospital?
>
> PATIENT: My wife, she's the wife of my life, no strife.

Echolalia. In answering a question, the patient unnecessarily repeats words or phrases of the interviewer. This can be fairly subtle, to the point that you may recognize it only after several repetitions.

> INTERVIEWER: How long were you in the hospital that time?
>
> PATIENT: How long were you in the hospital? I was in the hospital a long, long time, that's how long I was in the hospital.

Verbigeration. The patient continues to repeat a word or phrase without obvious purpose: "It was deathly still. Deathly. Deathly still. Deathly. Still deathly."

Incoherence. The patient is so disorganized that even individual words or phrases appear to have no logical connection: "Shovel . . . it wasn't the . . . best hatred . . . lifetime." Sometimes this is more colorfully termed *word salad.*

Neologisms. In the absence of artistic intent (such as in Lewis Carroll's "Jabberwocky"—" 'Twas brillig, and the slithy toves/Did gyre and gimble in the wabe . . . ")—the patient makes up words, often from parts of dictionary words. The resulting structure may sound quite authentic: "I didn't want him spinning cobwebs all over, so I hit him with my arachnosquisher [a shoe]."

Perseveration. The patient repeats words or phrases, or repeatedly returns to a point that has already been covered or mentioned.

> INTERVIEWER: And what was your girlfriend like?
>
> PATIENT: Oh, she had long, blonde hair and she wore it in a pony tail . . .

INTERVIEWER: Did you feel she supported you when you had that trouble with your ex-wife?

PATIENT: But she wasn't very tall. Just a bit over 5 feet.

INTERVIEWER: What I'd really like is to hear about your relationship with her.

PATIENT: She was pretty, really pretty.

Stilted speech. Accent, phraseology, or choice of words gives speech an unnatural or quaint flavor, as if the patient were someone else entirely. An American who affects a British accent or who frequently uses British idioms might be said to have stilted speech.

Rate and Rhythm of Speech

Patients who speak rapidly, and often at considerable length, are said to show *push of speech* (or *pressured speech*). Because these patients are often loud and hard to interrupt, they can pose a real challenge for interviewers. Push of speech is usually associated with *decreased latency of response*, in which the period of time between your question and the patient's response is markedly reduced. Sometimes the response seems to come almost before you have asked your question. *Push of speech and decreased latency of response are classically found in patients with mania, who may tell you that their words cannot keep up with their rapid thoughts.*

A patient with *increased latency of response* takes far longer than normal to answer or interjects long pauses between sentences. This speech pattern can mirror more general *psychomotor retardation.* When the statement is finally offered, it may be brief and delivered with excruciating slowness. *Increased latency of response is characteristic of severe depression.*

When the timing of syllables deviates from normal, disorders of rhythm of speech occur. *Stuttering* is one such disorder. In *cluttering,* the patient speaks rapidly and becomes tangle-tongued and disorganized. Patients with cerebellar lesions may utter each syllable at the same pace as the last, yielding a rate that is too precisely even. Those with some forms of muscular dystrophy may speak in clusters or have difficulty uttering syllables.

Other speech patterns occur that usually have no pathological significance at all. Whereas they may be quite noticeable to the listener, the individual who uses them can remain totally unaware of how often they occur.

The term *circumstantial speech* means that much extraneous material is included with the principal message. In this common speech pattern, the speaker eventually comes to the point, although often at considerable cost to the listener's time and patience.

In *distractible speech*, the speaker's attention may be diverted by stimuli that are extraneous to the conversation. Noise in the corridor or a moth fluttering against a window may send the conversation off in a new (though usually temporary) direction. Distractible speech is usually normal, but it can also be encountered in mania.

Verbal tics are conventional expressions that many people overuse from time to time, usually without realizing it. Such time-fillers are almost always normal, if boring.

"You know"
"I go" (for "I said")
"Basically"
"Really"
"Awesome"

Many of the terms with which we label speech patterns are confusing, and various experts will use them differently. Once again, I strongly recommend that you make your record as clear as possible by writing down *verbatim* examples of any speech you consider to be pathological.

Chapter 12

Mental Status Exam II: Cognitive Aspects

Nearly all of the findings mentioned in Chapter 11 are typically made by passive observation alone. In contrast, you must use active questioning to elicit most of the material presented in this chapter.

SHOULD YOU DO A FORMAL MENTAL STATUS EXAM?

Some clinicians still fail to assess—or to report—the cognitive aspects of the mental status exam, despite the critical importance of this information to the overall evaluation of any patient. Others feel that it is insulting to ask obvious, routine questions such as "What is the date?" and "Who is the president?" of an adult who seems clearly unimpaired. They choose not to do formal testing without a positive indication, such as a complaint by relatives that the patient has had a memory problem.

You probably wouldn't jump right in and ask an obviously unimpaired patient about hearing voices. But unless you ask, you can never be sure that any patient is unimpaired. This is why I strongly recommend, especially if you are just starting out, that you do a formal mental status exam on all patients. You can take some steps to reduce the likelihood of resentment for the patient and embarrassment for you.

• Start by explaining what you are about to do. Stress the fact that these questions are the norm and are not occasioned by something the patient has said or done:

"Now I'd like to ask some routine questions that will help me assess how you think about things. It will only take a few minutes."

Words such as *routine* and *normal* help pull the sting from questions that might otherwise be taken amiss.

- Use whatever degree of positive feedback seems warranted, as long as you speak no more than the truth:

"That's excellent! This is the best I've seen anyone do calculations all week."

- Respond attentively to any distress these questions seem to cause. If necessary, take a break and return later to any aspect that is troublesome:

"Subtracting sevens in your head is tough. Let's give it a rest and try presidents instead."

- In any case, everyone will feel far more comfortable if you get this portion of your evaluation out of the way during your first interview. If you delay asking until treatment is well underway, you increase the possibility of embarrassment for you and your patient.

Anyone who observes seasoned professionals doing the formal portions of the mental status exam will notice that they don't ask every question of every patient. With time and experience, clinicians learn which tests can be omitted for certain patients and which must be performed every time. While you are still learning, I recommend that you do the entire procedure each time. That way you will learn it all; you will also develop your own sense of what responses are normal for each test. Once you become expert (after your first several hundred exams), you can decide which tests to omit and when.

The mental status exam properly concerns only current behaviors, experiences, and emotions. However, it is often convenient to cover related historical data at the same time. This is the reason why so many of the screening questions begin with "Have you *ever* . . . "

One further thought: Some of the experiences covered in the following pages are unusual enough that your patient might feel reluctant to respond frankly. To address such reluctance, you can point out that people can have all types of strange experiences when they are stressed or ill or taking medications. Framing your inquiry this way can help reduce anxiety and encourage your patient to reveal what you need to know.

CONTENT OF THOUGHT

Whatever the speaker is focused on at the moment constitutes the content of thought. During the history of the present illness, this will usually concern the problems that caused the patient to seek treatment.

But it is vital that you cover several topics of thought with every exam you do. The patient is likely to mention some of these spontaneously, but you will have to discover others by asking screening questions. In order to do a systematic, thorough initial interview, you must keep all of these topics in mind and ask screening questions for each of these major thought abnormalities.

Whenever you are investigating abnormalities of thought, probe gently enough that the patient continues to view you as someone who is sympathetic and friendly. Don't make snap judgments or show surprise at the responses you hear. Remember that bizarre ideas like flying saucers or talking fish may seem as normal to the patient as your own closest-held convictions (even including religion and politics) do to you.

Delusions

A *delusion* is a fixed, false belief that the patient's culture and education cannot account for. All portions of this definition must be fulfilled. Others of the same culture must consider the belief or idea to be obviously false; it must be unshakable, despite evidence that it is wrong.

"I've been sent to guard the president." (At age 73, this patient had chronic alcoholism and hadn't worked in years.)

"My husband goes secretly to have sex with the woman across the street. He signals her with the venetian blinds." (Her husband sighed and admitted to the interviewer that he had been impotent for 15 years.)

"My initials are J. C. That means I'm Jesus Christ!" (Six brothers and sisters testified that he had been ill for years.)

You can test the strength of your patient's beliefs by asking:

"Is it possible that this feeling is due to some sort of nervous or emotional problem?"

If the patient replies, "No," and perhaps claims instead that the hospital staff has just joined the conspiracy, score the idea as a delusion.

Some patients, when similarly challenged, will agree that another explanation is possible; for them, you would not diagnose a delusion.

"It only seemed as if there was some sort of plot."

"Perhaps it was imaginary, after all!"

"My nerves have been bad lately."

Call it a delusion only when the patient maintains an obviously false explanation despite clear evidence to the contrary.

Because the cultural/educational criterion must also be satisfied, a traditional Navajo should not be called delusional for believing in witches, nor should children who write letters to Santa Claus.

Screen for delusions by asking questions such as the following (with appropriate pauses for responses):

"Have you ever had any thoughts or feelings that people were spying on you, talking about you, or trying to harm you in some way?"

"Have you ever gotten unusual messages?"

"Have you ever had any other thoughts or ideas that others might consider unusual?"

Patients are often aware that other people think their delusional ideas are unusual or strange; they may go to some lengths to hide these delusions. Usually a sympathetic, interested, nonjudgmental manner will relax tensions enough for your patient to discuss these problems about as freely as any others. You may be able to get your patient to elaborate on a delusion and perhaps to volunteer others by asking the noncommittal question:

"How do you know this [the delusion] is the case?"

If you challenge delusions, you risk upsetting the patient. If you accept them, you risk confirming these false ideas in the patient's mind. You may have to walk a fine line. Naturally, you wouldn't show disbelief, and you'll be safest if you can avoid stating any opinion at all. If pressed for an opinion, you can truthfully state:

"Many people would consider it [the delusion] unusual."
Because this is something the patient already realizes, it comes as no shock; the answer often seems to satisfy. If further pressed, you may have to respond more fully:

"I think that other explanations may be able to account for your discomfort. You could be mistaken, or it could be some form of nervousness."

Because you offer it tentatively, this sort of statement may not provoke much argument. If it does, perhaps you and the patient can amicably agree to disagree.

Once you have detected a delusion, learn all you can about it. The following questions should help:

"How long have you felt this way?"

"What actions have you taken as a result?"

"What other actions do you plan to take?"

"How do you feel about these goings-on?"

"Why do you think this is happening?" (More specific "Why . . . " questions—"Why do you think you were fired?"—are another way that you may be able to elicit delusions.)

Finally, is the delusion *mood-congruent?* In other words, is the content of the delusion in keeping with the patient's mood? Here is an example of a mood-congruent delusion:

> A middle-aged man hospitalized for a depression believed that he had literally gone to hell. He thought that the medical personnel clustered around his bedside were devils who had gathered to administer well-deserved punishment for his sins.

And an example of a mood-incongruent delusion:

> An elderly woman, chronically ill with psychosis for many years, also had ankle swelling due to heart failure. She rather blandly explained that her body fluids were being pulled into her legs by gravity machines installed in her basement by Nazis.

The presence of mood-congruent delusions should make you suspect a mood disorder; mood-incongruent delusions are more typical of schizophrenia.

Specific Delusions

In the course of interviewing many patients, you will probably encounter a wide variety of delusions. Here are some of the best known:

- Death. Also called *nihilistic* delusions, these rare symptoms are extreme cases of delusions of ill health.
- Grandeur. The false belief is that the patient is someone of exalted station (God, Paris Hilton) or has powers or gifts not possessed by other people (immense wealth, virtuoso musical ability, eternal life). Be sure to distinguish these ideas from joking references: Presidents, kings, and industrial chief executive officers sometimes assume the mantle of prescience or invincibility. To them, "I am God" may be a partly realized figure of speech. *Delusions of grandeur are typically found in mania, but may also occur in schizophrenia.*
- Guilt. These patients believe they have committed some grave error or sin, for which they may claim to deserve punishment. *Delusions of guilt are found especially in severe depression and in delusional disorder.*
- Ill health or bodily change. These patients believe they are afflicted by some terrible disease: Their insides have rotted; their bowels have turned to cement. *Delusions of ill health and somatic delusions are occasionally found in severe depression or schizophrenia.*
- Jealousy. The patient's spouse "has been unfaithful." *Delusions of jealousy are classically seen in alcoholic paranoia, but are also encountered in paranoid schizophrenia and delusional disorder.*

- Passivity or influence. Such patients believe that they are being controlled in unusual ways by outside influences, such as television, radio, or microwaves. As a result, they can deny responsibility for their behavior. By contrast, some may feel that they can control the environment: What they have for breakfast has influenced the secretary of state to mention Iran in a speech, or their thought waves cause rivers to rise. *Such delusions are typically found in patients with paranoid schizophrenia.*

- Persecution. Patients believe that they are being threatened, ridiculed, discriminated against, or otherwise interfered with. *Such delusions are typical of paranoid schizophrenia.*

- Poverty. Despite evidence to the contrary (money in the bank, a regular disability check), these patients believe that destitution will force them to sell the house and auction their property. *These delusions sometimes occur in severe depression.*

- Reference. People are spying upon patients, slandering them, or working against them in some other way. These patients "observe" that people whisper about them as they walk past; print or broadcast media contain messages that are intended specifically for them. For example, "On *The NewsHour* last night, Jim Lehrer said that a settlement was imminent. This means that I should agree to the property settlement with my former wife." *Delusions of reference are especially common in paranoid schizophrenia, but may be found in other psychoses as well.*

- Thought broadcasting. The patient's thoughts seem to be transmitted locally or across the continent. *Thought broadcasting is found in schizophrenia.*

- Thought control. Thoughts, feelings, or ideas are put into the patient's mind or are withdrawn from it. *Closely related to passivity feelings, these delusions have similar import.*

PERCEPTION

Hallucinations

Hallucinations are false sensory perceptions that occur in the absence of a related sensory stimulus. (For example, the patient hears voices speaking from the fireplace or sees a quartet of purple snakes floating in the bathwater.) Hallucinations can involve any of the five senses. Among mental health patients, auditory hallucinations are by far the most common; visual hallucinations are next.

Screen for hallucinations by asking:

"Do you ever hear voices or other sounds when there is no one around to produce them?"

"Do you ever see things other people cannot see?"

Some patients mistakenly respond "Yes" to questions about auditory hallucinations, when they mean only that they hear a voice right now (the interviewer's) or that they "hear" their own thoughts (though not spoken aloud as in audible thoughts, which are described later in this chapter). With careful questioning, you can usually distinguish these false positives from genuine hallucinations.

For example, when someone claims to hear noises or a spoken word or two, ask:

"Could this be something coming from you, like your conscience or your own thoughts?"

An admission that it could be "my imagination" or "sounds from out in the hall" doesn't fit with the sort of true auditory hallucination I expect from a person who has a serious psychosis. I'll sometimes ask a patient whether the voice is as clear as mine, and whether it speaks in complete sentences, again discounting "no" answers. Hallucinations that occur only when a patient is reliving trauma also suggest diagnoses other than schizophrenia. I may reassure such a patient that this sort of experience likely doesn't mean anything dire.

Hallucinations should be characterized as to severity. *Auditory hallucinations*, for example, can be graded on a continuum: Vague noises mumbling → understandable words → phrases → complete sentences.

Here are some additional questions that can help you learn more about auditory hallucinations:

"How often do you hear this sort of voice?"

"Is it as clear as my voice is now?"

"Where is it coming from?" (The patient's head or body? The microwave oven? The hallway?)

"Whose voice is it?"

"Is there more than one?"

"Do they talk about you?"

"What do they say?"

"Do they hold conversations with one another?"

"What do you think the cause is?"

"Can others hear these voices?"

"How do you react?" (Many patients are frightened by their hallucinations; some are only bemused.)

"Do the voices give commands?" (If so, does the patient obey them?) *This is an important point: patients will sometimes obey command hallucinations, and have been known to inflict harm on other people as a result.*

Audible thoughts constitute a special form of auditory hallucination, in which patients hear their own thoughts spoken so loudly that others can hear them.

Visual hallucinations can also be graded: Points of light → blurred images → formed people (what size?) → scenes or tableaus. Some of the questions recommended for auditory hallucinations, appropriately modified, should be asked of patients who admit to visual hallucinations. You especially want to know when they occur (only when the patient is using drugs or alcohol, or at other times?) and what the content is. How does the patient respond to these hallucinations? (It can be extremely frightening to perceive faces changing color or form; one woman looked into the mirror and saw that she had become a mushroom!)

Visual hallucinations are especially characteristic of cognitive psychoses. For example, small animals or Lilliputian people are commonly reported by patients who experience DTs when withdrawing from heavy, prolonged alcohol use. Trailing phenomena, in which images appear to linger on the patient's retina, sometimes accompany psychedelic drug use. But visual hallucinations can also occur in schizophrenia, early symptoms of which may include intensification of color or changes in the size of objects.

Tactile (touch), *olfactory* (smell), and *gustatory* (taste) hallucinations are uncommon in mental health patients. *These symptoms usually suggest psychosis due to such disorders as brain tumor, toxic psychosis, or a seizure disorder. Visual, auditory, and tactile experiences may also occur in normal people when they are falling asleep or awakening. They are easily discerned from actual hallucinations by their exclusive time of occurrence.*

A woman recently told me, "You're going to think I'm crazy. Early one morning last year, I saw the Devil standing over me in my bed. I was completely paralyzed—I couldn't move my arms or legs, but I was totally awake! I was so frightened, I shook for an hour afterwards." I was glad to be able to tell her that she was sane—that she had experienced a combination of *hypnopompic imagery* (images that occur upon awakening, not true hallucinations at all) with sleep paralysis, which also sometimes occurs when awakening.

Anxiety Symptoms

Anxiety is fear that is neither directed at nor caused by anything specific the patient can identify. It is usually accompanied by various unpleasant bodily sensations. Other mental symptoms may include irritability, poor concentration, mental tension, worrying, and an exaggerated startle response.

Screen for anxiety symptoms by asking:

"Do you think you worry about things excessively or out of proportion to their real danger to you?"

"Does your family tell you that you're a worry-wart?"

"Do you feel anxious or tense much of the time?"

If any answer is "Yes," follow up with some of the questions covered in the section on anxiety disorders in Chapter 13.

When intense anxiety occurs suddenly in a discrete episode, with a rapid increase in these bodily sensations, the patient is said to be experiencing a *panic attack*. Patients often report fearing disaster, madness, or impending death.

Screen for panic attacks by asking:

"Have you ever had a panic attack—a time when you suddenly felt overwhelmingly frightened or anxious?"

Follow up with the same sort of questions you would ask for other anxiety disorders (Chapters 13 and Appendix D). *Complaints of inner tension, sometimes accompanied by marked restlessness, can be associated with akathisia in patients who have been using even some of the newer anti psychotic medications.*

Phobias

A *phobia* is an unreasonable and intense fear associated with some object or situation. Common *specific phobias* are fears of various animals, air travel, heights (*acrophobia*), and being closed in (*claustrophobia*). Common *social phobias* include fears of public speaking, eating in public, using a public urinal, or writing when others might see the patient's hand tremble. *Agoraphobia* is fear of being away from home or of being in public places.

To the outsider, a phobia may seem every bit as unreasonable as a delusion. The difference is that whereas the phobic patient recognizes how unreasonable these feelings are, the delusional patient does not.

Screen for phobias by asking:

"Have you ever been afraid of leaving home alone, or being in crowds, or in public places such as stores or on bridges?"

"Have you ever had fears that seemed unreasonable or out of proportion to you, but that you just couldn't shake?"

In the case of social phobias (such as public speaking), be sure to ask about the development of *anticipatory anxiety*. In this condition, anxiety that is often intense and incapacitating is experienced prior to performing the act that the patient dreads.

Dysmorphophobia is a term sometimes used to describe excessive concern about slight (or imagined) defects in body appearance. Usually these flaws are facial (wrinkles, shape of nose), but they have been reported for nearly every imaginable body part. Of course, the patient cannot avoid the body part in question, so the condition is not really a phobia at all. It is now called *body dysmorphic disorder.*

Obsessions and Compulsions

An *obsession* is a belief, idea, or thought that dominates the patient's thought content and persists, despite the fact that the patient realizes it is unrealistic and may try to resist it. For example, a middle-aged man had the persistent thought of doing something embarrassing, such as standing up and screaming during a church service. Obsessions often involve dirt, time, or money.

Compulsions are acts performed repeatedly in a way that the patient realizes is neither useful nor appropriate. Often they are performed in response to (or to cope with) an obsession. Some examples:

Counting things repeatedly
Heeding groundless superstitions
Following rituals (such as a set bedtime routine that, if not followed to the letter, must be started all over again)

A key aspect of obsessions and compulsions is the fact that the patient realizes these ideas or behaviors are senseless and often tries to resist them.

Screen for obsessions and compulsions by asking:

"Have you ever had obsessional thoughts or ideas? I mean thoughts that may seem senseless to you, but keep coming back anyway?"

"Have you ever had compulsions—such as rituals or routines that you feel you must perform over and over, even though you try to resist?" (Be ready to cite examples, should the patient ask.)

Some people do not realize that their behaviors—excessive neatness, for example—are at all unusual. Careful questioning may be required to draw them out:

"How neat is your home, your personal belongings?"

"Have you ever gone to bed and left dirty dishes in the sink?"

"If someone sits on your bed after you've made it, do you feel the need to straighten it again?"

A minor degree of obsessional thinking is quite common, so it is important to judge severity. As with phobias, this is best measured in terms of the effects on activities such as school, work, and family life. In severe cases, patients may spend many hours a day occupied in pointless handwashing, dressing, or bathroom rituals. As with phobias, ask about onset, duration, and treatment, as well as severity.

Thoughts of Violence

Whether or not there have been previous suicide attempts or violence directed at others, you must learn what the patient is thinking now. Screen for *suicidal ideas* by asking:

"Have you any ideas or thoughts of harming yourself in any way or of killing yourself?"

Because most of us have had such a thought at one time or another, a positive answer could reflect merely a fleeting reaction to stress or an overwhelming life situation. But it would be an unwarranted, potentially tragic leap of faith to ignore any answer that is even equivocal. You must thoroughly investigate any such ideas you uncover.

Review all the material you have already obtained about past suicide attempts (see Chapter 9). Learn whether the patient has current plans and the means to carry them out. You should ask:

"What would it take to make suicide seems less attractive?"
Regard as serious and ominous any equivalent to the answer "Nothing could." If you encounter this sort of thinking, especially if it is bolstered with evidence of current drinking or depression (feelings of worthlessness, hopelessness, trouble with thinking, loss of energy, guilt feelings), you may have a situation that demands hospitalization—possibly even before the hour is up.

Ideas of homicide or violence present a similar, urgent call to action. The terror of violent ideas is mitigated only by the fact that they are encountered much less often than are suicidal ideas. Screen for thoughts of homicide or violence toward others by asking:

"Have you been feeling so angry or upset that you think about harming someone else?"

"Have you ever had trouble resisting the urge?"

Any positive answer must be followed up immediately and compared with the historical information you have already obtained. Are there plans or only ideas? Does your patient have the means (firearms, lethal drugs) to carry out this plan? Is there a timetable? (Be sure to review the detailed material on violence covered in Chapter 9.)

Symptoms That Are Worrisome, but Usually Normal

There are a number of symptoms you don't ordinarily have to ask about: Either they are normal or they have no diagnostic import. However, patients sometimes worry about them and bring them up during interview sessions. You should have explanations ready.

Illusions are misinterpretations of actual sensory stimuli. Usually visual, they most often occur when there is decreased sensory input (such as in dim light). The benign explanation is readily acknowledged as soon as the patient becomes aware of the mistake. You've probably had the experience yourself: A crack on the wall looks like a frightening snake; once you put on the light, you feel immediate relief. To distinguish illusions from hallucinations, obtain details about such matters as circumstances (dim light, etc.) and timing (perhaps only when going to sleep). Although usually normal, illusions can be encountered in patients with dementia or delirium.

Déjà vu, French for "already seen," is the commonplace sensation that a person has previously experienced a situation or locale when that is probably not the case. Most normal people have had this feeling more than once, although *déjà vu* can occur in temporal lobe epilepsy.

Overvalued ideas are beliefs that we continue to hold despite lack of proof as to their worth. Like delusions, they cannot usually be challenged by argument or logic; unlike delusions, they are not obviously false. Examples include the superiority of one's own gender, race, political party, or religion. Overvalued ideas are sometimes pursued to a point where they interfere with the individual's functioning, causing suffering to the person or to those around. A common example is racial hatred. Overvalued religious ideas can shade into religious preoccupation, and from there into religious delusions, and the dividing line can be hard to draw. In such a case, note the patient's exact words as a baseline for later review.

Depersonalization is an alteration in one's own perception of self. People usually experience it as a feeling of being detached from body or mind; they may have the sensation of viewing themselves or of being in a dream. In *derealization*, people feel that they are real, but that the environment is not. Screen for these experiences by asking:

"Have you ever felt unreal? As if you were a robot?"

"Have you ever felt that things around you are unreal?"

Derealization and depersonalization are reasonably common and usually normal; they sometimes develop during a period of profound distress or with sleep deprivation. When these experiences are protracted or repeated and severe enough to cause distress, the individual may be diagnosed as having depersonalization disorder. They also can occur during bouts of PTSD and with organic brain pathology.

CONSCIOUSNESS AND COGNITION

In the next section of the mental status exam, you test your patient's ability to absorb, process, and communicate information. The clinical tests are only approximate, but they can serve as a useful guide.

To introduce these tasks, you might want to restate the reassurance that you often ask these routine questions of new patients. I hope you'll avoid one common mistake of young clinicians, who, perhaps embarrassed at having to ask such questions, may describe them as "silly." Devaluing these tasks can diminish a patient's motivation. To someone who wants to know why you're asking, the correct answer is "To help evaluate you." Neither should you refer to them as "simple," which will only increase the discomfort for a patient who has difficulty answering. Remember that any test of mental functioning can be traumatic, especially when there is fear of failure. Doing poorly is always stressful, and the patient who stumbles may need some support:

"Most people can't perform at their best when they feel under pressure."

"Most patients have some difficulty with that task."

In any case, try to emphasize what the patient is able to do:

"You did well on those serial sevens."

"You're doing better than many others have on this test."

(Of course, you should never use this sort of supportive comment unless it is true.)

Attention and Concentration

At this point in the interview, you will already have a good idea of your patient's *attention* (which we'll define as the ability to focus on a current task or topic) and *concentration* (the ability to sustain that focus over a period of time). You can get at these qualities in a more formal way from calculations, which assess the ability to focus on a stimulus. Ask your patient to subtract 7 from 100. Once done, request another subtraction of 7 from the result, and so on toward 0. Most adults will finish in less than a minute with fewer than four errors. Remember to consider the patient's age, education level, culture, and degree of depression and anxiety when you assess the performance.

Personally, whenever possible, I prefer to evaluate attention during the body of my interview. This possibility can arise, for example, when a patient mentions a date years in the past. "Let's see," I'll say, "how old were you then?" I probably won't pursue this sort of testing any further if the patient can come up with the correct age and seems to focus well on our (perhaps prolonged) conversation.

If subtractions prove too difficult (they do assume some education and facility with math), ask your patient to count backward by ones from, say, 87 and to stop at 63. This test of attention is less culture-bound than serial subtractions. Spelling *world* backward is asked so often that some patients can rattle it off without thinking. Try a different word, such as *strap* or *watch,* but first make sure your patient can spell it forward. Recalling a series of five to seven digits forward, then backward, accomplishes the same task and is less educationally dependent. *Reduced attention is found in patients with conditions such as epilepsy, demen tia, and head injury, as well as in patients with schizophrenia and bipolar disorders. Because so much of mental processing hinges on the ability to focus, you should interpret cautiously the rest of your mental state exam findings when attention is impaired.*

Orientation

Whether patients know their own names (orientation to person) should be evident from the earlier portions of an interview. Test to be sure that your patient is oriented to time and place by asking:

"Where are we now [city, state, name of the facility]?" If this draws a blank, ask what type of a facility you are in. *An answer such as "a library" or "Ground Zero" suggests severe pathology, although you should beware of overinterpreting what you hear from a facetious or otherwise uncooperative patient.*

"What is the date?" *Not infrequently, patients will give the correct date and month, but miss the year. Be sure to ask for all components of orientation to time. Patients will often miss the date by a day or two. This is usually without significance, especially for hospitalized patients who, divorced from their usual routines, tend to lose track of time.*

If you detect confusion about time or place, ask about orientation to person:

"Would you tell me your full name again?"

Occasionally you will encounter a patient who is not only disoriented, but also tries to hide mistakes by making up responses that sound logical. This process of making up answers is called *confabulation,* and it does not signify lying; patients seem truly to believe these stories they tell. If asked whether you have met previously, such a patient might agree, even though it is the first time you have ever laid eyes on one another. *Confabulation is characteristic of patients whose ability to remember is severely impaired by such disorders as chronic alcoholism with thiamine deficiency.*

A student recently asked me the difference between a delusion and a confabulation. Good question, that! A confabulation is an attempt (not intentional) to fill in defects in memory, which are not typical of delusions. Delusional patients have been reported to confabulate, and at least one resource notes that the line between the two conditions is sometimes a fine one. Stay tuned.

Language

Language refers to the means whereby we understand and express meaning through words and symbols. The areas of language that are usually assessed include comprehension, fluency, naming, repetition, reading, and writing. Their routine assessment can be quickly done; it is especially important in older patients and in those who are physically ill. It is not uncommon for hysteria, dementia, and other mental conditions to be misdiagnosed when a patient actually has a disorder of language.

- The degree of *comprehension* should already be evident from the way your patient has responded to conversation during the interview. As a simple test, request some complex behavior, such as: "Pick up this pen, put it into your pocket, then return it to the desktop."
- *Fluency* of language should also be obvious from the patient's use of normal vocabulary and prosody to produce sentences of normal length. Be alert for hesitation, mumbling, stammering, and unusual emphasis.
- Problems with *naming* may be evident if, instead of their names, your patient uses circumlocutions to describe everyday objects. Examples of such a naming aphasia:

   Watch band: "The thing that holds it on your wrist."
   Pen: "A whatsis for writing."
Screen for aphasias by asking your patient to name the parts of a ballpoint pen: point, clip, barrel.
- To test *repetition*, ask your patient to repeat a standard, simple phrase, such as "Tomorrow will be sunny."
- *Reading* is quickly tested by asking the patient to read a sentence or two. Note that, even in advanced societies, a small percentage of adults are functionally illiterate. You will need to evaluate the results of this and other tests against what you already know about your patient's educational background. Be prepared to offer support for the embarrassment of the occasional patient who has trouble with this task.
- Test *writing* by asking your patient to write a sentence (you can dictate something if the patient has trouble thinking of one).

   Asking for the names of a pencil and watch tests for *expressive dysphasia*. So does the request to write out a sentence of the patient's choice.
- Test for *apraxia* (the inability to perform a voluntary act, despite intact motor pathways) by asking your patient to copy a simple geometric figure, such as this one:

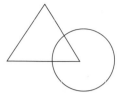

Inability to reproduce the basics of this figure (ignore shakiness and ro-tation) could indicate an *ideomotor apraxia*. Apraxias can stem from a le-sion on the right side of the brain.

If you encounter problems with any of these screening tests, you should ask for a neurological evaluation. Your patient's mental condi-tion may be complicated by a significant neurological dysfunction.

Memory

Memory is usually divided into three or four parts. For convenience we will discuss three: immediate, short-term, and long-term. If you feel un-comfortable with asking any of these questions, you can lead into them:

"Have you had any problems with your memory? I'd like to test it."

Immediate memory (the ability to register and reproduce informa-tion after 5 or 10 seconds) is more a test of attention, which you may have already accomplished with serial sevens or counting. But you can assess it again on your way to testing short-term memory. Name several unrelated items, such as a name, a color, and a street address. Then ask for a repetition of these items. This repetition not only assesses imme-diate memory, but also provides assurance that the patient has under-stood you.

Should you warn patients that you plan to ask them to repeat the three items later? There are two schools of thought. One advises you to give a heads-up, though I don't think I've ever read the reason why. The other cautions you that such a warning invites cognitive rehearsal, which could mean that some patients benefit from practicing while perhaps paying insufficient attention to the questions you ask in the meanwhile. Although I've always subscribed to the latter school, per-haps the issue is more cosmetic than cosmic—either method may be OK, as long as you are consistent. What you want is to gain a feeling for normal responses to the way you ask your questions.

Five minutes later, test *short-term (recent) memory* by asking your pa-tient to recall the three items. At 5 minutes, most patients should be able to repeat the name, color, and at least part of the address. When you are interpreting the results of this test, be sure to consider your patient's apparent degree of motivation. *Failure on all three tasks suggests se-rious inattention due to a severe cognitive disorder or to severe stress from de-pression, psychosis, or anxiety.*

You can best assess *long-term (remote) memory* from the ability to or-ganize the information necessary to relate the history of the present ill-ness. You will also have a good idea from your patient's facility with dates of marriages, births of children, and so forth—material that you will have elicited in the course of obtaining the personal and social his-tory. Experts disagree as to where the dividing line lies between short-term and long-term memory. Most agree that some sort of consolida-tion takes place between 12 and 18 months, so that memories stored long-term are not easily forgotten. *Although patients with severe dementias such as Alzheimer's typically retain long-term memories better than short-term memories, even long-retained information will eventually be lost if the disease progresses far enough.*

Amnesia, that temporary loss of memory often due to physical or psychological trauma, is very different from dementia. It can be found in head trauma, alcohol blackouts, PTSD, and dissociative disorders. Amnesia can be hard to ascertain—the natural answer to "Have you ever suffered from amnesia?" is "I don't remember." You might try:

"Have there been periods of time that you cannot remember at all?"

"Have others ever commented that you have trouble with your memory?"

If you encounter amnesia, try to determine whether it is fragmen-tary (the patient can remember isolated bits from the affected periods of time) or *en bloc* (there is complete loss of memory for that time). You might try to bracket the memory hole with the memories on either side of it ("What's the last thing you can recall just before the period of am-nesia begins? What's the first thing you can recall afterwards?"). You could also inquire: "Have you asked friends or relatives to try to help you reconstruct what happened then?"

Don't assume that a memory hole means that something bad hap-pened. Clinicians have come to grief persuading patients that amnesia implies assault or molestation—the so-called "false memory" syn-drome.

Cultural Information

Some texts no longer even mention cultural information tasks, which mainly assess the patient's remote memory and general intelligence. However, these are a traditional part of the mental status exam, so you should have some familiarity with the classical questions.

"Name the five most recent presidents [or prime ministers or other heads of state], beginning with the current one." Most patients can name four or five, working backwards. Ask them one at a time. Understandably, many patients find it daunting to be asked to "name the last five presidents in reverse chronological order." If a patient misses one, it's fair to try to jog memory: "Let's see, did you leave out anyone?" or "He's hiding between two Bushes."

"Who is the governor?"

"Name five large cities."

"Name five rivers."

Cautions about interpretation are the same as for subtractions and counting, mentioned previously. Alternatively, you might get quite an accurate picture of your patient's interest, intelligence, and memory by asking about current events: outcomes of major sports events, the names of those running in the next election, and other items of popular cultural significance.

Abstract Thinking

The ability to abstract a principle from a specific example is another traditional test that depends heavily on culture, intelligence, and education. This ability has nothing to do with sanity, as was once thought. Commonly asked abstractions include the interpretation of proverbs, likenesses, and differences. Here are typical proverbs to interpret:

"What does it mean when someone says that people who live in glass houses shouldn't throw stones?"

"Can you tell me what this means: A rolling stone gathers no moss?" Note that a given proverb may have more than one interpretation (gathering moss could be judged as either desirable or not). I accept any logical interpretation.

Similarities and differences are somewhat less culture-bound than proverbs, so you are probably better off asking some of these:

"How are an apple and an orange alike?" (They are both fruit; both are spherical; both have seeds.)

"What is the difference between a child and a dwarf?" (A child will grow.)

Mini-Mental State Exam

The Mini-Mental State Exam (MMSE), sometimes called the *Folstein test* in honor of its first two authors, extends and quantifies tests of cognition. It takes just a few minutes to administer and score, and for years it has been a staple of routine mental health evaluations. A score below

24 suggests dementia, though a highly educated, intelligent patient may score higher and require formal neuropsychological testing to reveal mild dementia. A good use for the MMSE is to follow the cognitive changes in a patient with dementia. The MMSE, which used to be freely available, can no longer be reproduced in its entirety. It is available for purchase from Psychological Assessment Resources (www. minimental.com), or you can look up the original article, a reference to which I've included in Appendix F.

Even the Mini-Mental State Exam yields only an approximation of the patient's cognitive abilities. For greater precision yet, you can request formal neuropsychological testing by a qualified psychologist.

INSIGHT AND JUDGMENT

Insight refers to your patient's ideas about what is wrong. In the context of the mental status exam, it has nothing to do with theories of etiology or psychodynamics. You could ask:

"Do you think there is something wrong with you?"

"What kind of illnesses do people come here to get treated for?"

"What strengths do you think you have?"

"Do you think you are impaired?"

Insight may be full, partial, or nil. For example, a patient with mania who has partial insight may realize that something is wrong, but may blame others for it. Insight also tends not to be static, but to deteriorate with worsening illness and to improve during remission. *Poor insight is typical of cognitive disorders, severe depression, and any of the psychoses (especially mania and schizophrenia). Patients' assessment of their own strengths—what they think they are good at—can be important for recommending treatment and estimating prognosis.*

You should also try to get a feeling for your patient's self-image by asking:

"What do you like about yourself?"

"How do you think other people see you?"

Judgment refers to the ability to decide upon an appropriate course of action to achieve realistic goals. Some writers still advise interviewers to assess judgment by asking hypothetical questions such as "What would you do if you found a letter with a stamp on it?" or "How would you react if a fire broke out in a theater when you were attending a performance?" Such abstract questions probably have little bearing on your patient's ability to get along in the world; you are better off avoiding them. There are several other questions you can ask to assess your patient's judgment:

"Do you think you need treatment?"

"What do you expect from treatment?"

"What are your plans for the future?"

In the final analysis, your best appraisal of judgment will probably come from the hour or more of history you have just obtained.

WHEN CAN YOU OMIT THE FORMAL MENTAL STATUS EXAM?

The obvious answer to the question posed in this heading remains "Never." The reason is that unless all your information comes from printed records, you make a great number of mental status observations every time you have a conversation. The question we are really asking is this: When can you safely avoid asking the questions contained in the cognitive portion of the mental status exam (the entire contents of this chapter)?

It is seldom risk-free to leave out any test; any time you do so, it must be with the idea of balancing benefits (your time and the patient's possible embarrassment) versus disadvantages (less diagnostic information). The disadvantages are usually inconsequential: Most tests are quick, and most patients will accept with reasonably good grace whatever questions you pose. Nonetheless, here are a few situations in which you could abbreviate your mental status exam by omitting some formal tests of orientation, knowledge, attention, and memory:

> You have a well-organized history. For example, an outpatient who consults you for a relatively nonthreatening problem (life stress, perhaps, or marital difficulties) clearly relates a story that is coherent and devoid of gaps or inconsistencies.
>
> Test results are available. You have a report of recent psychological testing, which will be far more precise than your approximate tests.
>
> The patient is distressed. If the patient has been quizzed recently by other examiners and is embarrassed or angered by repeated requests, you may want to abbreviate your exam. This may be especially true of patients who have trouble with certain of the tests.

You should not omit any portion of the formal mental status exam under the following circumstances:

Any forensic exam. Such reports may be scrutinized in a court of law; leave no stone unturned.

Any other legal requirements. Commitment proceedings, competency evaluations, and examinations mandated for certain procedures (such as electroconvulsive therapy) almost always require a complete report.

Any benchmark record. For example, if you know you'll need to evaluate the results of treatment later, you had better have a record of what the patient was like "before."

Any hint of suicidal ideation or threats of violence. Personal consequences for the patient and legal fallout in general mandate the complete exam.

Major diagnoses. Any major (Axis I or Axis II) diagnosis must be thoroughly investigated.

Inpatient status. Any patient who is sick enough to be hospitalized is sick enough to have a complete workup.

Possible brain injury. Always do a complete mental status exam when there is a history of head injury or neurological illness.

A beginning examiner. Performing the complete evaluation over and over will give you both familiarity and facility with it.

Chapter 13

Signs and Symptoms in Areas of Clinical Interest

The areas of clinical interest are simply a way of thinking about historical and mental status information. The eight groups that will be discussed here include most of the signs and symptoms a mental health professional can expect to encounter. The areas of clinical interest should help you focus your inquiry on the information you will need to devise a differential diagnosis.

Your job is to obtain the facts necessary to assess the importance of any of these areas you encounter to the overall evaluation. Remember that each of them comprises a number of clinical diagnoses that have symptoms in common. In order to decide which diagnosis fits best, you must inquire about symptoms of each of the disorders you have in mind.

As an example of how this process works, consider a patient who has complained of feeling depressed, blue, or down in the dumps. You would expect to find some of these additional symptoms of a mood disorder: crying spells, hopelessness, disordered appetite, change in sleep patterns, feeling worse at certain times of the day, low energy, poor concentration, pessimistic outlook, and suicidal ideas or behaviors. Most patients won't have all of these symptoms, but even a couple of them would suggest that your patient could suffer from some kind of a depressive condition. In that case, you should learn whether the symptoms and course of the illness will support one of the mood disorder diagnoses. In other words, first get the data. Later, when all the facts are in, you can decide which of the diagnoses best fits the facts.

In discussing each area of clinical interest, I will present these features:

1. Tip-offs, the "red flag" symptoms that should alert you to explore further.
2. The main diagnoses, a section that comprises the most important disorders covered by that area of clinical interest plus the principal differential diagnoses. I've marked with an asterisk (∗) those that I've included in the Appendix B paraphrase/ summary of diagnostic criteria from the *Diagnostic and Statistical Manual of Mental Disorders*, fourth edition, text revision (DSM-IV-TR).
3. Historical information, which briefly explains the importance of each bit of historical data you should ask about.
4. Typical features from the mental status examination. The current mental status is usually not as helpful as history in sorting out the differential diagnosis, so I have just listed the typical symptoms.

At times it is hard to know where history ends and the mental status begins. For that reason, you might find that some features mentioned under one section seem to belong in another. For example, a patient might report some moods that are not observed during the interview.

In Appendix D, you'll find a semistructured interview that includes most of the mental health diagnoses. I've included it mainly to give people who want it a way to ensure that they've "covered everything" in their interview. I do want to warn you, however, to be careful about interviewing *for* a particular diagnosis. The purpose of the initial interview is to determine what's wrong, not merely to find evidence that will reaffirm your preconceptions—or what another clinician has already claimed.

PSYCHOSIS

Psychosis means simply that the patient is out of touch with reality, as judged by the presence of hallucinations, delusions, or markedly loosened thought associations. This condition may be either transient or chronic, although with today's treatment methods it is unusual for a person to remain psychotic for extended periods.

Tip-Offs

Symptoms that would make you consider psychosis as an area of clinical interest include the following:

Affect that is flat or inappropriate
Bizarre behavior
Confusion
Delusions
Fantasies or illogical ideas
Hallucinations (of any of the senses)
Insight or judgment that is disturbed
Muteness
Perceptual distortions or misinterpretations
Social withdrawal
Speech that is incoherent or hard to follow

Main Diagnoses

A patient who presents with psychosis is likely to have one of three principal diagnoses: an organic psychosis, schizophrenia, or some sort of mood disorder (either depression with psychosis or severe mania). Of those, mood disorders and schizophrenia will be encountered most frequently. However, here is a more complete list:

Schizophrenia*
Major depressive episode*
Manic episode*
Cognitive disorders, such as delirium* due to a variety of causes
Substance-induced psychotic disorder* (e.g., due to alcohol)
Brief psychotic disorder
Schizophreniform disorder
Schizoaffective disorder
Delusional disorder*

Historical Information

Age at onset. Schizophrenia tends to begin early (late teens or 20s); delusional disorder starts in middle to late life.

Alcohol or drugs. Many psychotic patients use substances. Check the chronology. If the psychosis began first, schizophrenia with secondary substance misuse is the likely diagnosis. If substance use began first, the psychosis is probably a secondary diagnosis, and schizophrenia is less likely.

Depression. If there is a past or present severe depression, consider the diagnosis of a mood disorder with psychosis.

Environmental stress. Severe stress that precedes the onset of psychosis suggests a diagnosis of brief psychotic disorder.

Family history. Schizophrenia and mood disorders tend to run in families; having a relative with either condition increases the likelihood of that diagnosis for the patient.

Length of illness. The longer a psychosis has lasted, the more likely is schizophrenia to be the final diagnosis.

Loss of drive, volition, interest. These symptoms are typical of the later phases of schizophrenia.

Onset. Sudden onset (a few days to a few weeks) suggests a cognitive or mood disorder with psychosis. The longer and more gradual the onset—up to several years in some cases—the more likely is this psychosis to be schizophrenia.

Physical illness. Cognitive psychoses are associated with a number of health risk factors: endocrine or metabolic disorders, tumors, toxic substance exposure, trauma, and a variety of neurological and medical diseases.

Previous episode with recovery. Mood disorders tend to be episodic illnesses; these patients are more likely to recover completely than are those with schizophrenia.

Schizoid or schizotypal premorbid personality. Long-standing character traits such as aloofness, emotional withdrawal, few friends, or odd beliefs or behaviors sometimes precede the onset of schizophrenia.

Unemployment or reduced job level. If unemployment or underemployment has been present for years, and especially if the reduced job level continues after recovery from an acute episode, schizophrenia is more likely than if the patient worked at a high-grade, demanding job until just recently.

Note on first-rank symptoms. A much-discussed set of hallucinations and delusions is that of Kurt Schneider's *first-rank symptoms*, any one of which he believed was diagnostic of schizophrenia. Although subsequent research has shown that patients with other disorders may also report these symptoms, you will encounter the concept of first-rank symptoms often enough to warrant a brief listing.

Audible thoughts
Delusional perception, in which a normal observation has abnormal significance for a patient; for example, when a patient was served a grilled cheese sandwich for lunch, he "knew" that his aunt was about to die
Delusions of influence
Delusions of thought control
More than one voice talking about the patient
Voices commenting on the patient's actions

Somatic hallucinations (body sensations produced by outside influence)
Thought broadcasting

Mental Status Examination

Appearance and behavior
  Abnormalities of motion
    Reduced activity
    Pacing
    Posturing
    Rigidity
    Negativism
    Grimacing
    Stereotypies
  Clothing eccentric or
    disheveled
  Hyperalertness
  Neglect of hygiene
Mood
  Flat or silly
  Perplexity about identity
Flow of thought
  Speech restricted in amount
  Mute
  Incoherent
  Loosened associations
  Illogical ideas
  Preoccupied with fantasies
Content of thought
  Hallucinations: When?
    Where?

Hallucinations (*cont.*)
  Auditory
    Voices?
    If so, whose?
    Audible thoughts?
  Visual
  Tactile
  Taste
  Smell
Delusions
  Death
  Erotomania
  Grandeur
  Guilt
  Ill health or bodily change
  Jealousy
  Passivity
  Persecution
  Poverty
  Reference
Language usually not impaired
Cognition generally preserved
Insight often absent
Judgment may be impaired in
  the acute phase

MOOD DISTURBANCE: DEPRESSION

Depression means a mood that is variously described as blue, low, or melancholy—as well as depressed. This low mood must be persistent, usually lasting at least a week or two. It is often described as a marked change from the patient's normal mood. The information needed for the history of the present illness addresses both cause of depression (see later) and severity.

Tip-Offs

You should investigate depression if your patient presents with any of these symptoms:

> Activity level that is either markedly increased or decreased
> Anxiety symptoms
> Appetite changes
> Concentration poor
> Death wishes
> Depressed mood
> Interest decreased for usual activities (including sex)
> Sleeplessness or excessive sleepiness
> Suicidal ideas
> Tearfulness
> Use of drugs or alcohol
> Weight loss or gain
> Worthlessness

Main Diagnoses

Many of the same physical diseases that produce psychosis can also lead to depression. However, the principal problem with diagnosis is differentiating *primary* depression (i.e., depression that is chronologically the first disorder to appear) from *secondary* depression (i.e., depression that begins after and is caused by another mental or personality disorder). Principal diagnoses to consider are these:

> Major depressive episode* (as part of either major depressive dis-
>   order or bipolar I or bipolar II)
> Melancholia*
> Dysthymia*
> Seasonal mood disorder
> Secondary depression

Historical Information

Alcohol and drugs. Substance use is a principal finding preceding the onset of secondary depression.

Atypical features. Stress-related depression may have symptoms of excessive sleep (hypersomnia), increased appetite, and weight gain; patients may feel better in the mornings and when they are with people they like. These features are called *atypical* because depressed patients typically have insomnia, feel better in the evenings, and complain of decreased appetite and weight.

Change from usual self. Often patients who have severe bipolar depressed episodes or unipolar depression report that the way they feel is a "complete change from the way I used to feel."

Environmental stress. Any severe environmental stressor can be associated with depressed mood. A depression that remits as soon as the stressor lifts is sometimes called *reactive*. Reactive depressions are usually less severe than depressions that are not stress-related, and are less likely to require medication.

Episodic illness. Has there been a previous episode of depression? Did the patient recover completely? "Yes" answers suggest such forms of depression as bipolar depressed episodes, unipolar depression, and seasonal mood disorder. A chronic, low-intensity depression that has been present for years is typical of dysthymia.

Family history of mood disorder. This is a classical finding in severe depression; bipolar disorders, for example, are at least in part inherited.

Indecisiveness. Inability to make up one's mind, even regarding minor details, is also emblematic of severe depression.

Isolation. Withdrawal from friends or family suggests a severe depression such as melancholia.

Mania ever. The distinction between a bipolar depressed episode and major depressive disorder is easily made with the finding of previous episodes of mania.

Neglect of hobbies, activities. Loss of interest in usual activities accompanies severe depression.

Recent loss (bereavement). This is another common environmental stressor; grief reaction is not considered a mental disorder in DSM-IV-TR, but it is often the cause of depressive symptoms.

Seasonal pattern. Some patients report regular onset of depression at a particular season of the year (typically fall), with full remission later (typically springtime). Such patients may be diagnosed as having seasonal mood disorder.

Sex interest decreased. Loss of libido is a classical symptom of moderate to severe depression.

Suicide ideas, attempts. For any depressed patient, ask about psychological and physical seriousness of previous attempts. Are there current ideas about suicide or means for carrying them out?

Trouble thinking or concentrating. These symptoms are usually found in moderate to severe depression.

Vegetative symptoms. Classical for severe depression with melancholia are terminal insomnia (patient awakens early and cannot return to sleep), decreased appetite, weight loss, and low energy (fatigue). Patients tend to feel better in evenings than mornings, and don't improve much when with people whose company they normally enjoy.

Mental Status Examination

Appearance and behavior
  Tearful
  Decreased attention to
    appearance
  Decreased interest in usual
    activities
  Slowed actions
  Agitation
Mood
  Sad face
  Anxiety
Flow of thought
  Slowing
Content of thought
  Guilt feelings
  Ruminations
  Hopeless
  Worthless
  Loss of pleasure

Content of thought (*cont.*)
  "Better off dead"
  Death wishes
  Suicide ideas, plans
  Mood-congruent delusions
    Guilt
    Sin
    Worthlessness
    Ill health
    Poverty
Language not usually affected
Cognition
  Usually intact
  May have "pseudodementia"
Insight and judgment
  May deny feeling depressed
  May deny possibility of
    improvement

MOOD DISTURBANCE: MANIA

Manic patients describe their moods as high, hyper, exalted, excited, or euphoric; sometimes they are mainly irritable. Although mania is a condition that has been well recognized for more than 100 years, these patients are often misdiagnosed as having schizophrenia. Cognitive disorders can sometimes present with symptoms of mania.

Tip-Offs

Consider mania when confronted with any of the following symptoms:

Activity level increased
Distractibility
Grandiose sense of self-worth
Judgment deteriorating
Mood euphoric or irritable

Planning many activities
Sleep decreased (reduced need for sleep)
Speech rapid, loud, hard to interrupt
Substance use recently begun or increased
Thoughts moving rapidly from one idea to another

Main Diagnoses

Most manic patients also have episodes of (often severe) depression. Cyclothymia, a milder condition in which high moods that are *not* psychotic alternate with depressed ones, is the other principal possibility to consider. Differential diagnoses includes the following:

Mania* (bipolar I disorder, manic episode)
Bipolar II disorder
Cyclothymia
Organic mood disorder

Historical Information

Alcohol misuse. This may be an attempt to treat the uncomfortable feelings of being speeded up.

Concentration decreased. Manic patients often start projects that they do not complete.

Episodic illness. A previous episode of mania or depression with complete recovery usually clinches the diagnosis. If so, look especially for rapid cycling (four or more switches between highs and lows in the course of a year). These episodes, which may be as brief as a few days, have implications for the type of treatment that may be effective.

Insomnia. This is often experienced as decreased need for sleep.

Judgment poor. This appears as a history of spending sprees, legal troubles, or sexual indiscretions.

Libido increased. Manic exuberance can lead to promiscuity, pregnancy, and the risk of sexually transmitted disease.

Personality change. At the extreme, a normally quiet, unassuming person abruptly becomes boisterous, argumentative, or ill-tempered.

Physical conditions. Disinhibition similar to mania can be encountered after head trauma and in various conditions such as brain tumors and endocrine disorders.

Relationships disrupted. Friends and family have difficulty coping with a markedly changed behavior.

Sociability increased. Manic patients may excessively enjoy parties and other social gatherings.

Work-related problems. Loss of concentration and preoccupation with grandiose plans contribute to decreased performance on the job or in school.

Mental Status Examination

Appearance and behavior
  Excited, agitated
  Hyperactive
  Increased energy
  Loud speech
  Flamboyant or bizarre dress
  May be threatening or
    assaultive
Mood
  Euphoric
  Irritable
  Rapidly changing moods
Flow of thought
  Racing thoughts
  Flight of ideas
  Pressured speech

Flow of thought (*cont.*)
  Wordplay, jokes
  Distractible
Content of thought
  Self-confident
  Increased religiosity
  Full of schemes and plans
  Grandiosity that may be
    delusional
Language usually not affected
Cognition usually intact
Insight and judgment
  Lack of insight into the fact
    of being ill
  Poor judgment (refuses
    hospitalization, treatment)

SUBSTANCE USE DISORDERS

Substance misuse is defined by the culture in which it occurs. In most segments of our culture, the majority of adults use substances, if only caffeine. Whether we consider a person to be misusing a substance depends not simply on the amount or frequency of use, but also on the consequences of this behavior. These consequences may be behavioral, cognitive, legal, financial, and physical. Many of them also affect society as a whole.

Tip-Offs

The following symptoms should lead you to consider a diagnosis of a substance use disorder:

Alcohol use greater than one or two drinks per day
Arrests or other legal problems
Financial problems: spends money needed for other items
Health problems: blackouts, cirrhosis, abdominal pain, vomiting

Illegal substance use
Job loss, tardiness, demotions
Memory impairment
Social problems: fights, loss of friends

Main Diagnoses

In current diagnostic usage, these disorders are categorized as dependence (defined later) and abuse, which is a residual classification for patients who have some problems with substances but don't qualify for the diagnosis of dependence. Substance induced cognitive mental disorders, the brain syndromes that many people who heavily use substances also have at one time or another, will be considered in the section on difficulty thinking.

The classes of substances that are recognized as subject to misuse are given below. Many substance users will use more than one of these classes.

Alcohol*
Amphetamines*
Cannabis*
Cocaine*
Hallucinogens*
Inhalants*
Nicotine*
Opioids*
Phencyclidine (PCP) and related psychotomimetics*
Sedatives, hypnotics, anxiolytics*

Substance misuse can occur as a solitary diagnosis, but it is often associated with another major mental health diagnosis or personality disorder. Those to look for especially include the following:

Mood disorders (depression* and mania*)
Schizophrenia*
Somatization disorder*
Antisocial personality disorder*

Historical Information

Abuse. Substance abuse is a specific diagnosis applied to those users who are not actually substance-dependent (see below), but who continue to use despite at least one of the following: (1) physical danger (such as driving under the influence); (2) knowledge that they have problems resulting from substance use; (3) failure to fulfill obligations (job, home, school); (4) interpersonal problems (fights, arguments).

Activities used to obtain supply. These include drug sales, theft, robbery, and prostitution.

Age at onset. How old was the patient when substance use began? For alcohol use, women may have a much later age of onset than men.

Chronology. If there is an associated mental disorder, which came first? For example, if alcoholism chronologically precedes depression, the depression is regarded as secondary.

Dependence. Dependence on any substance is defined by three or more of the following symptoms within 12 months (numbers 1 and 2 don't usually apply to cannabis, the hallucinogens, or PCP):

1. Tolerance (the patient needs more drug to produce the same effect or obtains less effect with the same dose).
2. Withdrawal (the patient experiences withdrawal symptoms characteristic of the substance or takes more of it to avoid withdrawal).
3. More of the substance is used than the patient intended.
4. The patient tries unsuccessfully to control substance use.
5. The patient spends much time obtaining or using the substance or recovering from its effects.
6. Substance use causes the patient to give up important work, social, or recreational activities.
7. Despite knowledge that it has caused physical or psychological problems, the patient continues to use the substance.

Emotional/behavioral disorders. Complications that are especially likely include psychosis, mood syndromes, anxiety syndromes, delusional disorder, and delirium on withdrawal.

Frequency of use. How often has each drug been used? Has the pattern changed with the current episode?

Health problems. Has deteriorating health been suggested by evidence such as cirrhosis, stomach disorders, wasting, tuberculosis, or respiratory problems?

Legal problems. Have there been arrests or incarcerations for possession, sales, or criminal activities to finance supply? A history of criminal activity occasioned by the need to obtain money for drugs must be distinguished from antisocial personality disorder. Antisocial personality disorder may be the correct diagnosis if illegal activities have been undertaken when the patient was clean and sober.

Needle sharing. If intravenous usage is reported, has the patient *ever* used dirty needles? Had hepatitis? How recently has there been a test for HIV?

Pattern of use. Has there been continuous, episodic, or binge usage? If more than one drug is involved, what is the pattern for each?

Personality change. How has drug use affected the way the patient relates to others? Has there been a general loss of motivation (especially with long-term use of cannabis or hallucinogens)?

Relationship problems. These include divorces, separations, and fighting. Some couples stay together only *because* of a common interest in drug use.

Route of administration. Any of the following means can be used: swallowing, snorting, smoking, subcutaneous, intravenous.

Mental Status Examination

Appearance
  Red-faced
  Tremor
  Disheveled
Mood
  Depressed
  Anxious
  Belligerent
Flow of thought
  Often talkative
Content of thought
  Maudlin
  Demanding
  Hallucinations
    More often visual
    May be auditory

Language
  Fluency reduced (mumbling,
    slurred speech)
Cognitive
  May show cognitive signs if
    there is a concomitant
    cognitive disorder
Insight and judgment
  May reject the diagnosis
  Patients often refuse
    treatment or sign out
    against advice

SOCIAL AND PERSONALITY PROBLEMS

Personality *traits* are patterns of behavior or thought that persist throughout adult life. To be termed personality *disorders*, traits must be pronounced enough to cause the patient distress or functional impairment (social, emotional, or biological).

Tip-Offs

You should consider social and personality problems whenever your patient has any of the following characteristics:

Anxiety
Behaviors that seem odd or bizarre
Dramatic presentation
Drug or alcohol misuse
Interpersonal conflict
Job problems
Legal difficulties
Marital conflicts

Personality disorders must be distinguished from ordinary problems of living that are not mental disorders. The latter can include borderline intelligence, academic problems, marital and other family problems, job problems, and uncomplicated bereavement.

Main Diagnoses

Although many personality disorders have been proposed over the years, only the 10 given below currently enjoy official diagnostic blessing. Because they have features in common, they are usually presented in three clusters.

Cluster A. These people tend to be viewed as odd or eccentric. The cluster includes these three personality disorders:

Paranoid
Schizoid*
Schizotypal

Important differential diagnoses (aside from other personality disorders in this or other clusters) include the following:

Schizophrenia*
Delusional disorder*

Cluster B. These people are seen as dramatic, overly emotional, and erratic. The cluster includes these four personality disorders:

Antisocial*
Borderline*
Histrionic
Narcissistic

Important differential diagnoses (in addition to other personality disorders) are as follows:

Substance-related disorders*
Mania*
Somatization disorder*

Cluster C. These patients seem anxious or afraid. The cluster includes the following personality disorders:

Avoidant
Dependent
Obsessive–compulsive*

An important differential diagnosis (besides other personality disorders) is this:

Obsessive–compulsive disorder*

As indicated above, for any patient with any personality disorder, other personality disorders (or clusters) may come to the fore in the future.

Historical Information

Many traits have been linked to personality disorders. For purposes of description, I have used several common headings. This list makes no pretense of completeness; it does present traits that clinicians consider important in defining currently recognized personality disorders. This is some of the information you should pursue in the quest of a personality disorder diagnosis.

Callousness. Forces sexual activity on others; takes advantage of others for own gain; humiliates others publicly; uses harsh discipline; takes pleasure in suffering of others.
Carries grudges.
Childhood delinquency. Truancy; starts fights; fights with weapons; runs away; is cruel to animals or people; destroys property; sets fires.
Compliance is excessive. Volunteers for unpleasant tasks so as to be liked by others; agrees with people to avoid rejection.
Concern for others is lacking. Self-centered; unable to recognize how others feel.
Criticism is rejected. Resents useful suggestions; easily hurt by others.
Dishonesty. History of frequent lying; history of stealing, robbery, or conning others.
Impulsivity. Wanders without a fixed abode; sexual indiscretions; shoplifts; reckless disregard for personal safety.

Indecisiveness. Avoids making decisions or depends on others to make them; vague about goals.

Indifferent to praise.

Inflexibility. Reluctant to do things that differ from routine; perfectionism that interferes with task completion; preoccupation with rules, lists, order; misses the forest for the trees; resists letting others have their way; rigid about morality, ethics.

Insecurity. Feels uncomfortable when alone; won't get involved unless sure of being liked; fearful of self-embarrassment in social situations; exaggerates risks of doing something outside the routine; afraid of being abandoned; feels helpless or uncomfortable, so avoids being alone.

Irresponsibility. Defaults on financial obligations such as family support or debts; unable to hold a job; fails to do a reasonable share of the work; "forgets" obligations; puts things off.

Mood instability. Mood fluctuates more rapidly or more widely than is usually considered normal for the circumstances. May be quick to show anger; "hair-trigger temper."

Physical aggression. Fighting or assaults.

Saves objects of no value.

Sex drive is low.

Sociability is low. Is a loner (prefers solitary activities); uncomfortable in social situations or with strangers; avoids close relationships.

Stinginess. Shows lack of generosity with money or time.

Suicidal ideas or behavior.

Suspiciousness. Reluctance to confide in others; easily slighted; reads hidden meaning into innocent remarks or situations; expects to be exploited or harmed by others; questions loyalty of friends or fidelity of spouse/partner.

Trusts others excessively. Chronically chooses associates or situations that lead to disappointment.

Unstable interpersonal relationships.

Workaholism.

Mental Status Examination

Appearance and behavior	Appearance and behavior (*cont.*)
Lacks sense of humor	Cold or aloof
Hypervigilant	Sexual seductiveness that is
Argumentative	inappropriate
Appears tense	Overly concerned with
Reluctant to confide	appearance, attractiveness

Mood
  Hostile or defensive
  Temper; inappropriate, intense anger
  Exaggeratedly emotional speech, behavior
  Denies experiencing strong emotions
  Feels empty or bored
  Lacks remorse for hurting others
  Shallow, shifting emotions
  Apathy
  Restricted or inappropriate affect
  Cool, aloof, or silly
Flow of thought
  Vague speech
  Odd speech (vague, digressive, impoverished)
Content of thought
  Expects to be exploited
  Questions loyalty of friends
  Suspects hidden meanings
  Fantasies of success, power
  Ideas of reference (e.g., "as if" strangers talk about patient)

Content of thought (*cont.*)
  Odd beliefs, superstitions or magical thinking, illusions
  Uncertainty about identity (self-image, sexual orientation, long-term goals, values)
  Frequently requests reassurance or approval; fishes for compliments
  Fears being embarrassed
  Judgmental of self and/or others
  Unreasonably devalues authority figures
Language: no abnormalities are typical
Cognition: no abnormalities are typical
Insight and judgment
  Exaggerates accomplishments
  Lacks remorse for behavior
  Feels others make unreasonable demands
  Overvalues own work; self important; feels problems are unique; sense of entitlement

DIFFICULTY THINKING (COGNITIVE PROBLEMS)

A wide variety of physical and chemical insults can interfere with thinking. These causes include the following:

Brain tumors
Head trauma
Hypertension
Infections
Metabolic disorders
Postoperative complications
Seizure disorders

Toxic substances or withdrawal from psychoactive substances
Vitamin deficiency

Tip-Offs

Any of the following symptoms or signs should stimulate further investigation of cognitive problems:

Bizarre behavior
Confusion
Decreased judgment
Delusions
Hallucinations
Memory defects
Mood fluctuations
Toxin ingestion

Main Diagnoses

Physical or chemical brain dysfunction produces abnormalities of behavior or thinking that can be either temporary or permanent. The types of problems include these:

Amnestic syndrome*
Anxiety syndrome
Delirium*
Delusional syndrome
Dementia*
Dissociative disorders
Intoxication* and withdrawal*
Psychosis of intoxication or withdrawal*
Mood syndrome
Personality syndrome

The important differential diagnoses include the starred diagnoses in the previous group, plus these:

Depression*
Schizophrenia*
Substance use disorders*

Delirium and dementia may coexist.

Historical Information

Age at onset. Dementia is most commonly encountered in elderly persons; delirium is common in children *and* in older people.

Course. May be stable, fluctuating, deteriorating, or improving. If the damage is structural (such as following massive brain trauma), there tends to be some permanent dysfunction, even though improvement may occur. Patients with dementia (such as Alzheimer's) tend to deteriorate.

Depressive disorder. It is especially important to know about a history of depression and current depressive features, because *pseudodementia*, one of the possible presentations of severe depression, is a completely treatable mood disorder that is no dementia at all.

Difficulty caring for self. Often this is what drives family members to bring demented patients for care.

Fluctuating symptoms and mental status. Such fluctuations are especially characteristic of delirium.

Head trauma. Recent trauma can produce a subdural hematoma, which produces symptoms days to weeks later. Bleeding inside the skull can also cause an epidural hematoma, which leads to symptoms within hours or days. Also be alert for loss of memory that can result from concussion.

Impulsivity. Demented patients lose the ability to judge what is acceptable behavior; consequently, they act on impulses they previously would have suppressed. Delirious or demented patients may try to run away, as a reaction to either fear or confusion. Spending money thoughtlessly can occur, as it does in mania, though in demented patients it may lack the grandiose quality it has in mania.

Laboratory testing. This should be consistent with the suspected cause of any cognitive syndrome.

Memory loss. Defective memory is characteristic of the dementias. Recent memory is affected most often, though in severe dementia long-term memory can also be involved. Some patients try (though not consciously) to compensate for defects in memory by *confabulating*—making up stories.

Onset. The development of symptoms may be rapid or insidious, depending on the cause and nature of the disorder. Rapid onset is characteristic of disorders caused by infectious processes or brain trauma; vitamin deficiencies and brain tumors may develop gradually.

Personality change. Many of the symptoms of cognitive syndromes involve a change from the patient's previous personality. These include outbursts of rage or combativeness, social withdrawal, coarsening of behavior (crude jokes), and neglect of grooming or hygiene. One patient with Alzheimer's dementia who had always welcomed racial diversity shouted racist comments. Excessive neatness (known as *organic orderliness*) sometimes develops.

Psychotic symptoms. Delusions, usually persecutory, occur in dementia (patients with Alzheimer's often believe that people steal from them). Delusions may be indistinguishable from those of schizophrenia. Hallucinations commonly occur in delirium, but they are usually visual.

Sleep–wake cycle changes. Delirious patients are typically drowsy, although some have trouble falling asleep; vivid dreams or nightmares occur.

Suicide attempts. The presence of suicidal behavior should cause you to consider the diagnosis of major depression, although attempts (and completions) can occur in the dementias.

Mental Status Examination

Appearance and behavior
  Disheveled
  Tremor
  Restlessness
  Picking at bedclothes,
    clothing
Mood
  Affect bland or shallow
  Anger
  Anxiety
  Apathy
  Depression
  Euphoria
  Fear
  Irritability
Flow of thought
  Slurred speech
  Perseveration
  Rambling, incoherent
  Loosening of associations
Content of thought
  Suspiciousness
  Current suicidal ideas
  Illusions
  Psychotic features
    Delusions
    Hallucinations (especially
      visual)

Language
  Comprehension decreases
    with advancing dementia
  Fluency is often preserved,
    even with moderately
    severe dementia
  Naming: aphasias
Cognition
  Drowsy, hard to stay awake
  Disorientation
    Not knowing the date may
      be an early symptom of
      delirium
    Disorientation to place,
      person are later
      symptoms (especially
      dementia)
  Impaired abstract thinking
    (similarities)
  Low attention span (easily
    distractible) is found
    especially in delirium
  Impaired memory
Insight and judgment
  Impaired judgment

ANXIETY, AVOIDANCE BEHAVIOR, AND AROUSAL

Conditions in this area of clinical interest have in common anxiety symptoms that result in attempts to avoid the stimulus.

Tip-Offs

Symptoms that would cause you to explore this area include any expression of anxiety or fear, as well as somatic symptoms that suggest breathing or heartbeat problems when there is no known basis for concern.

Anxiety
Chest complaints (pain, heaviness, trouble breathing, palpitations)
Compulsive behavior
Fear of objects, situations, dying, impending doom, going crazy
Nervousness
Obsessional ideas
Panic
Trauma (history of severe emotional or physical experience)
Worries

Main Diagnoses

The principal disorders covered by this area of clinical interest include:

Panic*
Generalized anxiety*
Phobic*
Obsessive–compulsive*
Posttraumatic stress*

Although anxiety symptoms are found in nearly every mental disorder, the important differential diagnoses include the following:

Depression*
Substance-related disorders*
Schizophrenia*
Somatization disorder*

Historical Information

Age at onset. Most of these conditions begin when the patient is relatively young. Animal phobias begin in childhood; situational phobias usually begin in the 30s.

Agoraphobia. May occur with or without panic disorder. Occurs in situations from which escape is difficult or embarrassing, such as being away from home, in a crowd, in a car, or on a bridge.

Alcohol or drug use. This could be either a cause or an effect of anxiety symptoms.

Anticipatory anxiety. Common in phobias, this sensation of dread is experienced for minutes to hours before the arrival of a feared stimulus (such as speaking in public).

Caffeine intake. Excessive coffee (or tea) drinking can cause anxiety symptoms.

Circumstances of panic attacks. How many attacks have there been, and in what period of time? Were they unexpected? (Panic attacks tend to come out of the blue.)

Compulsions. The most common compulsions are handwashing, checking, counting, and routines that *must* be followed (e.g., at bedtime). They may occur as rituals (rules) or as "antidotes" or responses to obsessions.

Depressive symptoms. Determine whether these came before the anxiety syndrome, suggesting primary depression, or after, suggesting that the depression is secondary.

Duration of panic attacks. Individual panic attacks last only a few minutes, but they may recur over a period of weeks, months, or years.

Frequency of panic attacks. They usually occur several times a week.

Lifestyle constriction. As a result of anxiety, does the patient stay at home or avoid specific situations or objects? This may be true for phobic disorder, obsessive–compulsive disorder, PTSD, agoraphobia, and panic disorder.

Mental content of panic attacks. Patients may fear they are going to die, lose control, or lose their minds.

Obsessions. Most common are ideas of (1) harming or killing and (2) swearing (blaspheming). These ideas persist despite the fact that patients recognize the ideas are senseless and foreign to them.

Physical symptoms of anxiety. Most of the same physical sensations occur in panic attacks and in anxiety disorder:

Breathlessness	Heart palpitations
Chest pain	Lump in throat
Chills or flushes	Muscle tension
Dizziness	Nausea
Dry mouth	Restlessness
Fatigability	Sweating
Frequent urination	Tremor

Prescription medication use. Clinicians often prescribe, and patients with anxiety often resort to, drugs in an attempt to keep symptoms in check.

Social phobias. These phobias typically involve performing, speaking, or eating in public; using a public toilet; and trying to write when someone is watching.

Specific phobias. Formerly called *simple phobias*, the most common are fear of air travel, animals, blood, closed-in places, heights, and injury.

Stressors. A severely traumatic physical or emotional experience is a required precipitant for PTSD.

Worry. Unwarranted or excessive concern about multiple real-life circumstances is characteristic of generalized anxiety disorder. Examples are losing the house to the bank 2 months before the mortgage is paid off; being fired when one is the favorite of the company president.

Mental Status Examination

Appearance and behavior
  Hypervigilance (scanning the environment)
Mood
  Depression
  Anxiety
Content of thought
  Obsessional ideas
  Killing
  Blasphemy
Insight and judgment
  Insight retained that the fear or behavior is unreasonable
  Tries to resist

PHYSICAL COMPLAINTS

Physical illness (anatomically demonstrable heart attacks, asthma, ulcers, allergies, and the like) must always be a prime concern of any clinician whose patient voices somatic complaints. But many patients come to mental health care complaining of physical symptoms for which no basis in physiology, chemistry, or anatomy can be found. Such symptoms are commonly called *hypochondriacal* or *psychosomatic*. Often, by the time a patient finally seeks help from a mental health clinician, there has already been a full range of medical tests and evaluations. Because certain demographic and symptom features are held in common, I have included anorexia nervosa and bulimia nervosa in this group.

Tip-Offs

Consider this area of clinical interest if your patient presents any of the following problems:

> Appetite disturbance
> Depression that is chronic
> History that is complicated
> Multiple complaints
> Physical symptoms unexplained by known illness (especially neu-
>   rological symptoms such as pain, convulsions, sensory loss)
> Sexual or physical abuse in childhood
> Substance misuse in a woman
> Treatment failures that are repeated
> Vague history
> Weakness that is chronic
> Weight changes (up or down)

Main Diagnoses

The principal diagnoses in this area include the following:

> Anorexia nervosa*
> Body dysmorphic disorder (dysmorphophobia)
> Bulimia nervosa
> Hypochondriasis
> Pain disorder (chronic pain syndrome)
> Somatization disorder*

Other disorders that should be considered in patients who complain of physical symptoms are these:

> Depression*
> Panic disorder*
> Physical illness
> Substance-related disorders*

Historical Information

Age at onset. Most of the mental disorders in this group begin early (childhood or adolescence). Hypochondriasis usually begins in the 20s, and pain disorder in the 30s or 40s.

Childhood physical or sexual abuse. Common in patients with somatization disorder, abuse should always be inquired about.

Chronic pain. In pain disorder there is no known basis for pain, or the pain is out of keeping with a known physical cause.

Doctor shopping. A relentless search for a cure frequently accompanies somatization disorder. It may lead to repeated, fruitless medical evaluations.

Environmental stress. Social problems (marital, job, interpersonal) may impel patients with somatization disorder to seek mental health treatment for what they perceive as physical problems.

Fear of medical illness that is not present. The nondelusional idea that the person is ill persists despite (often repeated) reassurances to the contrary. This is the cardinal symptom of hypochondriasis.

Operations. Patients with somatization disorder often have a history of multiple surgical procedures during which organs may be removed.

Medical illness in childhood. Did the patient receive attention for being ill as a child? In some cases this factor may underlie the somatization.

Physical defect (imagined or exaggerated). The essential symptom in body dysmorphic disorder, this idea is not of delusional intensity. Patients with anorexia nervosa typically regard themselves as appearing overweight, even when they are obviously emaciated.

Review of systems. This is a specialized review of four symptom categories; eight symptoms are required to diagnose somatization disorder. The complete review of systems is given in Appendix B.

Secondary gain. This occurs when a person receives attention or support from being ill; it is classical for somatization disorder and other somatoform disorders.

Suicidal ideas, behavior. These patients often threaten or attempt suicide; occasionally they do kill themselves.

Substance use. Misuse of alcohol or drugs frequently complicates somatization disorder and other disorders in this group.

Mental Status Examination

    Appearance and behavior
      Dramatic presentation
      Flashy dress
      Ingratiating manner
      Exaggerated mannerisms
      Marked wasting
    Mood
      Indifference toward symptom (*la belle indifférence*)
      Anxiety
      Depression
    Flow of thought: no abnormalities are typical

Content of thought:
  Centers on physical (sometimes imagined) mental illness
Language: no abnormalities are typical
Cognition: no abnormalities are typical
Insight and judgment
  Overinterprets physical symptoms

Chapter 14

Closure

An hour usually provides enough time to explore the reasons for seeking treatment and to obtain a great deal of personal background information about your patient. During this time, you should also have conducted a formal mental status examination. Even though there is still much you would like to know, you probably shouldn't push the interview too much further. You're conducting an interview, not a test of everyone's endurance, and you need to be fresh enough to keep evaluating what you hear and see. Perhaps another patient appointment dictates that you will have to finish next week, or the hour of the day could suggest that you return tomorrow. Or, if both you and your patient still have time and the inclination, just take a coffee break before continuing.

THE ART OF CLOSING

Closing an initial interview is a minor art form that requires some care. A good closing does not just summarize the interview; it also prepares the patient (and clinician) for the sessions that lie ahead. Your patient, who has just invested considerable hope and confidence in the time you have spent together, quite reasonably expects some information to carry away from the encounter. The content of that message will depend in part upon your relationship with the patient.

If you are a practicing clinician responsible for this patient's care, you will probably follow these steps: (1) Summarize your findings; (2) with the patient's collaboration, develop a plan for future management; and (3) set a time for your next meeting. Whenever it is justified, you should also (4) include a message of hope for the future. Here is an example:

"From what you've told me, it seems that both you and your husband have had a lot of trouble adjusting to the death of your daughter.

It's something you haven't talked much about, and you're suffering from the lack of communication. I think I can help, but before we decide on a plan of action I'd like to talk with your husband. You said you thought he'd be willing to come in. Could you ask him to make an appointment for next week?"

The closing phase of your initial interview as a trainee might sound something like this:

"Thank you for spending so much time with me. You really helped me understand about your type of depression. I agree that your therapist is doing everything possible to help. Tomorrow I'd like to ask you more about your family background, if that's all right with you."

You shouldn't expect to anticipate everything the patient needs to hear. In any session as intense as a typical initial interview, you are likely to leave unspoken something that is important to the patient. Therefore, it is usually a good idea to learn whether you've omitted anything that should be covered right away. Before you quit, say something that invites comments or questions about your interview:

"What questions do you have about what we've said so far?" (Note: By assuming that the patient does have questions, you encourage their expression. For some patients, the alternative "Do you have any questions?" may shut down this avenue of communication.)

"Are there any important issues we haven't covered?"
You may find that something you've left out needs action now—such as additional information about proposed treatment, uncertainty as to the time of the next appointment, or reassurance about prognosis. Try to respond factually to any substantive issues.

Of course, you won't be able to cover everything in a single interview session. Most patients will accept this and will be content to delay other concerns, questions, and items of historical information until a subsequent appointment.

Occasionally, something comes up right at the end of an interview that would require considerable time to cover adequately. Examples:

"What does the future hold for someone like me?"

"What do you think I should do about my son's alcoholism?"
If neither you nor the patient has any time constraints, you can deal with these questions when they arise. But scheduling conflicts often require that you delay further inquiry until your next interview.

In either case, consider the possible reasons for this new question so late in the interview. Some patients habitually save important information for closing time. Perhaps they need nearly an entire session to get up the courage to discuss important problems—are they afraid of what you might suggest? Others may find their sessions so valuable that they unconsciously try to prolong them.

You can deal with most of these last-minute items by expressing interest and promising to discuss them during your next session:

"I'm glad you mentioned that. It's something I want to learn more about. Let's make it our first order of business next time."

If the last-minute information is of life-threatening proportions (suicidal or homicidal ideas), you have no choice but to run overtime. If this happens habitually to you, you should train yourself to raise these sensitive topics earlier in your interviews.

QUITTING EARLY

A rare patient may try to break off the interview before you've finished. Usually this will be someone who is exhibiting a character disorder, a psychosis, intoxication, or extreme stress (perhaps from sleep deprivation or physical illness). Sometimes all of the above apply! Whatever the cause, you suddenly find yourself trying to get information from someone who is putting on a coat to leave. How should you react?

If it is close to the end of the session, point out that you will need only a few more minutes to finish. Then try to accommodate your patient's agitation by selecting only the most important remaining questions to ask.

With a new patient, you don't have much leverage, so try to avoid direct confrontation. If it is early in the interview, especially right at the beginning, the patient might not fully understand the reasons for the interview. Try explaining again. At the same time, you can offer some empathy:

"I can see that you have been pretty upset. I'm sorry to be adding to your discomfort, but we do need to talk. It's the only way I can get the information I need to help you."

Your appeal to reason may succeed about half the time. If it doesn't, try switching gears to a discussion of the feelings that have blocked cooperation. As before, lead with an empathic statement:

"You seem pretty uncomfortable. Could you tell me what you are feeling?"

You may learn quite a lot about your patient's fear, anger, or discomfort. By pursuing what you have just heard, you may be able to ease back into the interview.

INTERVIEWER: I can see this has upset you. Could you tell me what you're feeling right now?

PATIENT: *(Rising to leave)* I can't stand it. It's just like the last time!

INTERVIEWER: Were you pretty upset then, too?

PATIENT: You bet I was! You'd be, too, if your therapist treated you the way mine treated me.

INTERVIEWER: It must have made you terribly uncomfortable.

PATIENT: *(Sitting down again)* I was humiliated. And scared.

As in this example, you may hear a good deal about previous attempts at therapy that have gone awry. Be prepared to spend considerable time (both in the initial interview and later) digging out the facts about the previous treatment, even though it may have little or nothing to do with the actual reasons the patient has come in at this time. (Take care not to criticize or otherwise disparage the previous clinician—your information so far may be pretty one-sided.)

If all your best efforts fail, respect the comfort and privacy of your patient. Specifically, don't plead, threaten, or imply shame or guilt. If your patient gets up to leave the room, don't use physical restraint. Instead, acknowledge the patient's right to make this decision and your intention to respect it. But promise to have another try soon at this important task of gathering information:

"I can see that we'll have to break it off for now. That's OK—you have a right not to be bothered when you're feeling this bad. But it's really important that we figure out what difficulties brought you into the hospital. I can come back this afternoon, after you've had a chance to rest up."

Occasionally, you may decide to quit early, well short of an hour. This alternative will seem especially attractive when:

- It is late at night, your patient has just been admitted to the hospital, and both of you are exhausted.
- Because of severe psychosis or depression, your patient cannot focus on the interview situation for longer than a few minutes at a time.
- Anger renders your patient unwilling to cooperate.
- You have squeezed a brief interview into an already hectic day. By agreement, you will talk just long enough to discover the major issues and to decide how soon you should meet again.

Chapter 15

Interviewing Informants

Most patients can tell you nearly everything you need to know, but you can often enrich the tapestry of your database with third-party information. However, some situations virtually demand that you seek additional information or verification of data from informants. Here are a few of them:

- Children and adolescents often lack adequate perspective on their own behavior.
- Even some adults don't know certain important items of family history.
- Patients with mental retardation often require help in relating their own information.
- Patients of any age who feel ashamed of past behavior may conceal historical information that you can learn from family or friends. Examples include sexual indiscretions, substance misuse, suicide attempts, violence, and criminal behavior of any type.
- Patients with psychosis may present delusional interpretations of fact, rather than the facts themselves.
- Childhood health history, often unknown to the patient, can be relevant to mental retardation or specific learning disorders. There may be a history of obstetrical complications during the birth of patients who have a sporadic form of schizophrenia.
- Patients with cognitive disorders such as Alzheimer's dementia may be unable to give a good history.
- Informants can tell you about cultural norms. This may be the only way to learn that it is normal in your patient's family to believe in astrology or to speak in tongues in church.
- Some patients with character disorders (especially antisocial personality disorder) do not reliably tell the truth.

- Some personality disorders don't much bother some patients; their families and friends are the ones who suffer.
- For some, safeguarding a family secret may be more pressing than telling you things that could help with diagnosis or treatment.
- For obvious reasons, it is unwise to rely solely on self-report in forensic situations.

So whenever possible, I like to obtain information about a patient's present illness from other sources, such as relatives, friends, previous clinical records, and other clinicians. By verifying existing information and providing new facts, you can obtain a clear, comprehensive, balanced view of both patient and milieu. Collateral information can reveal characteristics that will help you better understand or manage the patient. For example, high levels of emotional expression in relatives may predict relapse in a patient with schizophrenia who lives with these relatives.

You will almost always interview the patient first; this helps ensure that the patient will give a complete and honest account. The only significant exceptions, besides children and younger adolescents who are brought in by their parents, are adults who lack the capacity to speak for themselves. These include regressed patients with schizophrenia, patients with dementia, some individuals with mental retardation, and persons with whom you do not share a common language. But even when you and your patient communicate well with one another, a little time spent with relatives will usually improve your perspective on the patient's disorder. This is especially true when a relative comes along for the first visit—often a sign of the relative's fear that, without help, the entire story may not be told. Rarely, an insecure patient needs the support of a relative while telling you the reasons for needing to be seen.

OBTAINING PERMISSION FIRST

Before you talk to friends or relatives, you must usually ask permission from the patient. Most patients will consent willingly. The few who demur may worry that you will let slip something they have been trying to keep secret. You can often quiet these fears by pointing out that your main job is to seek information, not to dispense it, and that to help the most you need another person's perspective. Here's how you might phrase your reassurance:

"What you've told me is confidential, and I'll respect that confidence. You have that right. But you also have a right to the best help I can give. For that I need to know more about you. That's why I'd like to talk with your wife. She'll naturally want to know what's wrong and what we plan to do about it. I think I should tell her, but I'll only tell what you and I have already agreed upon. I won't tell her about anything else we've discussed, unless you give me permission in advance."

Once you have reached such an agreement, be scrupulously careful not to divulge additional information. Revealed secrets have an uncanny way of identifying their source. On the rare occasion when you are denied permission, you might suggest that the patient sit in when you talk to the friend or relative. This will address any fears that you might use the meeting to hatch some sort of plot behind the patient's back.

As a rule, though, you should try to interview the informant when the patient is not present. The privacy will improve your chances for obtaining complete, accurate information, and both you and the informant will feel more comfortable.

There are only a few significant exceptions to the requirement to obtain the patient's consent first. These include patients who are:

Minors
On conservatorship or unable to give consent
Violent
Mute
Acutely suicidal
Experiencing any other medical or mental health emergency

Then, when it is clear that a patient does not have the judgment to exercise autonomy, it is your duty to step in and make a decision as to the best course of action. To accomplish this, you will usually obtain information in any way you can.

What about the friend or relative who calls with information and requests that you withhold it from the patient, or at least that you not reveal its source? To give such a promise makes you complicit in weaving a tangled web—a situation I would try to avoid. To be sure, there's no point in creating problems by blabbing stuff needlessly. But you can drive yourself nuts trying to keep straight whom you've promised to keep what secret from whom.

CHOOSING AN INFORMANT

Because your goal is to obtain as much pertinent material as you can, you will naturally choose an informant who knows your patient well. A spouse or partner is usually the most up to date, so if the patient is married or has an intimate relationship of long standing, that is the person you will probably speak with first. But the sort of information you need may dictate a different choice. For example, if you want to know about childhood hyperactivity, you should interview a parent. Another consideration: Studies show that relatives who have had an illness similar to the patient's are better able to recognize its symptoms. (Perhaps this is because they have been sensitized to the symptoms and course of illness.) Finally, as we shall discuss later, yours could end up being a group interview with several relatives, friends, and even coworkers or spiritual counselors.

WHAT DO YOU ASK?

You should start by briefly explaining the purpose of this interview. Relatives will readily accept that you need to verify history or to give them information. But they may worry that as a clinician you have another agenda, such as blaming them or asking them to assume increased responsibility for the patient.

Your earlier interview with the patient should have given you a considerable knowledge base, so your discussion with informants can usually be comparatively brief—anywhere from a few minutes to half an hour. Even if you think you know exactly what questions you want answered, you could be surprised with new information about a problem you hadn't recognized before. That's why you should begin with a brief fishing expedition to learn what the informant knows. Use an open-ended question as bait.

In the example that follows, the patient had spent much of the initial interview talking about her previous episodes of depression. So, when her husband came in, the interviewer was ready with questions about depressive symptoms, treatment, and response. Fortunately, the leading question was open-ended.

INTERVIEWER: What can you tell me about your wife's difficulty?

PATIENT'S HUSBAND: Well, I just hope you can do something about her drinking. She's drunk nearly every afternoon when I get home from work, but she refuses to admit she's got a problem.

Once you've determined that the patient and informant(s) identify the same set of problems, you can get down to the business of obtaining the additional specific information you need. It will be of two sorts: (1) questions the patient was unable to answer; and (2) items about which there is some confusion in your mind, often due to inconsistency in the patient's story. Here are a few examples of each:

History of mental illness in a parent
The patient's own developmental history
A reappraisal of your patient's drug or drinking history
The patient's symptoms during a psychotic illness
The ability of a patient to provide self-care
Relatives' willingness to provide care after discharge from hospital
A spouse's view of the reasons behind marital discord
Behavior that suggests a possible criminal career
An appraisal of the patient's personality characteristics
Effects on the family of any change in behavior

Even if you don't learn much that is new about the patient, an open-ended session with an informant may help you learn the answers to these questions:

How well does the family understand the illness?
What has the patient told the informant about the symptoms?
How has your patient interpreted the facts?
Has the patient distorted what you have said?

If the information from an informant conflicts with what you have obtained from your patient, you must decide which (if either) story to believe. You are by no means safe if you automatically accept the informant's version—status as a mental health patient should not automatically discredit anyone's testimony. Rather, when you evaluate conflicting stories, weigh the following factors for each informant, including the patient:

How much contact has the informant had with the patient?
How much does the informant appear to remember?
Does the informant seem to be protecting someone (self, patient, or others)?
Does family taboo appear to prevent the informant from discussing sensitive material?
How much is the story being distorted by wishful thinking (for example, the imagined happiness of a faltering marriage)?
Is there evidence of a halo effect that puts a spin (positive or negative) on all the patient's behavior?
Does your informant seem well motivated to give you a complete and accurate story?

Afterwards, it's a good idea to discuss the session with your patient. You should provide some idea of what was said, so as to provide reassurance that you have broken no confidences, but how specific or general you will be depends on your patient's needs and your own taste. You should also take care not to break any confidences from the relatives.

Here is an example of the sort of feedback you might give your patient:

"I had a very good talk with your wife, Mr. Crenshaw. Her information confirmed what you told me last week about your depression, and I think we all see eye to eye on the need for treatment. As you requested, I didn't say anything to her about the cocaine use, but I do think you'll feel better once you've gotten up the nerve to discuss it with her yourself."

GROUP INTERVIEWS

If the patient's family is large and many members live nearby, you may find yourself interviewing whole groups of relatives. Some clinicians find this difficult, especially when the family is unhappy and expresses itself forcefully. Although it can be difficult to manage a large group of relatives, there are advantages to this approach.

- It is far more efficient than trying to talk with them individually. Although you might sometimes get the family to agree on one spokesperson with whom you will meet, information can be lost or distorted that way.
- The family is an important part of your patient's environment. A group interview gives you the chance to observe how the relatives interact with one another and, by logical inference, with the patient. Do they treat one another considerately? Do you detect accusations, scapegoating, or guilt in one or more of your informants? Is their concern generally for the patient or for their own comfort?
- In some cases, you may elect to interview family and patient together. This obviates all problems with confidentiality, because all hear what all say. It also gives you the chance to observe directly how the patient and family interact. Do relatives ignore or answer for the patient? Do they disagree a lot? Fight?
- If you determine that family dynamics contribute in part to your patient's difficulties, meeting with everyone can help lay the groundwork for eventual change in the home milieu, as an adjunct to therapy.
- You could lay the groundwork for later family therapy, if it seems that this might be a useful approach to your patient's difficulties.

When you are meeting with more than one informant at a time, be sure to encourage all relatives to have their say. Often someone will be passive and silent; this is the individual you should try to draw out. It is better to have everyone's input at the beginning, rather than leaving them all to sort out their perspectives later, when you're not around to help. You shouldn't make decisions for them, and you shouldn't take sides. Your goal should be to facilitate the discussion so that all can understand the patient and their common problems.

OTHER INTERVIEW SETTINGS

Telephone Calls

Several studies have shown that you can obtain good-quality information from telephone interviews. If there is no other way to speak with a relative, it is certainly better than nothing. But it is a challenge to meet someone for the first time without face-to-face contact. If you must rely on words and tone of voice alone, you can't extract the nuances of meaning that body language so readily conveys. Furthermore, unless you are participating in a video conference call, on the telephone relatives cannot size *you* up. A personal interview can so much better convey the warm feelings that allow relatives to know that you are some one they can trust with secret or sensitive information. Finally, consider confidentiality laws. Without visual contact, it is more difficult to be sure whom you are speaking with. If you give out information to someone you think is a spouse, but is actually an employer, you could harm your patient's career and your own reputation.

House Calls

Although the house call has generally gone the way of insulin coma therapy, it can still be a useful tool for the clinician who wants maximum information about all aspects of a patient's milieu. There you can get a feeling for the environment (type of dwelling, neighborhood) *and* the family, which, when relaxed at home, may behave more "normally."

Chapter 16

Meeting Resistance

In most interviews, two individuals work together to achieve a common understanding. The vast majority of patients will be cooperative, knowledgeable, and (to some degree or other) insightful. But all patients have their own agendas, and sometimes these conflict with the usual goals of the initial interview. That's why many patients will in some manner resist giving complete information. The result can be behavior that frustrates your attempts to obtain a complete database while building rapport.

Resistance is any conscious or unconscious attempt to avoid a topic of discussion. Because nearly everyone feels uncomfortable with some topic or other, resistance is perhaps the most frequent problem behavior clinicians must learn to deal with. For a number of reasons, then, it is important to address resistance when it appears, and not simply to move on without trying to determine (and remedy) its causes.

RECOGNIZING RESISTANCE

To counter resistance, you must first recognize it. Sometimes this is easy, especially if it comes in the form of such an obvious statement as "I'd rather not talk about that." But many patients feel uncomfortable with open defiance; they may resist you in ways so subtle you will be hard-pressed to detect them. Watch for any of these behaviors that could indicate that your interview may be in trouble:

Tardiness. Being late for the interview is a classic sign of resistance. It is perhaps less common during an initial interview than during subsequent ones.

Voluntary behaviors. Poor eye contact, glancing at the clock, answering a cell phone or pager, or shifting uneasily while seated suggests that your patient may feel uncomfortable with the topic currently under discussion.

Involuntary behaviors. Flushing, yawning, or swallowing also implies discomfort. The blank stare of a patient with PTSD experiencing a flashback falls somewhere between voluntary and involuntary behavior.

Forgetfulness. Some patients develop a "convenient" poor memory and respond to certain questions with "I don't know" or "I can't remember."

Omissions. The patient leaves out certain information. Unless reliable informants are consulted, even experienced clinicians find this sort of resistance difficult to detect. "I don't have any problems" may be an overt attempt to bury issues that should be exhumed.

Contradictions. Information that contradicts what you thought you learned earlier is relatively easy to spot but may be difficult to reconcile.

Changing the subject. Shifting to another topic of conversation may be an attempt to draw you away from a subject the patient would like to avoid. For example, you ask Mr. Blocker how he feels about his impending divorce; he responds by telling you that his wife's attorney has been bleeding him dry.

Exaggerations. Puffing up their own accomplishments is one way some people avoid facing the truth about themselves. Perhaps you can't detect an individual exaggeration, but with time you may begin to discern a pattern of improbable claims.

Diversionary tactics. These include telling jokes and asking to get a drink or to use the bathroom. Some patients may try to control the interview by asking about the interviewer's personal life.

Silence. This can be a major indicator of resistance. It should not be confused with the time some patients need to think before responding to a complicated question.

A slight hesitation. Most subtle of all may be just a slight hesitation before answering certain questions.

WHY DO PATIENTS RESIST?

Patients may resist telling the whole story to a clinician for a variety of reasons. Understanding these reasons can provide the key to breaking up the resistance.

- Preventing embarrassment is probably one of the most common reasons; it may operate especially during an initial interview. This is certainly understandable: Baring your soul to a total stranger is the unnatural antithesis of self-protection. It is especially hard for some peo-

ple to reveal sensitive material about sex, illegal activities, and any behavior that demonstrates a lapse of judgment.

• Some patients (or their families) fear criticism or worry that you
may be shocked by their stories. They have learned to avoid disapproval
simply by not risking it: They keep material they consider blameworthy
to themselves.

• Some patients may withhold information because they are too
afraid of its implications for diagnosis, prognosis, or treatment. The
stigma of mental illness—perhaps being thought "crazy"—is one example.

• Your new patient may not yet feel enough trust to communicate
fully with you, especially about thoughts or behavior that might damage an intimate relationship or jeopardize a job or legal status. Unhappily, a previous experience may have instigated the fear that a mental health professional might violate confidentiality.

• A patient might altruistically seek to protect a friend or loved
one from any of the consequences mentioned previously.

• Some incidents or thoughts may seem too trivial to relate.

• The patient may unconsciously be testing you to see whether you
are smart enough or persistent enough (do you care enough?) to dig
out the information that is being withheld.

• Patients may withhold information because of anger, conscious or
unconscious, that could have any of a number of causes. You may have un-
intentionally said something upsetting, or the patient may be reenacting
with you feelings held for someone else in the past—a behavior called
transference. Transference is by no means limited to feelings of anger.

Whatever the cause, you must not allow resistance to persist unexplored and unchallenged. You must try to determine the cause and to
remedy it. It can be a serious error to skip important topics or just passively to follow the patient's lead.

HOW TO COPE WITH RESISTANCE

Above all else, it is most important that you try to understand (and correct, if you can) the reasons behind the behavior. The first step should
be to consider whether you have done anything to provoke the resistance. There may be something obvious that you can deal with directly.

INTERVIEWER: I notice that you seem to have grown quiet all of a
sudden. What seems to be the problem?

PATIENT: Oh, I don't know.

INTERVIEWER: I'm wondering if you're upset that I said I wanted to talk to your husband.

PATIENT: *(Long pause)* Well, I don't understand why you want to.

INTERVIEWER: Could you tell me what you're afraid of?

PATIENT: He wouldn't understand about that affair I told you about. He isn't a bit broad-minded.

INTERVIEWER: Ah, I can see why you're unhappy. I think anyone would be, who worried that her therapist might break a confidence like that one. But that wasn't what I had in mind. The reason I want to talk to him is to learn how he views the marital problems you two are having. I think it would help me to understand the whole picture better. Do you think that you could ask him to join you for your next appointment?

This clinician's explanation told the patient three things: (1) that the clinician understood her, (2) that she had a right to her feelings, and (3) that her fears were groundless. Finally, it suggested that they continue with the plan.

All too often, however, you will be unable to identify anything specific that can be quickly corrected. Then the approach you take will depend on several features of the resistance itself.

Its cause
Its severity
The form it takes
The importance of the information you are seeking

Managing Silence

A common example of mild resistance is the embarrassed silence. You may encounter this reaction to questions about sex (see Chapter 9), but it could occur in nearly any interview situation. Your best first response may be a little silence of your own. You might try glancing away for a few seconds to emphasize your willingness to wait. By saying nothing for a few moments, you give your patient some extra thinking time. (Maybe that's all the silence signified in the first place. But if instead it's early resistance, you allow the patient time to try to resolve the conflict.)

However, a prolonged lack of response may establish a precedent for withholding further information later in the interview, and that is not in the patient's best interests. If a decent interval (no more than 15 seconds or so) fails to produce any response, you should probably intervene.

During the brief silence, your patient's thoughts may have wandered, so your next step should be to refocus the question by asking it again in a slightly different form. From the top, here's a brief example:

> INTERVIEWER: How has your sexual adjustment been?
>
> PATIENT: *(Silently looks at the floor for 15 or 20 seconds.)*
>
> INTERVIEWER: I was wondering whether there had been any problems with your sex life.

If the question seems important (the patient's inability to answer suggests that it might be), you should probably persevere. Start by giving the patient control over what will be said and by offering reassurance.

> INTERVIEWER: Tell me what you feel comfortable saying about your sex life.
>
> PATIENT: This is really hard for me.
>
> INTERVIEWER: That's all right. It's safe to talk about it here.

Another tactic combines multiple approaches. You might word it something like this:

"A lot of people have difficulty with sensitive issues like this one. I'm really sorry that I have to put you through this, but to help you most, I need all the information I can possibly get. Please try to help me."

In this single speech you have (1) expressed sympathy, (2) underscored the normality of your patient's feelings, (3) reemphasized the importance of obtaining a complete database, and (4) issued a personal appeal.

Yet another approach is to try to name the emotions your patient might be having. If you do so correctly, you will enhance your image as an empathetic, perceptive interviewer who can be trusted with secrets. You will maximize your chances of success if you name several possible emotions, as in this example:

"I can see you are having a real problem with that question. Sometimes people have trouble with questions when they feel ashamed. Or sometimes it's anxiety or fear. Are you having any of those feelings now?"

Although you have now asked something that is different from your original question, the two are related. Your patient may be able to respond more readily to the second one.

You want to reinforce in your patient the habit of responding to you, and even a nod is better than nothing at all. Once you have obtained any response, even a silent shrug or frown, you can often parlay it into a renewal of speech.

INTERVIEWER: You must be feeling pretty upset about this. Am I right?

PATIENT: *(Nods.)*

INTERVIEWER: I think maybe we should move on and talk about your education instead. Does that seem like a good idea to you?

PATIENT: *(Nods.)*

INTERVIEWER: Is that something you think you can talk about?

PATIENT: Yes . . . I think so.

INTERVIEWER: That other subject is pretty important, but this clearly isn't the time to talk about it. We'll come back to it later.

Delaying the discussion of difficult material, as in the example just given, is probably one of the most often used methods of dealing with moderate to severe resistance. The technique sacrifices information for the sake of rapport and the integrity of the interview, so you should use it sparingly. It is important for the patient to understand that the matter isn't closed, only postponed.

An answer of "I don't know" gives you no more information than does dead silence; if repeated often, it can cause an interview to grind to a halt. Occasionally, you might succeed in getting the patient off dead center by responding:

"Well, what do you *think* about it?"

Unfortunately, often this only elicits the obvious (and maddening) rejoinder, "I don't know."

If you're not getting much information anyway, you won't take a big risk by forcing a rare confrontation. You may get some clues as to the reason for the resistance. In this example the patient confronted is Julie, a 16-year-old girl:

INTERVIEWER: *(Leans forward and smiles.)* Several times when you've said, "I don't know," it's been about questions that I think you know the answer to. What do you think might happen if you didn't hold back?

JULIE: I don't know.

INTERVIEWER: A lot of kids don't like to talk because they're upset about something. Have you been feeling upset?

JULIE: Maybe.

INTERVIEWER: *(Smiles.)* Maybe we should try to understand that. What were you feeling just a moment ago?

JULIE: My dumb mother made me come. *(Pauses.)*

INTERVIEWER: So it was your mom's idea to come?

This example demonstrates confrontation and naming of feelings, which we have already mentioned. It also suggests several other techniques that can help break through resistance:

• Focus on describing the symptoms; just for now, don't worry about what they might mean.

• Switch from facts to feelings. Resistance usually has an emotional basis. This interviewer recognized that feelings had to be explored before getting on with the history taking.

• Emphasize the normal. Patients sometimes conclude that they must be pretty bizarre, just to be under the care of a mental health clinician. Julie may have felt better once she learned that her interviewer had encountered this behavior before and didn't find it strange.

• Reject the behavior; accept the person. By leaning forward and using warm words and tone of voice, the interviewer clearly indicated both (1) unconditional acceptance of the patient as a person and (2) the desirability of a different response.

• Use verbal and nonverbal encouragements. Once the patient began to speak, the interviewer encouraged further efforts by a smile and making a suggestion that took off from her "Maybe." Praise the patient for giving a response. Other encouragements (nods, paraphrasing) have been discussed in Chapter 4.

• Focus on the patient's interests. As soon as it became clear that this patient was angry about being forced to come, the interviewer shifted the focus to her relationship with her mother. Subsequently, the session became much more productive.

• Still another technique is to look for a less affect-laden model of the behavior or feelings in question, and discuss the model first. Often this is a similar episode that happened to the patient long ago, but it could be one that affected a friend or relative. Here's how the process works:

INTERVIEWER: Have you been feeling so bad you've thought about harming yourself?

PATIENT: I—I can't say.

INTERVIEWER: It's a pretty upsetting subject, isn't it?

PATIENT: *(Nods.)*

INTERVIEWER: Didn't you say you made a suicide attempt several years ago?

PATIENT: Yes. *(Long pause)*

INTERVIEWER: What happened then?

PATIENT: I overdosed on my wife's heart tablets. But I threw them all up.

INTERVIEWER: You must have been feeling pretty desperate.

PATIENT: *(Nods.)*

INTERVIEWER: Are you feeling that way now?

PATIENT: I guess so. But I don't like to talk about it. It scares my wife.

With variations, this technique can sometimes ease you into a fruitful discussion after a more direct approach has failed. But if the only result is more resistance, you should probably change topics completely—as long as the delay doesn't pose possible danger to the patient.

Sometimes patients will spontaneously fall into this technique of changing to a less affect-laden model. When that happens, hear out the past example, then ask:

"Can you see any connection between what happened then and the way you have been behaving just recently?"

Most patients will see the point. For those who do not, you can gently draw the comparison yourself.

Tardiness

With only one interview in your sample, you don't know whether lateness is going to be a chronic problem. If the patient is late to the first interview, and if you have the next time slot available, it wouldn't be amiss to run long and complete your evaluation. If not, your best option is to say, "Let's make the best use of the time we have," and get right to work.

But the patient who is often late to appointments is the bane of many a mental health practice. If it only happened once or twice, you could perhaps ignore it. Some people are habitually late everywhere, but it isn't especially useful to accept that as a reason; chronic tardiness gets in the way of more than just mental health care. I don't recommend giving additional time to someone who is always late—it sends the message that it's OK not to fulfill personal obligations, and it's unfair to the patient who has the next appointment. Here is behavior you have to deal with as resistance.

First, make sure the patient doesn't think that you are offended. And you shouldn't be: It isn't about you; it's about your patient's problem (perhaps the very one that prompted treatment in the first place). Rather, your words and your demeanor should say, "I'm concerned that you aren't getting the help you need." Invite the patient to explore with you the possible reasons—"What are you afraid might come up during our session?"—but then focus your efforts on correcting the behavior. "What can you think of to help get yourself here on time?" You'll probably find yourself discussing the use of alarm clocks, postcards, and, nowadays, reminders the patient can get from dozens of free Internet reminder services.

Special Techniques

Several other interview techniques are sometimes useful in countering resistance. For the most part, these strategies apply in specific situations or to particular types of patients. Novice interviewers will rarely use these specialized techniques.

• Offer an excuse for unfavorable information. By helping out with plausible reasons, you may encourage your patient to be frank about embarrassing or distressing problems.

INTERVIEWER: How much have you been drinking just recently?

PATIENT: Not much. I really don't keep track.

INTERVIEWER: What with all the stress surrounding your husband's death, I thought you might have started drinking heavily again, like what happened several years ago when your mother died.

PATIENT: You're right. I've been so overwhelmed. If I didn't have three or four doubles every evening, I wouldn't be able to get to sleep at all.

• Exaggerate negative consequences that *didn't* happen. By emphasizing the worst possible outcome of a behavior, you diminish the patient's anxiety about what actually did happen.

INTERVIEWER: During that fight, did you really hurt your wife?

PATIENT: Well . . . (*Silence*)

INTERVIEWER: Well, did you kill her?

PATIENT: Nah, I just knocked her around a little bit.

• Induce your patient to brag. Rarely, a patient withholds information about an exploit but seems secretly proud of it. Some interviewers try to encourage frankness by subtly implying admiration for some aspect of the behavior in question.

INTERVIEWER: How much were you drinking then?

PATIENT: Gee, that's hard to say.

INTERVIEWER: You're a pretty good-sized man. You look like you could really put it away.

PATIENT: I've hoisted a few in my day.

INTERVIEWER: I'll bet you could drink them all under the table!

PATIENT: Yeah, I suppose I've won my share of chug-a-lug contests.

This technique can build rapport while it obtains information. Although it is probably innocuous enough when applied to substance misuse, I worry that it might send a message of approval to a patient with personality disorder whose activities include sexual misconduct, fighting, or criminal behavior. If you ever use this technique, be careful not to condone or encourage the behavior itself.

PREVENTION

As with any other problem, no remedy for resistance is as satisfactory as preventing it in the first place. The following strategies should help you avoid having to use the more devious techniques we have just discussed.

• If you can obtain information before the interview begins about your patient's character or style of interacting, you may be better able to modify your approach to difficult topics. Resources include word-of-mouth information from referring clinicians and records from previous hospitalizations.
• Sometimes you can tell right away that your patient is reluctant to talk. A scowl, a sigh, or an upturned gaze may tip you off, even before you begin to speak. If so, perhaps this is the time to break my Chapter 1 rule and start with small talk. A few moments of conversation about some thing you share (the weather or sporting interests)

might help identify you as "friendly" and reduce your patient's antago-
nism. The purpose of small talk—to grease the skids for productive
conversation with a potentially difficult patient—suggests two warnings: (1) Politics and religion are never "small" topics; avoid them like a
dirty needle. (2) For any subject, avoid taking a position that might be
considered strong or controversial. It could throw you into confrontation that your already challenging interview hardly needs.

• Carefully monitor your reactions to the information you obtain.
If your speech or facial expression hints of surprise or disapproval, you
may seriously damage rapport and limit both the quantity and quality
of your information.

• Answer questions as completely and honestly as you can. This is
the obvious approach to take with any patient, but your open, careful
discussions of your intentions and the possible benefits of cooperation
might especially help reduce the suspicions of someone who is paranoid or even psychotic.

• Individualize your history-taking technique. Some patients simply won't be hurried. They aren't psychotic or demented; they simply
have to tell their stories in their own way. When you encounter such a
patient, you might as well forget about your time schedule, relax, and
enjoy the ride. You'll get your history—a little at a time—and you'll preserve rapport.

• Preface your mental status exam questions about delusions, hallucinations, and orientation with the remark that these "routine questions" are part of your usual thorough evaluation. This should help to
defuse any concern that you suspect your patient of being mentally
slow or psychotic.

• If you encounter psychotic material such as delusions or hallucinations, don't argue. You won't win points by refuting what your patient "knows" to be true. But neither should you agree with something
you know is false: You don't want to reinforce the psychosis. Instead,
ask how long the patient has felt that way, or emphasize your concern
for the accompanying discomfort. For example, the patient may be
frightened by the content of the hallucination.

YOUR ATTITUDE

As we have noted before, with all patients it is important to understand
your own feelings. If you find yourself feeling bored, angry, or disgusted, ask yourself, "Why?" Is there someone this patient reminds you
of, such as a supervisor, parent, or spouse? (When therapists' feelings
toward patients are carried over from their own relationships, this is

called *countertransference.*) Perhaps there are features of this patient's personality that remind you of some of your own less admirable traits. Do you have anxiety about your own health, marriage, or family? These feelings are ubiquitous, so even experienced therapists must take care that they do not intrude into their relationships with patients.

A patient who is uncooperative or difficult in other ways creates a special challenge. As a clinician, you must not let passive–aggressive behavior, sarcasm, or anger precipitate an outburst from you. Such negative affect, especially when it comes early in the relationship, can imperil an interview and seriously damage future rapport. If you find yourself feeling uncomfortable during an interview, ask yourself:

"Why should I be feeling so upset?"

"What message am I missing?"

"Whom does this patient remind me of?"

The answers to these questions should help determine what corrective action to take.

Chapter 17

Special or Challenging Patient Behaviors and Issues

All patients are special, and each is unique. But the behaviors of some can be especially challenging: They may be vague, hostile, untruthful, confused, or even violent. And certain other characteristics of patients besides behaviors may require particular attention as well. Such behaviors and issues offer us the opportunity to hone our skills of accommodation and persuasion, and to practice the virtues of patience and tolerance.

VAGUENESS

Instead of information, a patient may give you only empty words. Here are a few examples:

The unfocused chief complaint. A variety of concerns may be stated, but none of them seems an adequate reason for seeking treatment.

Overgeneralizations. A single episode of illness may be treated as typical when it is not; one example of a friend's behavior is labeled as "usual." The words *always* and *never* may tip you off to overgeneralization.

Approximate answers. Often this means that the patient gives you adjectives when you want numbers.

> INTERVIEWER: How long have you been drinking?
>
> PATIENT: A long time.
>
> INTERVIEWER: Can you give me an idea of how long?
>
> PATIENT: Well, quite a while.

Sometimes a patient simply seems unable to give precise descriptors.

INTERVIEWER: How did you feel when your stepdaughter arrived for that long visit?

PATIENT: Lousy.

INTERVIEWER: Well, can you describe your feelings then?

PATIENT: I felt terrible.

Dealing with Vagueness

Try first to determine why the patient is being vague. Sometimes it may be a function of the particular mental disorder: Vague speech is especially characteristic of patients who have mental retardation, psychosis, or personality disorders. You could also encounter it in almost anyone who is unaccustomed to thinking in precise terms. Perhaps this is the first time your patient has tried to express troubling feelings. It may also indicate resistance to the interview—does this person have something to hide?

As you might imagine, it won't be helpful to accuse the patient of being "unclear." If you have to label the behavior, try "overgeneralizing." You can ask, "Help me to understand." You can also deal with vagueness by providing structure: Indicate clearly what type of answer or degree of precision you expect.

INTERVIEWER: How much time did you serve in the penitentiary?

PATIENT: Oh, quite a while.

INTERVIEWER: How long was that in months or years?

To the patient who persists in using general descriptions such as *terrible*, you might respond:
"What is your interpretation of *terrible*?"
"Could you give me an example of what you mean by *terrible*?"
You may have to pin down some patients with specific questions, perhaps based on the areas of clinical interest (see Chapter 13) or on what you know about specific mental disorders.

INTERVIEWER: What do you mean by *terrible*?

PATIENT: I don't know. I just felt bad.

INTERVIEWER: Can you give me an example?

PATIENT: *(Pauses.)* Just really awful.

INTERVIEWER: Well, were you depressed?

PATIENT: Sometimes.

INTERVIEWER: Did you feel anxiety?

PATIENT: Yeah, that's it! I was wound up like a clock!

Whatever technique you use, once you have clarified your patient's meaning, summarize to be sure you have understood:

"So when you said you felt 'terrible' when your stepdaughter arrived for a visit, you were a little depressed, but mainly you felt this sense of overwhelming anxiety."

It may require a lot of prompting to teach the habit of precision to a patient who prefers approximate answers. You could find yourself resorting to multiple-choice questions. Early in the interview, the unfocused, rambling patient may require you to use focused, short-answer questions. If the vagueness persists despite your best efforts, suspect some source of underlying resistance. To explore the reasons for this resistance, you might have to risk a confrontation. Try:

"In order to help you, I really need a more definitive answer. Is there some reason you are having trouble answering my questions?"

Inability to Generalize

A problem related to vagueness is that some patients cannot generalize experiences. When you ask them to give you a broad picture, they respond with specific examples and tiny vignettes.

You can try to deal with this by redefining what it is you are after. Using words like *common*, *often*, and *usually* may help you teach your patient what you want.

INTERVIEWER: Do you have a lot of trouble dealing with anger?

PATIENT: Last week I got really burned at my mother-in-law, threw a fit.

INTERVIEWER: Here's what I'd like to know: Is this pretty common for you?

If your patient cannot generalize, you may have to make do with several examples from which you distill the generalization yourself. Then summarize aloud to make sure that you've got it right.

LYING

As a part of the therapeutic contract, the patient agrees to tell the truth. At the beginning of your relationship with any patient, you should assume that this will be the case. Unfortunately, for a variety of reasons, it doesn't always turn out this way.

Patients may lie when they are frightened, ashamed, worried, or angry. To a degree, these emotions probably apply to most people who seek the help of mental health professionals. Other patients may lie for social gain: to get or keep a job, to avoid punishment, or to feel more respected. Those who habitually lie without discernible cause, popularly termed "pathological liars," probably constitute a small minority.

A variety of clues could warn you that your patient might not be telling the truth:

• The history is inconsistent with the known course of the disorder you suspect. For example, your patient denies ever being hospitalized, despite a long history of severe manic symptoms.

• You ask about any behavior that would make most people feel ashamed or guilty. Common examples include drug use, sexual issues, suicidal behavior, and violence—any of which could provide an incentive for shading the truth.

• The patient tells a story that is internally inconsistent; for example, someone who never passed eighth grade claims to have held high-level executive positions.

• You notice some of the behaviors that have been associated with lying. These can include shifting gaze with poor eye contact, yawning, stammering, sweating, hyperventilating, motor restlessness, flushing, raised vocal pitch, rapid speech, and a delay in answering to sort out the impression the patient wants to give. Because any of these behaviors can have other causes, you shouldn't leap to conclusions. Rather, try to confirm your suspicions with information from other sources.

• You suspect a severe personality disorder. A childhood history of delinquency progressing to adult criminality would make you suspect antisocial personality disorder. These patients often display little regard for the truth.

• Despite ample opportunity and objective justification, your patient denies all negative personal attributes. For example:

An embittered 40-year-old woman is a college graduate stuck in a dull secretarial position. Her life has apparently been loveless and friendless. But when you ask her what she would change about herself if she had it to do over again, she replies, "Nothing."

• Your patient seems to exaggerate lifetime accomplishments.

Dealing with Lying

As with other forms of problematic behavior, dealing with suspected lying requires a delicate touch. You need accurate information to make a diagnosis, but open confrontation risks early rupture of the relationship. (In ongoing therapy, you would eventually have to deal with the need for trust in your relationship. Although treatment is not the principal goal of the initial interview, neither do you want to say anything that will impede your later ability to work constructively with your patient.)

Before settling on any course of action, it is often worthwhile to ask for a restatement of what your patient just said:

"Could you run that by me again?"

Perhaps you misunderstood; perhaps the patient misspoke; but added details could clarify the issue. Another obvious approach is to ignore the lie and seek the truth elsewhere—from records or informants, for example. You may be able to arrive at the truth by piecing together a careful, year-by-year history of work, education, and social activities. Although it takes time, I've always found life history detective work to be interesting and rewarding.

Should you conclude that a confrontation over the issue of misinformation is warranted, formulate your questions in a way that avoids making accusations. Couch them in terms of resolving a misunderstanding or clearing up your own confusion:

"Something puzzles me. You just said that you hadn't had any problems with drinking, but your health care record here mentions two emergency room visits in the past year for intoxication. Can you help me out with that?"

To someone whose response indicates a willingness to fight ("You calling me a liar?"), you can answer that your problem isn't with the patient but with the story:

"Help me to understand some of the contradictions."

Something of the same approach—a gentle request to help you understand—may help you cope with the related behaviors of exaggerating and minimizing symptoms.

HOSTILITY

Of all the problem behaviors, hostility—anger directed toward someone—is usually the easiest to spot. The patient's feelings are clearly shown in a scowl, clenched fist, angry tone of voice, or sarcastic content of speech. Even those patients who resolutely smile despite their negative emotions may betray these underlying feelings by a set jaw or by tension in the voice. Whatever its manifestations, hostility must be dealt with immediately and effectively. To do less jeopardizes your entire interview.

The possible causes of hostility are numerous. Here are a few, some of which have already been mentioned as causing other problem behaviors:

Fear of illness. These patients reject the notion that they are ill by rejecting their need for a caregiver.

Displaced emotion. Perhaps it isn't you or the present situation, but a boss, spouse, or previous mental health professional, that lies behind the hostility. You become the innocent target of negative transference.

Fear of intimacy. This reason may be especially relevant in a mental health interview, where hostility could serve to "protect" the patient from making unwanted revelations.

Fear of dependence. Some patients resent having to seek help for any problem. For them, hostility may be a mechanism for keeping a safe distance from people they view as wielding power. Perhaps this stems from previous experiences of being socially "one-down."

Habit. Whatever the initial cause, some people have become habitually aggressive and hostile in their social interactions. They may have learned this as a way of maintaining control over others.

Apparent lack of interviewer empathy. In addition to the foregoing "patient-centered" causes, consider the effect of an interviewer who appears uninvolved or uninterested. Most mental health patients already bear a considerable burden of negative emotions. If they must also cope with someone who is supposed to behave therapeutically, yet doesn't come across as empathic, the natural reaction might well be added hostility.

Negative emotions usually make their owners feel uncomfortable; hostility makes friends and acquaintances feel that way as well. Because this reactive discomfort also applies to mental health interviewers, your first impulse may be to change the subject quickly. That strategy could succeed if the problem is anger or resentment stirred up by your line of questioning. But true hostility tends to be generalized more than anger; you're unlikely to deal with it successfully by ignoring it.

Handling Hostility

Any evidence of hostility warns you that before continuing, you must confront your patient's feelings. To advance your interview effectively, you must make your confrontation nonthreatening and nonjudgmental. Here's how you might accomplish it:

INTERVIEWER: Why did you come here?

PATIENT [a tall, heavy-set, 28-year-old man]: Why was I brought here, you mean. And why should I tell you? You're the third one I've talked with this afternoon!

INTERVIEWER: I'll bet you're getting sick of talking about it. I don't blame you.

PATIENT: You don't blame me; you just bug me.

INTERVIEWER: I don't mean to bother you. I can see that anyone as upset as you are must have a lot on his mind.

PATIENT: You've got that right.

INTERVIEWER: What is it? It must be pretty awful to get you this stirred up.

PATIENT: It's that, all right. *(Pauses.)* My wife left me.

Although this patient's angry words were directed toward the interviewer, the underlying reason for the hostility was much more personal. By excusing the behavior and sympathizing with the feelings, the interviewer could side with the patient and break through to the core of his hostility. Responding to the fear behind the hostility is often an excellent counter to hostility. Notice how this interviewer also drew the patient away from invective and into conversation by requesting details.

Different reactions from the interviewer would probably only have produced additional negative feelings:

"Look, I'm only trying to help you." (Guilt)

"If you don't talk about it, you'll never get over it." (Anxiety)

"Don't bark at me! I haven't done anything to you." (More hostility)

This last response brings up a point that we sometimes forget. Hostility is contagious; if you aren't wary, it can infect you. However natural a sharp retort from you might seem under the circumstances, it could ruin your interview—perhaps the outcome your patient was trying to provoke all along. It may help you maintain your composure if you remember that you have known your patient too short a time to have provoked any personal animosity. Any verbal attack must therefore be the product of your patient's own problems.

If you are talking to a voluntary patient who demands to leave, it is possible that you will never complete the interview. But if your patient is being held involuntarily on a closed hospital ward, time will be on your side.

A 20-year-old man was admitted against his will. In the following dialogue, notice how the interviewer didn't argue, but instead agreed with the patient's every statement, giving each request a twist that required the patient's cooperation:

> PATIENT: Look, I don't want to talk to you or any other shrink. Just get me the hell out of here!
>
> INTERVIEWER: That's what I'm trying to do. My job is to help you get out of here. But the law says that I can't let you go until I've decided it's safe. And I . . .
>
> PATIENT: Don't give me any of that crap. I want out of here now!
>
> INTERVIEWER: *(Gets up to leave.)* I'll be glad to start working on it as soon as I get the information I need from you.
>
> PATIENT: You mean I've got to stay here all night?
>
> INTERVIEWER: *(Moves toward the door.)* Well, it could be several days.
>
> PATIENT: Wait a minute! You can't just leave me here!
>
> INTERVIEWER: I'll be glad to come back when you're ready to talk.
>
> PATIENT: I'm going to sue you for every nickel you've got!
>
> INTERVIEWER: We'll help you get legal representation tomorrow. But it would be quicker if you'd just decide to cooperate.

This interviewer left the room but returned 20 minutes later at the request of the patient, who subsequently did cooperate fully—and was released a few hours later. The confrontation was defused when the interviewer adopted an attitude of being on the same side as the patient, who could only get what he wanted with a change in behavior.

Defusing hostility can be a supreme test of any interviewer's professionalism. To pass it, you must continually monitor your own feelings and respond in ways that address your patient's emotional needs, not your own.

POTENTIAL VIOLENCE

Patients are only infrequently hostile to the point of violence. Although it's uncommon that a mental health worker is severely injured by a patient, most of us have been shaken up or struck at least once during our careers. At best, this is an unsettling experience—one that we must keep alert to prevent.

Unfortunately, predicting who will become violent is pretty hard. Although the vast majority of seriously mentally ill patients present no danger to others whatsoever, they do account for about 5% of homicides in the United States. In addition to psychoses due to schizophrenia and mood disorders, you could encounter violence in those with cognitive disorders, personality disorders (especially antisocial personality disorder), and acute substance intoxication. You should be especially vigilant when you are interviewing either a male or a female who has any of these diagnoses.

Regardless of diagnosis, an actuarial approach uses the presence or absence of several factors to help predict who will become violent. These factors include relative youth, previous history of violence, a history of being physically abused in childhood, and command hallucinations that order the person to commit violent acts (other sorts of hallucinations do not predict violence). When any of these factors obtains for a given patient, I tend to be extra vigilant.

During any interview, keep in mind several safety principles. They apply to anyone but are especially relevant for female interviewers, whom some patients will treat as vulnerable targets. Remember that no one cares as much about your safety as you do. Here are some of the preventive measures you should adopt:

- Review any documentation before you interview your new patient. Be especially wary of those with a history of past violence or who seem to have a condition that suggests poor impulse control. Again, psychosis, current intoxication, and antisocial behavior are obvious candidates.
- Ideally, an interview room in a mental health emergency facility will have two doors, both of which open outward. Even if this is not the case, arrange the seating in any office you use so that the patient is never between you and your escape route.
- When you are meeting a new patient for the first time, try to have a security guard available, especially if it is late at night and there are few other people around.
- Many clinics have panic buttons installed under the desktops in their offices. If your setting is one of those, be sure to familiarize yourself with its workings and the expected response.
- In doubtful circumstances, leaving the door to the interview room open will also provide you a sense of security and give the patient an added reason for restraint.
- Watch carefully for these signs of heightened tension: clenched fists, loud or quavering voice, angry words, narrowed gaze, or sudden bursts of activity.
- If your patient becomes agitated or otherwise intimidating, remain calm. "Please, just take your seat," you might say quietly. Although some situations can only be met with a show of force, evidence

of your own quiet competence may keep the lid on a cauldron threatening to boil.

You must be prepared to cope with potential harm to person or property. Some people get through life by bullying others; often their threats work without their ever having to follow through on them, but it is hard to know in advance just who will carry out a threat of bodily harm, or in what circumstances. It is therefore vital to have a three-part plan:

1. With the principles listed just above and the strength of a backup force, ensure your own safety and that of those around you.
2. Maintain your composure as you inform the patient about the consequences of further threats or actual acting-out behavior.
3. Be fully prepared to follow through with the limits you've set, should the need arise.

Suppose that despite your best efforts at forming rapport, your patient displays evidence of unremitting hostility. Then you may have to break off the interview, but try to do it in such a way that you preserve some basis for a future relationship. You might say something along these lines:

"I'm sorry. I'd really like to work with you, but right now you seem to be pretty upset. Perhaps we can get together again later."

Then leave the room quickly and notify the security staff. Remember that it is nobody's job to face single-handedly a hostile, possibly violent patient. It is trite but true that there is security in numbers, and it is always your responsibility as a mental health clinician to promote safety—your patients', your coworkers', and your own.

CONFUSION

Patients with confusion resulting from dementia or delirium present an unusually vexing challenge to the interviewer. They may think and speak slowly, mix up the chronology of events, forget important facts, or have difficulty following your instructions. Their own frustration with their poor performance sometimes precipitates hostility. Because the data you obtain from them are too few and too unreliable, it is hard to make a valid diagnosis. Sometimes you will conclude your interview with little to show for your efforts.

The best solution to this frustrating experience is prevention. Before the interview, obtain all the information you can from collateral sources (such as relatives, physicians, other mental health workers, and previous hospital records). According to a recent study, for some disorders such as a long-standing psychosis, medical records may provide the vast bulk of the information you need. Then you can concentrate on your thorough evaluation of the patient's mental status.

Even without collateral information, you can take several steps to facilitate your interview with a patient who is confused:

Introduce yourself slowly and distinctly. Before you begin your questions, make sure the patient understands who you are and why you are there.

Try not to rush. You're better off with a few reliable facts than a jumble of inaccuracies.

Use short sentences. Long speeches only compound the confusion.

Choose your words carefully. Jargon and slang may be especially treacherous for the confused patient.

Avoid shorthand phrases. For instance, a confused patient may take your question "Have you been hearing voices?" in its most literal sense.

Ask for repetition. If you wonder whether your question was understood, ask the patient to repeat it.

Ask about the events of a single day. If you aren't having much success with your usual questions, ask your patient to tell you about the day's activities, or about a typical day's schedule.

You may want to conduct your interview with a relative present. Especially for a patient with moderate dementia, it can increase the reliability of your information and provide support for the patient.

Don't move too quickly to the formal mental status evaluation; some patients with mild dementia may see the connection and take offense.

Keep smiling. At a time when you lack information, you don't want the appearance of irritation to rob you of rapport.

OLDER PATIENTS

Being old does not by itself constitute a disability. Too often interviewers forget this and assume that patients who are older are also confused, deaf, or feeble. Although you should always try to show appropriate concern, older patients justifiably resent being patronized, physically moved around, or shouted at. Don't let their advanced age deter you from asking questions about activities usually associated with youth. These people are old, not extinct. Many of them still enjoy sex, misuse drugs or alcohol, and even worry about caring for their own parents.

However, there are a number of special considerations to keep in mind when you interview older patients:

- You will probably need more interview time just to get through the sheer volume of material. During a lifetime that spans many decades, the average older patient has accumulated more experiences, both good and bad, than has the average younger patient. You'll especially need to allow more time for your older patient's personal and social histories. And because the mental health problems of senior citizens are more likely to be complicated by medical disorders, you'll need to spend extra time obtaining general health information.

- A stylistic change seems to take place somewhere during the seventh or eighth decade of life: Personality traits become accentuated. In addition, older patients tend to reminisce a lot—perhaps they feel better when they review happier periods of their lives. Young interviewers should try to accommodate themselves to this slower pace. Speak distinctly, allow more response time, and suggest additional interview sessions if you need them to finish gathering data.

- Older patients have some unique problems that young interviewers may have difficulty relating to. Trying to fill many leisure hours is an example of a problem with which many young clinicians have had no personal experience; the stress of a fixed, reduced income may be another. Even such ordinary activities as meal preparation and arranging for transportation can burden someone who has become isolated or withdrawn.

- Watch out for instances of elder abuse. This problem—which can include neglect, exploitation, and rights violations, as well as physical and psychological abuse—probably affects more than a million people over the age of 65 each year. It is especially likely to occur when an older person has recently become more dependent on a caregiver, who is often the one who does the abusing. You can screen for instances of elder abuse by asking the following questions:

"Are you afraid of anyone at home?"
"Has anyone at home ever harmed you?"
"Has anyone made you do things you didn't want to do?"

Abuse should be reported to the appropriate adult protective service for your state. In some states, failure of health care practitioners to report the physical abuse of older patients is a misdemeanor punishable by a fine or jail term.

• Older patients have suffered a variety of losses, which multiply with the passing years. These include loss of health, job, income, status, friends, and family members. Children have moved away; homes of many years have been sold when the owners move to retirement communities. Perhaps there is no telephone, producing loss of contact with others. Each of these losses demands special sensitivity. That means not only being sympathetic, but also keeping alert to the possibility of denial. Some patients will have difficulty admitting, even to themselves, the waning of their capabilities and prospects. The result may be overgeneralization or vagueness that you must counter with careful requests for more complete information. Here is an example:

INTERVIEWER: How often do you see members of your family?

PATIENT: Oh, pretty often.

INTERVIEWER: For example, when did you last see your son? I understand he lives just across town.

PATIENT: Well, it's been about 6 months, actually.

OTHER ISSUES AND BEHAVIORS

A variety of situations, attitudes, and behaviors can affect the success of your initial interview. Although you probably won't often encounter these characteristics, your response to them can modify their effect on your interview. My overall approach is to regard any issue or behavior that threatens to come between me and the patient as a problem that we should face together. In effect, I frame the issue so that the problem is on one side, confronted on the other side by the patient and me, working as a team.

Patient Demands

Whether due to narcissism or some other issue—anxiety about loss of status, anger at a spouse or boss, or the accustomed status of a VIP—some patients feel they should have special treatment. This can take the form of demanding a different room, the ability to smoke or eat, the privilege of taking notes on (or recording) the interview, or a special time for the appointment. Such patient demands can go against the grain, and clinicians may feel the urge to push back. Here is a place where I try to evaluate the individual situation. Where I can, I will make accommodations to increase the patient's level of comfort, so long as I don't feel that this will lead to a spiraling sense of entitlement.

> Rodney brought a tape recorder to his initial interview, so he could include excerpts in a biography he was writing. His clinician explained that he did not record interviews, because it could lead to discomfort and possibly loss of information. Rodney put away the tape recorder, and the interview unfolded normally.

> Elaine asked if she could take notes during her initial interview. She said that one of her concerns was that she couldn't remember things as well as she used to; she was afraid that she would forget some vital concept that was being discussed. Her clinician said it would be OK, as long as she kept note taking to a minimum. By the end of the hour, she had accumulated only a few lines of notes, and her clinician had a good grasp of her emotional issues.

You would apply similar, rational approaches to patients demanding VIP treatment. Whereas you may acknowledge their special status, you should also emphasize that the opinion they will get from you will be every bit as honest and thoughtful as for any regular patient.

Blindness

Blind patients can communicate just as well as people who can see. What they can't do is read the body language clinicians normally use to help convey concern and directions. With blind patients, you will have to use your tone of voice to indicate that you care, and take extra pains to put into words what you want them to do. If you get up or change positions, describe your movements. This will help answer questions before they are asked and tell these patients that you are a considerate interviewer who is sensitive to special needs.

Deafness

Most deaf patients will communicate quite well if you speak distinctly and slowly, while looking right at them (this facilitates lip reading). Don't hide your mouth behind your hand or a piece of paper. Of course, you wouldn't ordinarily smoke, eat, or drink anything during any interview, but here is one more reason not to. In addition, don't shout: Most patients with a significant hearing impairment use hearing aids, and loud noises only distort the sound. Whether or not they have any residual hearing at all, it is vital not to talk down to them; they may be deaf, but they are not children.

Also keep in mind that many hearing-impaired people bridle at the medical model of deafness, which implies that they suffer from pathology. These people adhere with pride to the cultural definition of deafness—that is, a community bringing people together through a common physical characteristic and a common language (sign). You should ascertain which point of view your patient holds; many culturally deaf persons vigorously deny that they have a disability at all, and may bitterly resent any implication to the contrary. You could ask for information this way: "I understand that many people regard their deafness as a cultural issue. Is this something you can tell me about?"

A Background That Is Different from Yours

As a general approach, asking a patient to teach you about issues of custom, ethnicity, language, and ritual has much to recommend it as a way both to gain information and to solidify rapport. It shows how much you are interested in the patient, who will also benefit from a sense of enhanced competence and worth. If the patient is foreign-born, find out early how recently the patient came to this country (it may help you avoid giving the impression that the answers you hear to questions are somehow deficient).

If you must communicate through an interpreter, be sure to look at the patient when speaking. As you would with a deaf patient who communicates through sign language with a hearing person, don't say, "Ask him if he . . . " Rather, ask the patient directly, and then let the translator speak.

Crying

Beginners sometimes worry that they'll have trouble coping if a patient cries. To be sure, tears can slow things down for a while, but in the long run they may even facilitate the flow of information about emotions. A quick touch on the arm (one of the few times I recommend physical contact other than a handshake between patient and therapist) lets the patient know of your concern. Offering a fresh facial tissue serves the same purpose. A few moments of silence may be enough to allow the patient to regain composure with dignity. If the patient cannot see your concern (because of crying), be sure to voice it:

"I can see this upsets you. Would you like to have a couple of minutes to collect yourself?"

Humor

Jokes can go a long way toward reducing tension, but patients will sometimes shroud their concerns in humor. This may be a way of conveying a concern in such a way that the clinician won't give it serious (and therefore potentially threatening) consideration. In any case, listen carefully when your patient treats sensitive material with a light touch: There may be more cause for concern than is first apparent.

Excessive Talking or Rambling

Some patients can be remarkably circumstantial. Left to their own devices, they will tell you far more than you want to know. Sometimes, especially if your patient isn't usually overtalkative, this could be an attempt to avoid confronting unacceptable feelings or revealing sensitive material, but much of the time it's just habit. Although circumstantial speech is not usually pathological, it carries with it too much chaff for the amount of wheat it provides. Rapport may also suffer when you endure talking that has no purpose, so you should probably intervene if your patient rambles. To attempt a graceful transition, try to let your intervention take off from something your patient has said. For example, in response to a question about drug usage, this patient spent several minutes discussing the drinking habits of a cousin:

> PATIENT: . . . So I don't think I've ever seen her after 6 P.M. when she wasn't in the bag. Another thing . . .
>
> INTERVIEWER: *(Interrupting)* But what about *your* drinking?

This clinician had to intervene and restate the desired responses several times before the patient could finally stick to the point.

Patients who are overtalkative seem to dominate an interview, even if they don't intend to. (Those with mania are notorious in this respect.) You may be able to handle irrelevant comments by only smiling an acknowledgment as you continue with your line of questioning. A more explicit gesture, such as a finger to your lips, may help even a boisterously manic patient talk less. Sometimes you may have to set firm limits, perhaps in the form of a direct confrontation:

"You have a lot to say that is very interesting. But our time is short, and we still have a lot of work to do. Let's try hard to stick to the subject."

"These details are interesting, but our first job should be to understand the broad outline."

Suppose the patient harps on one theme, even when you try to change the subject: You'll need to reevaluate the importance of this theme to the patient. Confrontation is the most direct method, but it should be phrased diplomatically:

"It seems to me that the subject of sex is difficult for you. Am I right?"

"We seem to be stuck on the issue of your son's accident. What else about it is important to you?"

For a patient who is extremely garrulous, you may be forced to ask only yes–no questions and to resist vigorously any attempt at amplification.

Somatic Concerns

Some patients, even those who do *not* have somatization disorder, firmly believe that their symptoms are physical in nature. Despite what their physicians have told them, they cling to the idea that their problems can be solved by drugs or surgery. There is little value in explaining the probable emotional origin of these complaints: Even after repeated failures, such a patient may continue to search for medicines and operations that will produce relief. Without arguing—one of your goals, remember, is to become the patient's ally—you can point out that physical approaches haven't helped (not enough, at any rate), and that talking about the patient's feelings may relieve some of the anxiety that inevitably accompanies illness. Also, you'll want to work with the patient's medical care provider to ensure that neither physical nor emotional/behavioral issues are overlooked.

Psychosis

In emergency rooms and admitting wards of hospitals, you will often encounter patients with such severe psychosis that they cannot communicate well. Their thinking is tangential or otherwise disordered, and the connections they make between ideas are so illogical that you cannot make much sense of them. You should certainly ask such patients to try to explain their thinking, but the answers may be of interest more for the psychopathology they show than for any historical information they contain. For history that is accurate and relevant, rely on informants or a chart from a previous admission. You should also ask the patients later, after the psychosis has abated.

When talking with someone who is extremely psychotic, you can focus on behaviors and feelings without buying into the patient's suspicions or convictions:

"I can understand how frightening it would be to feel you were being followed—can you tell me what went through your mind at the time?"

You can also offer reassurance that you believe the patient is being truthful in reporting experiences just as perceived:

"I know you've done your best to tell me exactly what happened. I wonder if there is any other possible interpretation as to the cause."

Other patients may not have psychosis, but may lack insight into being ill because of a severe character disorder (such as antisocial personality); still others may be in denial about heavy substance use. Patients without insight often feel no compelling reason to be interviewed. Unless you have some leverage (legal mandate, family pressure), you probably won't obtain much in the way of useful information from them.

Muteness

Like deafness, blindness, and other physical attributes, muteness can exist to varying degrees and can have a number of possible causes.

Neurological. A number of neurological problems can cause patients to be mute. Be sure that the patient is fully conscious and alert.

Depression. In the case of severe depression, the patient may not be completely mute, but just showing a long latency of response.

Conversion. A patient with mutism as a conversion symptom (so-called "hysterical mutism") may be able (willing) to produce a grunt or throat-clearing sound. With patience, coaxing, and praise for progress, you might eventually parlay these sounds into syllables, words, phrases, and sentences.

Psychosis. Someone with severe psychosis may heed voices that threaten reprisals for talking with real people. Head nods and shakes in answer to your "yes–no" questions may help you make this diagnosis. This same patient, given a pencil and paper, may be willing to write answers to your questions.

Gain. Could this patient have a reason to *appear* mute, either completely or partially? Motives such as avoiding punishment and achieving financial gain (insurance, workers' compensation) are the most obvious. If your patient has been overheard speaking normally with other patients or staff, this would tip you off that the muteness is voluntary—I hesitate to use the word *malingering*, because it is pejorative and hard to prove. To assess muteness, ask any friends or relatives present to leave before you continue your interview. In private, patients sometimes reveal secrets that they could never bear to share with their families. You might coax some people to talk by pointing out:

"I can get information about you from records, previous caregivers, or from friends or relatives. But I thought you might like to have me hear your version."

A relative paucity of speech, when it doesn't indicate actual muteness, may indicate fear, shame, confusion, lack of understanding, or perhaps a reluctance to contradict an authority figure (that's you). I'd probably try this approach:

"You seem pretty quiet in a situation where most people have a whole lot to say. I wonder if you can tell me why?"

A somewhat related difficulty is a patient's speaking extremely slowly. Often this is due to depression, in which case you have to strike a balance: Allow enough time to formulate an answer, but don't let the patient twist in the wind with a sense of helpless embarrassment. In such a case, I might ask if the patient would prefer that I ask some "yes–no" questions. Otherwise, prepare to make a long afternoon of it.

Rarely, you may encounter a patient who sits not only speechless but with a fixed facial expression—possibly one of perplexity. Later, there may be amnesia for the incident. This behavior would put me in mind of two main possibilities: some sort of seizure disorder, such as temporal lobe epilepsy, or a dissociative state. Such patients have probably had other episodes of the behavior, but these may not be accessible through an interview. Try asking:

"Do you sometimes become absorbed in your own thoughts or daydreams? If you do, can you tell me about it?"

Any such episodes require thorough investigation, perhaps with a neurological consultation. And, certainly, you should seek confirmation from informants.

Seductive Behavior and Other Inappropriate Behaviors

Seductive behavior is less likely to be a problem during the initial interview than during subsequent therapy sessions. However, the potential for seduction is always there, especially when the interviewer is male and the patient is female. (Studies have shown that the vast majority of health care workers who become involved with their patients are male, although female clinicians are by no means immune.)

If you find that seductive behavior is being directed toward you, ask yourself the usual questions: Why is this patient behaving this way? Is it a need to feel attractive? Over the years, has aggressive sexual behavior been reinforced with material or emotional rewards? The answers may be buried beneath memories too remote to uncover in a year, let alone in a single interview.

Seductive behavior may be as subtle as a sideways glance, as suggestive as provocative clothing, or as direct as a request to be held or kissed. Regardless of its form, the meaning of seductive behavior is always the same: danger for the interviewer and danger for the patient. This is because the overt message of seductive behavior ("Embrace me") is often quite different from what the patient really feels ("Help me; protect me"). If a health care professional responds literally to the request for physical contact, the patient may ultimately feel outraged and retaliate accordingly.

The best preventive approach to seductive behavior is to maintain appropriate distance. Address each patient by title and last name, and expect your patients to do the same for you. You can also discourage excessive familiarity if you stick to business and avoid discussing matters personal to you. If you are a male who does physical exams as a part of your job, be sure that a female attendant is in the room with you at all times when you are examining a female patient of any age. If you are a female examining a male, have a male attendant with you.

Other inappropriate behaviors may occasionally rear their heads—a patient's asking to use the telephone, opening books from your shelf, sitting in your chair, or bringing in lunch. Often the patient's evident diagnosis (I know, that's what you're trying to figure out) and the nature of the infraction will determine your response. For example, I'd try to redirect a patient with mania, repeatedly if needed—perhaps even using a gentle hand on the shoulder. To someone already suspected of personality disorder, I would probably request (perhaps a little sharply), "Please don't do that." In most cases, you would strive to be directive; early in your fact-finding phase with the patient is not a good time to be making interpretations.

Mental Retardation

Even without formal testing, you can often pick out the patient who is operating on the lower fringes of what is often called *general intelligence*. Research has shown that open-ended questions can lead to errors of reporting, whereas many patients will show a bias toward answering "yes–no" questions in the affirmative. It is often better to phrase your questions in a multiple-choice sort of way ("Was the voice you heard that of a stranger, or someone you know?"). Even then, it's more important than ever to check the facts with someone who knows the patient well. As you might expect, higher-functioning people with mental retardation are more reliable interviewees.

Patients with mental retardation can often communicate better about events than about feelings. They may interpret speech literally (without talking down as to a child, you'll want to speak clearly and avoid using metaphor), and tend to focus on the present (they may have relative difficulty talking about the past or future plans). You may also need to cut them some slack as regards their feelings; for a lifetime, these persons have watched siblings, schoolmates, and nearly everyone else they know enjoying more autonomy than they themselves can lay claim to. Small wonder if they have feelings of resentment that lie not too far beneath the surface—feelings that can pop out in unexpected ways. For example, a woman with mental retardation who refused to attend her younger sister's wedding was painfully aware that she herself would probably never marry.

Persons with mental retardation may also copy other gestures they have witnessed in others and bring them out at inopportune times—an attempted "high-five" at a moment of general sorrow, for example. I knew one young man who attended a game played by his favorite baseball team, though in another town in the opposing team's stadium. Becoming incensed when fans cheered wildly as his team fell behind, he stood and yelled at those around him, "Hey! What's the matter with you?"

Still another risk is that people with mental retardation may report as fact that which they themselves cannot verify. For example, a young man was thought by a clinician to be psychotic when he reported that an angel had touched him on the head and blessed him during one long winter night. He clung persistently to that belief; only with prolonged effort was it finally revealed that his mischievous roommate had originated the story. "Well, I didn't actually see it happen; that was Jeremy [his roommate] who told me," he eventually admitted. In the same vein, not all self-injury is evidence of a suicide attempt—it may be self-punishment or an attempt at controlling others.

Impending Death

Patients who expect to die soon, either immediately or in the near future, are often angry or depressed; sometimes they may deny what is happening to them. It is sad if friends and relatives begin to shun them; it is a tragedy if their therapists also refuse to talk frankly about death and the future.

Always invite a patient who is dying to verbalize feelings and reactions to this universal experience. Besides a full range of (often conflicting) emotions, you will also find a full range of everyday emotions, including fear, envy, love, hope, and joy. Such patients may have many regrets; some feel lonely. And each has a lifetime of memories and emotions that must be sorted out as carefully as if this person was going to live forever.

HOW TO RESPOND WHEN THE PATIENT ASKS . . .

Patients are forever asking questions, which is all to the good. Questions offer rich opportunities to provide reassurance, relieve anxieties, and reinforce good resolutions. Some questions also offer you a chance to put your foot in it, if you don't think carefully.

• "How do you feel about me?" This question is usually a request to be reassured that you like or accept the patient. You can give it, but try to throw in some information or instruction that might provide more substantive help. Here are two examples:

"I think you're a very nice person who is having a terrible problem with her marriage. It's going to be very important to get your husband to come in for some sessions."

"I think it took a lot of courage to sign yourself into the hospital. Now let's work together hard on that drinking problem."

• "Do you think I'm crazy?" The answer to this can be hard or easy, depending upon whether the patient has psychosis or not. If the latter, say so. If the former, try to avoid a direct confrontation (your claim that this is psychosis would probably only be rejected, anyway). Instead, you could respond with a question of your own:

"Why do you ask that?"

"Are you afraid of that?"

You could give an answer that sidesteps the question:

"I think you are clearly troubled by what has happened to you."

"You are having some unusual experiences, but we can help this."

If pushed to the wall ("Look, do you think I'm having a psychosis?"), I'll opt for the truth, but with the statement that I realize this may be hard for the patient to accept.

• "What should I do about [any concern the patient has]?" If this question can be answered simply, then do so. However, it may be a request for more help than any clinician can reasonably provide during an initial interview session. In that case, try to define what will be necessary (more information, more time) and when you might be able to provide it.

• "What's wrong with me?" (and you don't know). First of all, try not to feel insecure. No firm diagnosis can be made in about 20% of initial interviews, and even experienced clinicians are sometimes baffled initially. If you think there are some good possibilities that won't frighten or threaten the patient, state them. If you need more data, say so. A good generic response would go something like this:

"It's clear you're having a serious problem with [patient's chief complaint]. We need to get more information, so that together we can work out the best plan for you."

• "Can you help me?" The response should be some variation on "I hope so, but first we need more information . . . "

• "Why don't people like me?" Sometimes the answer seems clear to you, even on first acquaintance—the patient is self-centered, overbearing, prejudiced, hateful, or harboring a host of other attitudes and behaviors that you find off-putting. That's exactly the time not to venture an unvarnished opinion. For one thing, first impressions are often wrong; you may have sampled the behavior on an especially bad day. For another, remember your two main goals of the first interview: to get information and to form a relationship. Rather than answering the question directly, you can instead express sympathy for the unhappiness and offer hope for the future:

"I can imagine how much it would hurt to feel that way, but I don't know whether it's true or not. Together let's try to find out whether we have a real problem."

• "Have you ever experienced anything like this yourself?" Most patients are interested in their therapists' personal lives, and sometimes you may feel tempted to share something of yourself with your patient. That temptation may increase after the first few interviews, when you have come to know your patient better. Although I am not one of those who believes that a clinician should reveal nothing personal under any circumstances, I do agree that self-revelation can be fraught with difficulty, especially for the beginner. Certainly in an initial interview you will progress further and feel more comfortable if your own life and personality are not at issue. You can answer any personal question by gently redefining the purpose of the interview. At the same time, be careful to show that you are not upset that your patient has asked the question:

"A lot of patients wonder about the people who interview them. It's perfectly normal to be curious. But we should concentrate on getting the information we need to help you with your problem."

• And for any other question to which you don't know the best answer, here's a workable response that I use: "I can't tell you that right now, but here's how I plan to find out." I would then lay out my plan for a search of the Internet, discussions with colleagues, or whatever other approach seems reasonable.

Once again, the take-home point is the importance of figuring out how to work with, not against, the patient. Usually that's easy, but sometimes it requires a considerable helping of ingenuity, flexibility, and patience.

Chapter 18

Diagnosis and Recommendations

With all interviews completed, you face the task of evaluating your information. It should be organized in a form that is useful for making recommendations and for communicating with patients and other professionals. These tasks will be our concern in the final chapters of this book.

DIAGNOSIS AND DIFFERENTIAL DIAGNOSIS

Historically, some practitioners have called diagnosis "pigeonholing" and claimed that it denies the individuality of the patient. Such views now appear to have died down in favor of the majority opinion, which recognizes that diagnosis is an important guide for recommending treatment, predicting the course of illness, advising relatives, and communicating with other mental health professionals. Whether this opinion is consistent with your usual way of thinking, current mental health practice—hospital record rooms, third-party payers, and sometimes patients themselves—will often require you to make a diagnosis. Regardless of your professional discipline, it will pay you to learn to make the best diagnosis possible.

The importance of *accurate* diagnosis can hardly be overstated. At best, incorrect diagnosis will delay treatment; at worst, ineffective (or even dangerous) treatment may result. Inaccurate diagnosis also risks giving a prognosis that is either too gloomy or too optimistic for the individual patient. Planning then will suffer—planning about marriage, jobs, childbearing, buying insurance, and the myriad other tasks that mental illness can interdict.

Once made, diagnostic errors can be difficult to reverse. (That may help explain the reluctance of mental health clinicians to state a definitive diagnosis in the case of Cho Seung-Hui, the individual who shot and killed over 30 people at Virginia Tech in April 2007.) Diagnosis is passed along from one clinician to another, from one chart to the next; errors are abetted by patients and their families, who carry them along, sometimes for decades. It may be many years before a clinician with fresh perspective takes the time to review a chronic mental patient's history. Yet you can often avoid all of these difficulties if you take the utmost care to make the right diagnosis in the first place.

Accurate diagnosis usually poses few problems. Most patients clearly meet the criteria for a major diagnosis with which the majority of professionals would agree, and most do not meet criteria for other, confounding diagnoses. But about 20% of the time, the situation is less clear-cut. You may have insufficient information to make any diagnosis, or your patient may seem to meet the criteria for several diagnoses.

That is why most health care professionals state their impressions in terms of a *differential diagnosis*—a list of diagnoses that are possible and should be considered for any given patient. You should include in your differential diagnosis every disorder you consider even remotely possible. This is true all the more if you are in some doubt as to the correct diagnosis. You will have a better chance of selecting the right diagnosis if your working list is broad and inclusive.

In constructing your differential diagnosis, you should arrange all the possible diagnoses in decreasing order of likelihood, beginning with the one you consider to be most important. Sometimes called the *best diagnosis*, this is the one that most satisfactorily explains all of the historical data, signs, and symptoms of illness. Ideally, all elements of the history and the mental status examination should support your best diagnosis. Even if you believe there is only a small chance that your best diagnosis is incorrect, you should list other diagnoses to "rule out" or disprove. That list, with your reasoning behind the order in which you have placed the various possible diagnoses, is what creates the "differential."

I've provided a great deal of structure for the diagnostic process in my book *Diagnosis Made Easier.*

CHOOSING TREATMENT

Fortunately, mental health patients and their therapists today can draw upon a variety of effective biological, psychological, and social treatments. Most of these are not specific for any one diagnostic category; rather, they can be applied across a spectrum of diagnoses. Some of the available somatic and nonsomatic treatments are listed in Table 5.

TABLE 5. Outline of Mental Health Treatment Modalities

Psychological	Biological
Individual	Drugs
Cognitive-behavioral	Electroconvulsive therapy
Insight-oriented	Transcranial magnetic stimulation
Analysis	Vagus nerve stimulation
Short-term	Light therapy
Group	Psychosurgery
Disease-oriented (e.g., Alcoholics	
Anonymous, lithium clinics)	Social interventions
General medication clinics	
Family therapy	Vocational rehabilitation
General support groups	Social skills training
Behavioral	Education of family
Simple reassurance	Placement in a facility for acute,
Systematic desensitization with	intermediate, or chronic care
reciprocal inhibition	Involuntary commitment
Mass practice	Conservatorship
Ward token economies	
Thought stopping	

Note. Adapted from *Boarding Time: A Psychiatry Candidate's New Guide to Part II of the ABPN Examination* (3rd ed., p. 110) by J. Morrison and R. A. Muñoz, 2003, Washington, DC: American Psychiatric Press. Copyright 2003 by the American Psychiatric Press, Inc. Adapted by permission.

For most diagnoses, there are one or two treatments that are more effective than others. Current textbooks will spell out which treatments are most likely to help in specific diagnoses.

Let me underscore how important I feel it is to have a well-organized plan for how you will approach each patient's problems and issues. For one thing, it will help the patient understand what you think is the problem and how you are going to proceed. For another, it will help *you* keep these same issues in mind. Further, having a treatment plan that you can refer to from time to time offers you and the patient a set of benchmarks to gauge progress, or, alternatively, to help you both recognize when a different tack should be tried. Following are a number of questions to assist you in formulating a treatment plan that should help your patient:

- First, is any treatment likely to reverse the course of this disorder? Unhappily, the answer is sometimes "no." That may be the case for disorders such as the dementia of Huntington's disease. Although many such patients can be made more comfortable, and the social consequences of their symptoms can be lessened, there is no specific treatment to stay the ultimate outcome of disease. On the other hand, using one of the cholinesterase-inhibiting medications such as donepezil can slow the progression of Alzheimer's dementia—for a time. In antisocial personality disorder, a chronic disorder of character that affects perhaps 1% of young men (and far fewer young women), no treatment has yet proved superior to the passing of time.

• How certain is the diagnosis? Treatment has the greatest chance for success when it is based on clinical studies of reliably diagnosed patients. Your confidence in any treatment program will rise in proportion to the certainty that you have made the correct diagnosis. In general, treatments that are risky, complicated, expensive, and/or time-intensive should be reserved for well-diagnosed patients who have not responded to simpler measures.

What about the use of experimental treatments? Here's my rule, which you may find useful: It is acceptable to use proven treatments in uncertain diagnoses, and experimental treatments when diagnosis is certain; it is rarely acceptable to use unproven treatments when the diagnosis is uncertain.

Diagnosis is important in deciding treatment, but it is by no means the only determining factor. Some patients are so ill that treatment must be started even without a definite diagnosis. Acute psychoses provide the most frequent examples: Even while clinicians argue about bipolar I disorder versus schizophrenia, antipsychotic drugs must be started for the patient's safety and comfort. Some problems may merit intervention, even though no well-defined diagnosis is likely ever to be made. Marital discord is an example.

• How urgent is treatment? For most hospitalized patients, the answer is "urgent enough to begin at once." For outpatients, the need may be less immediate. In general, the urgency for treatment will increase under any of the following three conditions:

1. The number of symptoms is increasing. For example, the patient, who has had anxiety attacks for years, has recently also complained of depression, loss of appetite, and trouble sleeping.
2. The symptoms are getting worse. For example, in the last few days this same patient has had recurrent thoughts of suicide.
3. The symptoms lead to consequences that are more alarming. For example, for the past week this same patient has felt unable to go to work and has now resigned after 13 years with the same firm.

The three rules just cited can also help you decide which disorder to treat first, in the event that your patient has multiple concurrent diagnoses.

• How costly is the treatment? The patient's ability to pay must be considered. You wouldn't recommend prolonged psychotherapy for a self-supporting student who has no medical insurance. Someone who is fully covered by a health maintenance organization (HMO) or a private or government insurance program may be able to afford the latest in antidepressant medication, whereas a self-pay patient may request an older, generic drug.

You will probably have insurance information in hand even before you meet the patient. VA and other government facilities and HMOs set their rates in terms that patients are already familiar with. And if you are a private practitioner, your office will probably have included information about fees and other "housekeeping" matters in an initial packet of information sent to the patient in advance of the first appointment. If not, toward the end of the initial interview is an excellent time to go over this information, so as to avert unpleasant surprises down the road.

When selecting treatment, you must also consider whether the wanted effects of the treatment outweigh its unwanted effects. This warning applies especially to prescription medications: Will rapid heartbeat or wakefulness cause your patient to "forget" the evening dose? Can some other side effect result in injury or even death? What about interactions with other medications?

• Does the therapy you are considering have relative contraindications? These are problems that might make you reluctant to use a treatment, but that do not absolutely prohibit it. Common examples are drug allergy, the possibility of interaction with another medicine, and the use of electroconvulsive therapy for patients with known heart disease. You would also be reluctant to recommend intensive psychotherapy for patients who have a low capacity for insight or who are unreliable about keeping appointments. In fact, a history of noncompliance with treatment reduces still further the desirability of any treatment that is risky or complicated.

• Have you considered all feasible treatment modalities? Therapists of all professions feel most comfortable recommending those approaches they themselves use. Although this is understandable, it breeds the danger that a given patient might not be offered a treatment that could work well, but with which the therapist has had little experience. The best prophylaxis against the therapeutic rut is an attitude of flexibility.

> Psychiatrists expert in psychopharmacology must ever be alert to the possibility that for a given patient, family therapy might prove quicker, safer, and more effective than drugs.

Social workers, psychologists, and others who provide psychotherapy should keep in mind the indications for which drug treatment can be effective.

The fact that most mental and emotional disorders probably have multiple causes should encourage all clinicians to consider using more than one therapeutic modality for individual patients.

ASSESSING PROGNOSIS

The term *prognosis* has Greek roots meaning "to know in advance," which is, of course, impossible. But scientific progress over the past few decades has greatly improved our ability to predict outcome for individual patients. We'll discuss this in a few moments, after first defining what it is we are trying to predict.

Areas Defined by the Term *Prognosis*

The term *prognosis* commonly implies a number of meanings:

> *Symptoms.* Will they be relieved partly or completely, if at all?
> *Course of illness.* Will it be chronic or episodic? If the latter, will there be one episode or many?
> *Response to treatment.* How rapidly will this occur? Will it be slight, moderate, or complete?
> *Degree of recovery.* Once the acute episode has been arrested (either by treatment or by the passing of time), will the patient's previous personality be completely restored, or will there be residual deficits?
> *Time course of illness.* How long will recovery take? If the illness is episodic, how long is the patient likely to remain well between episodes?
> *Social consequences of the illness.* What will be the effects on the patient's job performance? Family life? Independence? Will financial support be needed? If so, for how long? Does this illness imply the need for conservatorship or other special legal proceedings? How will it affect the patient's ability to vote, to drive a car, to enter into contracts?
> *Are other family members at risk for this illness?* If it is hereditary, what degree of risk do you predict for first-degree relatives? How should you advise the patient who asks about having children?

Factors Affecting Prognosis

A number of factors help us make accurate predictions. Unfortunately, no one knows how strongly any one factor will influence the outcome in any given case. Because each can be important, I have simply tried to list them all, in no particular order.

- *Principal diagnosis.* Axis I diagnoses are usually more important than those listed on Axis II (the personality disorders and mental retardation); they are more traditional and generally better substantiated. Axis II diagnoses may be especially important for prognosis if no Axis I diagnosis exists or if none can be made with certainty. If your patient has more than one diagnosis, it is important to keep them all in mind when you are discussing the various aspects of prognosis.
- *Availability of treatment for the primary disorder.* If effective treatments exist, are they likely to be used? Geography can be an important factor: Does the patient live close enough to a center where effective treatment is offered? Another factor is the patient's financial condition, as demonstrated by this widely discussed example: Clozapine, a drug effective for schizophrenia, was introduced in the early 1990s at a cost of nearly $10,000 per patient per year. Many patients could not afford it until heavy pressure was brought to bear on the manufacturer to reduce the cost of laboratory monitoring.
- *Duration and course of illness.* Past behavior predicts future behavior.

> If there have been past episodes of illness (such as a mood disorder), you can predict with some confidence that there will be future episodes.
>
> Barring correction of a previous misdiagnosis, a patient who has been ill for many years stands scant chance of complete recovery.

- *Previous response to treatment.* As a predictor, previous treatment response is only as good as the previous treatment. If in the past your manic patient has been treated only with antipsychotics, you can upgrade your prognosis by an order of magnitude once mood stabilizer therapy is begun.
- *Compliance with treatment.* Even highly effective treatment is worthless if the patient refuses to accept it. Be sure to consider both Axis I and Axis II diagnoses, as well as treatment history, in estimating treatment compliance.

- *Available social supports.* Prognosis varies directly with the number of bridges the patient has left unburned. Consider all of these resources for help: family of origin, spouse/partner, children, friends, support groups, social agencies, physicians, and religious organizations. Besides providing comfort, they can help to ensure that the patient continues in treatment and avoids harmful influences such as drugs or alcohol.
- *Premorbid personality.* Premorbid personality is directly related to prognosis. Once patients recover from an acute episode of mental disorder, they tend to resume premorbid levels of functioning. Those who have maintained friendships, worked well at their jobs, and provided adequately for their families will probably do so again. All else being equal, parallel predictions are usually warranted for those who previously functioned at lower levels.
- *Highest recent level of functioning.* If productively engaged in work or school during the past year, your patient will probably regain that status once the current episode of illness has been resolved. Of course, this assumes that a deteriorating or chronically debilitating illness has not supervened. In Table 6 I've reproduced the Global Assessment of Functioning, which provides a convenient scale for evaluating a given patient's progress.
- *Other factors.* Within diagnostic categories, individual factors can often affect the outlook for a particular patient. For example, here are a few features that suggest a relatively good prognosis for a patient with schizophrenia: relatively late onset (30s or later), being married, female gender, education beyond high school, brief duration of untreated symptoms, and good previous response to treatment.

RECOMMENDING FURTHER INVESTIGATION

Further study may be necessary to confirm or rule out specific diagnoses. Resources for this information include the following:

A review of prior hospital and other records
Laboratory tests, including radiographic studies
Formal neuropsychological testing
Interviews with relatives

Further interviews and study of existing records usually cost nothing. They often provide new or corroborative information that can rapidly advance your understanding of your patient. Because testing costs both time and money, its use should be justified by the facts of each in-

TABLE 6. Global Assessment of Functioning

Code	Description
100 ⋮ 91	Superior functioning in a wide range of activities, life's problems never seem to get out of hand, is sought out by others because of many positive qualities. No symptoms.
90 ⋮ 81	Absent or minimal symptoms (e.g., mild anxiety before an exam), good functioning in all areas, interested and involved in a wide range of activities, socially effective, generally satisfied with life, no more than everyday problems or concerns (e.g., an occasional argument with family members).
80 ⋮ 71	If symptoms are present, they are transient and expectable reactions to psychosocial stressors (e.g., difficulty concentrating after family arguments); no more than slight impairment in social, occupational, or school functioning (e.g., temporarily falling behind in schoolwork).
70 ⋮ 61	Some mild symptoms (e.g., depressed mood and mild insomnia) OR some difficulty in social, occupational, or school functioning (e.g., occasional truancy, or theft within the household), but generally functioning pretty well, has some meaningful interpersonal relationships.
60 ⋮ 51	Moderate symptoms (e.g., flat affect and circumstantial speech, occasional panic attacks) OR moderate difficulty in social, occupational, or school functioning (e.g., few friends, conflicts with peers or co-workers).
50 ⋮ 41	Serious symptoms (e.g., suicidal ideation, severe obsessional rituals, frequent shoplifting) OR any serious impairment in social, occupational, or school functioning (e.g., no friends, unable to keep a job).
40 ⋮ 31	Some impairment in reality testing or communication (e.g., speech is at times illogical, obscure, or irrelevant) OR major impairment in several areas, such as work or school, family relations, judgment, thinking, or mood (e.g., depressed man avoids friends, neglects family, and is unable to work; child frequently beats up younger children, is defiant at home, and is failing at school).
30 ⋮ 21	Behavior is considerably influenced by delusions or hallucinations OR serious impairment in communication or judgment (e.g., sometimes incoherent, acts grossly inappropriately, suicidal preoccupation) OR inability to function in almost all areas (e.g., stays in bed all day; no job, home, or friends).
20 ⋮ 11	Some danger of hurting self or others (e.g., suicide attempts without clear expectation of death; frequently violent; manic excitement) OR occasionally fails to maintain minimal personal hygiene (e.g., smears feces) OR gross impairment in communication (e.g., largely incoherent or mute).
10 ⋮ 1	Persistent danger of severely hurting self or others (e.g., recurrent violence) OR persistent inability to maintain personal hygiene OR serious suicidal act with clear expectation of death.
0	Inadequate information.

From *Diagnostic and Statistical Manual of Mental Disorders* (4th ed., text rev., p. 34), by the American Psychiatric Association, 2000, Washington, DC: Author. Copyright 2000 by the American Psychiatric Association. Reprinted by permission.

dividual case. Tests ordered as a part of an admission routine and not in response to a perceived need are only rarely cost-effective.

When laboratory or psychological testing is involved, it should be justified on the basis of these factors:

- *Cost of the test.* The range can be enormous, from nothing at all to thousands of dollars.
- *Risk of the test.* Pencil-and-paper psychological tests have essentially no risk; some invasive procedures carry a risk to health and even to life itself.
- *Value of the test.* How strongly confirmatory will the results be? A costly lab procedure that has a good chance of nailing down a difficult diagnosis may well be worth the expense; a routine urinalysis that has no bearing on the diagnosis is too expensive by far.
- *Prevalence of the disorder.* Routine testing for rare disorders is not cost-effective. However, this does not mean that you should avoid ordering confirmatory tests for uncommon disorders that seem possible on the basis of history or physical exam.
- *Complexity of the question to be answered.* If the patient's illness is relatively simple and straightforward, you may well be able to omit laboratory testing completely.
- *Will the procedure facilitate treatment?* It is well and good to know what's wrong; it is better to learn how to fix it.

MAKING REFERRALS

You are likely to recommend mental health therapy that is directed specifically at your patient's complaints. You should also keep in mind the range of other treatments and referrals that may be needed, either to help manage the presenting complaints or to deal with social, psychological, and biological problems that are incidental to the main problems.

Many organizations and individuals can help you manage nearly any problem you may encounter. This is fortunate, because no clinician has the training and experience to do it all alone. It is vital that you know the limits of your own capabilities and refer for outside help those portions of each patient's difficulties that can be better treated by others.

How much outside help will be needed will depend on these factors:

Type of problem. A clinician whose training neglected behavior therapy techniques may need some assistance with a patient who presents with obsessions or phobias.

Severity of the problem. Mild depression may respond to cognitive therapy; a severe depression may require the services of a clinician skilled in psychopharmacology.

Strength and extent of support network. To give the most obvious example, a homeless patient will require far more in the way of social services than one who lives with relatives.

Degree of patient's desire and cooperation. Obviously, a patient's refusal to be hospitalized limits the scope of services that can be brought to bear.

The clinician's training, experience, and available time. I strongly recommend that students try to gain familiarity and experience with as many types of treatment as possible.

Although many of the resources mentioned in this chapter have traditionally been provided or arranged by social workers, all mental health professionals should be aware of the type of services that are available in the geographic area where they work. Too, clinicians in private practice will often find that they must arrange for their own referrals. Of course, you can use only the services you know about; hence this listing.

Other Therapists

No one can know everything; wise clinicians know their own limitations. If you practice group therapy and your patient needs olanzapine, of course you will refer the patient to a physician for medication. If drug therapy is your forte, it is important to refer your patient for cognitive-behavioral therapy when indicated, assuming you don't provide it yourself.

Mental Hospital

Although laypeople often consider hospitalization to be a last resort, in several situations the modern mental hospital is the most sensible recourse:

For patients who are dangerous to themselves
For patients who are dangerous to others
For patients who are unable to care for themselves

When the desired treatment is only available there
When the patient must be removed from the environment
When intensive evaluation/observation is required for medical or
legal purposes

Clinicians tend to be quite conservative when it comes to protecting their patients' lives. At least regarding suicidal ideas, which are probably the most frequently cited reason for hospitalization, most clinicians would agree that it is better to err on the side of overhospitalization.

Shelters

Shelters are vital resources for patients who do not need to be hospitalized, but who for various reasons cannot live at home. Specialized shelters are operated for the protection of children, battered women, runaways, and the homeless (men, women, and families).

Legal Assistance

Legal help may be needed for problems that might either cause or grow out of the mental disorder; sometimes the legal problems may be unrelated. If your patient has inadequate resources and needs services as varied as drawing a will or fighting criminal charges, a referral to a legal aid society may be necessary. If the problem concerns elder abuse or child abuse, refer to adult protective services or child protective services, respectively. The numbers of these agencies can usually be found in the county government listings in the telephone books of most major cities.

Support Groups

Many support groups are modeled after the famous Alcoholics Anonymous Twelve Steps. Most groups cost nothing to join, and many are nearly ubiquitous, having chapters throughout the country (in some cases throughout the world). The name of a group usually describes its function. Although a complete listing of support groups is impractical here (their name is legion), here are a representative few:

Adult Children of Alcoholics
Adults Molested as Children United
Al-Anon (for families)
Alateen
Alcoholics Anonymous

Batterers Anonymous
Gamblers Anonymous
Narcotics Anonymous
Overeaters Anonymous
Parents Anonymous (for parents who have abused their children)
Parents Without Partners
Recovery Inc. (for those with emotional problems)

Other Resources

Acute substance use treatment. Detoxification services are usually
available through referral from county mental health centers.

Medical evaluation. Available at county, state, city, and private hospitals for evaluation of rape, trauma, HIV status, and diseases
of any type.

Vocational services. Including evaluation for disability, job training,
and unemployment compensation, these services can be ac-
cessed through state and county employment offices.

Chapter 19

Sharing Your Findings with the Patient

Clinical findings and recommendations are useful only insofar as they are shared with others. The most important instance of this sharing is with the patient, and often the family as well.

CONFERRING WITH THE PATIENT

Whether or not you see an outward indication of nervousness, your patient will probably be feeling apprehensive about the results of your findings. This is why you should plan to discuss them just as soon as you can. Many clinicians do this at the end of each initial interview. Complicated problems may require more interviews or time to review materials. Even then, some sort of interim report will be appreciated, even if it is only a few sentences.

What you say will be governed to some extent by the patient's capacity to understand; this in turn may be heavily influenced by the disorder itself. But most patients can understand and appreciate the truth, which is what you should always try to communicate. I used to feel reluctant to give a patient or family the diagnosis of schizophrenia, because it often carries an ominous prognosis. But after a few such encounters, I discovered that patients tend to accept this diagnosis about as well as any other, and I stopped worrying.

If you follow a few simple rules when communicating your findings, your message will stand a better chance of being both heard and accepted.

Summarize the problems. By doing so, you give assurance that you really do understand why the patient has come for help. In the event that you don't understand as completely as you thought, the patient has the opportunity to educate you further.

Give a diagnosis. State your best diagnosis in terms appropriate for this patient. If you are unsure of the diagnosis, say so. Then lay out your plan for resolving your uncertainty (more tests? a therapeutic trial?).

Keep it simple. Bear in mind what the patient really needs to know, and convey that. This isn't the time to teach a graduate course in diagnostics.

Don't use jargon. The information should be transmitted in terms the patient can understand. If you use a lot of four-dollar words, you risk losing part of your message while the patient deciphers the code.

Keep asking for feedback. You'll get better compliance with recommendations and greater patient satisfaction when you assure through questions that the patient understands your explanation of the problem and the proposed approach:

"How do you feel about this?"

"Do you have any questions so far?"

Emphasize the positive. With the many therapeutic approaches mental health professionals have at their disposal, even gravely serious problems such as schizophrenia and bipolar I disorder can be helped. Even if you can't do much for a patient who is rapidly sliding into dementia, you may be able to help the family cope.

Show your compassion. Watch for changes in the patient's affect as you give information. Acknowledge the patient's feelings, and offer sympathy and suggestions as to how things might improve. Remember that all people need the feeling of hope.

Discussing Treatment

First and foremost, the treatment plan you arrive at should be structured as a collaborative effort between clinician and patient. Although this approach to treatment planning requires more initial effort, in the long run everyone will benefit. A plan shared with the patient is an important part of the initial interview.

What do patients want from their clinicians? I tend to answer this important question with another question: Exactly what would I want if I were the patient? I would want a sensible plan that linked diagnosis to rational treatment, and a clear explanation of the treatment process, its possible pitfalls, the alternatives to treatment, and an honest appraisal of the likelihood of its success.

A concrete plan for further investigations, as well as treatment, would help me feel hopeful for the future. Because it would put me back in control, I'd be more enthusiastic about it and less likely to drag my feet about implementation. A patient who buys into the plan is more likely to cooperate with it enthusiastically. I'd also want a clinician who was so keen to ensure my understanding that, if I asked questions, they would be treated not as challenges to authority but as opportunities to engage me in the treatment process. My compliance would be enhanced: I'd probably remember my appointments, try to do assigned exercises, and miss few doses of medicine. My improvement wouldn't be delayed, and I'd avoid treatment failures and dropouts from therapy. If something went awry and treatment didn't work, I'd be far less likely to lay blame on my clinician if I had signed on to the plan.

In the negotiated approach to treatment, patient and clinician together formulate the plan. This doesn't mean that the patient gets everything that's wanted, but that the clinician does listen to the patient. You can encourage your patient to "want" or choose the plan that you think would be best, but you must listen and react appropriately if the choice goes a different way. I've often felt, for example, that a teenager chose wrong when rejecting medication for depression. "I want to do it myself" is the typical response. But I've always accepted the decision with the best grace I could muster—and very often, several appointments down the road, the patient volunteers the opinion that "this isn't going as well as I'd hoped, and maybe I should try your pills after all."

When you are drawing up the treatment plan together, here are several points to consider:

• *Discuss the options.* It is human nature to feel more in control when there are choices; therefore, you should run through a complete list of the possible treatment options. One obvious choice that is seldom mentioned is no treatment at all. I often start with this one, because it allows me to discuss in concrete terms what I foresee as the outcome of no treatment (or inadequate treatment). This serves as a useful benchmark against which to measure the potential drawbacks and benefits of the other choices.

• *Mention the drawbacks.* No treatment is free of them: Medicines have side effects, psychotherapy takes time, group therapy involves other people, and behavior modification requires a lot of effort and anxiety. All of them are expensive. Negative aspects of treatment are unpleasant to contemplate, but patients need to know these things so they can make a rational choice. Many states have laws that require patients to be told about alternatives to somatic treatments, such as drugs and electroconvulsive therapy.

• *You can favor one option.* Most of the time you will probably convey your opinions directly. But for patients who feel the need to defy authority or who strongly desire a particular form of therapy, you may want to exert your influence more subtly. For example, you can find good news about drug therapy for the patient who needs it:

"You won't have to wait forever to gain control of your symptoms." You can also find good news for the patient, perhaps one with a personality disorder, who *doesn't* need drugs:

"You won't have to give up control of your own body."

Neither of these statements is untrue, and they can both promote one of the goals of mental health professionals: to encourage patients to accept what will help them.

• *Make sure the patient understands the options.* Most patients will, but under stress people can have difficulty focusing their full attention on what they are being told. If you have any doubts that your instructions about treatment were heard, ask the patient to repeat what you have said—"to see if I've been as clear as I should be." Providing a brief written summary of your recommendations is another way to help your patient understand you.

• *Avoid making promises, other than that you will do all in your power to help.* Of course, you cannot see into the future, and on some level patients know this. But patients (and families) are also often so worried about the future that they invest us mental health clinicians with powers we don't possess. Clinicians have gotten themselves into serious difficulties by painting a view of the future that is rosier than the data and the experience of others will support. When you offer hope, it should be in the context of a realistic view of the situation and a rational plan for the future. It should emphasize the importance of the patient's cooperation with all aspects of treatment—including questioning any of your conclusions or directions that might not be understood.

Motivating the Patient

Of course, without implementation, the best treatment plan in the world will accomplish precisely nothing. And far too often that is the outcome of a mental health consultation. Despite the best efforts of a clinician, a patient may forget to take medication, neglect behavioral exercises, or go ahead and drink or use drugs anyway.

Why do so many patients appear unwilling to improve? Often it can be traced to a lack of hope, perhaps based on long experience with the mental health system. Or disorders of personality or substance use may motivate people in ways that compete with the therapeutic plan. Or perhaps education, often cloaked in exhortation, has already been tried. Although greater knowledge about mental disorder may illuminate the source of the problem, it doesn't necessarily give the individual a sense of control, and studies have shown that education alone doesn't go far toward motivating change.

Enter *motivational interviewing* (MI), a client-centered approach for persuading people to change behaviors they need to adopt for health care (or other) reasons. Instead of confrontation, MI emphasizes collaboration; for education it substitutes *evocation*, which means unlocking resources for change the patient already has. MI helps get people off the dime and past ambivalence, to identify their own inner motivation. Time and again in controlled studies, MI has been demonstrated useful—even in the vast majority of patients with schizophrenia.

MI is based on the principle that it's easier to get people to do what you want than it is to prevent them from doing what you don't want—it's the "catch more flies with honey than with vinegar" approach. A patient doesn't have to commit to global change, just specific behaviors. Although whole manuals have been written about MI, it can be summarized in four basic steps:

1. *Empathize.* Without criticizing, you will help the patient express feelings and viewpoints. Note that beyond facilitating its expression, you don't have to agree with the patient's point of view.

2. *Help the patient recognize how current behavior is frustrating longer-term wishes.* The perception of that discrepancy is what will motivate the patient to seek behavioral change.

3. *When you encounter resistance, don't argue with it.* Instead, use it as an opportunity to explore the patient's feelings further. In MI, resistance means that the clinician needs to adopt a different approach.

4. *Show that you believe the patient can succeed,* thus providing hope.

Here, somewhat condensed, is a conversation with a young woman who has mild mental retardation, lives with a roommate, and has a job stocking shelves at a local grocery store. A long-time client, Misty has once again been having difficulties with her budget.

CLINICIAN: I understand that you've had a letter from your bank.

MISTY: Right, they said I was overdrawn again. And Janice [the resident manager at Seaview, the patient's independent living facility] says I could lose my account.

CLINICIAN: That would be too bad.

MISTY: Yeah, I'm bummed.

CLINICIAN: I can imagine. Anyone would be. What happened to get you overdrawn?

MISTY: I guess I wrote too many checks.

CLINICIAN: What were they for?

MISTY: You know—my cable, bottled water, rent, telephone. That's all.

CLINICIAN: That doesn't seem like a lot.

MISTY: It isn't. I always pay them on time.

CLINICIAN: I know, you've done a wonderful job with those responsibilities. I'm always so proud of you.

With praise for Misty's previous success, the clinician reaffirms their past connections and expresses confidence in her abilities. Step 4—support—shouldn't wait for new actions from the patient.

MISTY: And I bought some stuffed animals. I have a collection.

Misty and her clinician further list income and expenses; the clinician learns that since the holidays, Misty has been working fewer hours, and her paychecks have been reduced.

CLINICIAN: So you have less money right now.

MISTY: Right.

CLINICIAN: What do you think you can do?

MISTY: I could ask my mom for money.

CLINICIAN: And would she help? What happened last time?

MISTY: She said no, I'd have to spend less.

CLINICIAN: How would that work?

MISTY: Well, I have to pay rent.

CLINICIAN: Of course. What about the other items on this list?

They talk about the other bills, and agree that the telephone is essential. The clinician wonders about Misty's bottled water.

MISTY: It's crystal pure.

CLINICIAN: Do others at Seaview have bottled water?

MISTY: No, just me and Arlene [her roommate, whose finances are, if anything, even more straitened than Misty's].

CLINICIAN: And what would happen if you didn't have it?

MISTY: We'd have to drink tap.

CLINICIAN: Like the others.

MISTY: Yeah.

The clinician interprets the prolonged silence as evidence of significant resistance, and decides to approach it obliquely.

> CLINICIAN: I guess you'd rather not change, right?
>
> MISTY: Right.
>
> CLINICIAN: Bottled water is nice, and you're used to it.
>
> MISTY: Right. We use it for cooking, too.
>
> CLINICIAN: You're used to your cable TV, too.
>
> MISTY: Well, sure. We both like the cooking shows a lot.
>
> CLINICIAN: You're lucky; you both like cooking and the cooking shows.
>
> MISTY: We like to eat.
>
> CLINICIAN: You'd like to keep them both.
>
> MISTY: Yeah, we need them.

It develops that Misty and Arlene subscribe to every premium service their cable TV provides, including full sports, HBO, and Showtime.

> CLINICIAN: You know, I used to have HBO and Showtime, too, but I cancelled one of them. I thought I didn't need both.
>
> MISTY: Mm-hmm.
>
> CLINICIAN: What do you think?
>
> MISTY: I think people who live in a house have money. They can choose if they want.
>
> CLINICIAN: I see, and you feel that you don't have much of a choice, is that it?
>
> MISTY: Right!

Misty has made her point—a perhaps surprisingly insightful one that describes and explains her resistance to having a choice forced upon her. Realizing that Misty recognizes the discrepancy between what she can afford and what she wants, but needs time to work out what to do, the clinician backs off and says that they can work some more next time on solving the problem. This expression of support leaves Misty with the feeling of being heard and of having some hope for the future. Later in the week, she calls to say that she and Arlene have decided to get by on tap water for a while.

Although MI itself is relatively new, clinicians have negotiated with patients for generations; the technique was advocated by psychiatrist Adolf Meyer over 80 years ago. Clinicians who avoid parentalism and empower their patients in pretreatment decision making often find that they promote greater patient satisfaction. Furthermore, patients who have positive relationships with their clinicians are more likely to be happy with treatment and to find it helpful, even in the case of electroconvulsive therapy. Other research has demonstrated that patients accept treatment and follow through with it better when clinicians express empathy, are willing to explain and share information, and are accessible to patients on their own terms.

Obviously, the benefits of MI will not hold in the face of advanced dementia, blatant psychosis, acute suicide plans, or life-threatening anorexia nervosa. But as Misty and her clinician have shown, it can work even in patients with serious intellectual impairment.

DISCUSSION WITH THE FAMILY

A close-knit family will want to know what can be done for the patient. Many relatives have had considerable experience in dealing with mental health professionals, and this experience has not always been a happy one. The quality of their experience this time will usually be in direct proportion to the following:

The amount of contact they have with you
The degree to which they feel they have input
How caring you appear to be
The patient's opinion of you and of the treatment plan

You can avoid problems of confidentiality if you and the patient meet together with the family. Of course, if you need more information than your patient can provide, a portion of your family session will have to take place with the patient absent. If that is to be the case, I'd at least mention the meeting to your patient—who, you can point out, has had plenty of opportunity for confidential sessions.

If this is your first family conference, you might start out by asking what the members already know about the disorder. This helps you learn about their prior assumptions and therefore avoid discomfiting them with information that directly contradicts what they may have been told earlier. For example, if a previous therapist has diagnosed schizophrenia and you believe that the diagnosis should be bipolar I disorder, you might want to emphasize the psychotic symptoms that both clinicians have regarded as key.

Subsequently, your approach to the relatives should be pretty much the same as the one you have used for the patient. Let them know that you have negotiated an agreement about treatment. Describe the treatment plan, including its strong and weak points. It is especially important for relatives to know what to watch for: Side effects and wanted effects of treatment may be even more apparent to them than to the patient. Be sure to tell relatives how to get in touch with you, and emphasize that you want all three groups—the patient, relatives, and you—to work together as partners in problem solving.

WHAT IF THE PLAN IS REJECTED?

With the stress of mental illness in the family, it is not uncommon for someone—usually the patient, but sometimes a relative—to object to the treatment plan. If it is a relative or friend, and you and the patient agree about how to proceed, move ahead with the plan. But say something to the relative that shows you have considered the dissenting point of view:

"I'm glad you told me that you don't want your brother hospitalized. But he and I both feel it is the safest thing to do right now, so I think we should go ahead with it. I hope you'll visit him. You know him better than just about anybody, so I'll need your eyes and ears to help me judge how he is progressing."

If your patient is the one who balks at treatment, proceed with a series of steps that might resolve your impasse:

1. Try to discover what about it is not acceptable, and then offer reassurance. For example, side effects of treatment may be tolerable if the patient can be reassured that they are likely to be short-term.

2. Identify the areas that you do agree about. If it is the need for *some* treatment, proceed with the next step.

3. Learn what therapeutic measure the patient will accept. If it is something you feel will not be harmful, just not helpful (such as psychotherapy alone for a moderately severe depression), you may agree to try it for a specified period. At the end of that time, the patient may agree to proceed with your original recommendation.

4. You may agree to an experimental trial, with the proviso that you will monitor the results carefully and stop or change treatment if the patient feels dissatisfied.

5. Offer to arrange for a second opinion. This may be especially helpful if a trusted friend or relative is influencing the patient to reject your recommendation. But keep an open mind: Your consultant may recommend something helpful that is different from what you had in mind.

6. Finally, it is possible that either the patient or the family may reject treatment you consider to be essential. Here's my rule: I might proceed with a course of treatment that I believe is fully warranted against the wishes of either the family or the patient (in the case of a patient who is involuntarily hospitalized). But if both patient *and* family reject my advice, I will usually feel unable to work effectively with this patient. In such a case, I will try to help the patient find another clinician.

Chapter 20

Communicating Your Findings to Others

Somewhere, sometime, a mental health clinician might conceivably do an evaluation and provide a complete course of treatment without saying a word to anyone but the patient. If ever it happened, this rare event would probably take place in the office of an isolated private practitioner. But the demands of insurance carriers, government agencies, and HMOs make it increasingly likely that, regardless of where you work or who your patient may be, you will have to communicate your findings to someone.

THE WRITTEN REPORT

Even the most expert of clinicians collect their data somewhat haphazardly. It is therefore necessary to organize your findings before reporting them. For written and oral reports, the organization of material will be about the same. Written reports are usually the more complete, so they will be discussed first, and in far greater detail. Appendix C provides a complete interview and written report for a sample patient

Identifying Data

The identifying data provide the reader with a framework upon which to construct a mental image of the patient whose history you are reporting. In the first line or two of the report, you state the basic demographic data, including name, age, sex, race, marital status, religion, and any other item that seems relevant. In the military services, identifying data also include the patient's rank; in a VA hospital, you might note whether the patient has a service-connected disability.

In any case, you should note that the patient either is new to your facility or has been seen there before.

The Chief Complaint

As described in Chapter 2, the chief complaint is the patient's stated reason for coming to treatment. It is often written as a direct quote, but sometimes you'll want to paraphrase or summarize it—especially if it is vague, long-winded, or multifaceted. Occasionally a clinician cites two chief complaints: one from the patient, and another (suitably identified) from a relative, friend, or other informant. This double reporting is especially useful for patients who are too confused or too uncooperative to respond appropriately when you request the information.

Informants

Briefly state the names of those from whom you have obtained your information, and estimate the reliability of each. Besides the patient, mention relatives, friends, other health care workers, and old charts—anything or anyone you have used to help round out your picture of the patient.

History of the Present Illness

This section is the most important of the entire report. When you are writing up the history of the present illness, keep in mind several rules.

- This should be a chronological history. Like all good stories, this one should have a beginning, some development, and an ending. In most cases, it will begin with the onset of the first episode of illness. Some clinicians carefully mark that point with an opening phrase something like this:

> "Mr. Turner was well until age 32, when he suffered the first of several episodes of depression."

Note that in this single economical sentence, the reader is alerted to (1) the principal area of clinical interest (mood disorder: depression), (2) the age of onset, (3) the fact that Mr. Turner's problem is not a new one, and (4) the patient's good health during the decade of his adult life prior to the onset of this illness. Once your narrative is underway, it should proceed more or less chronologically, ending with the reasons that prompted your patient to enter treatment at this time.

Patients who have been repeatedly admitted to one facility for the same condition may prompt an interval note, abbreviated to avoid needless, lengthy repetition from one chart to the next:

"Since age 32 Mr. Turner has had five admissions to this medical
center for severe depression, each of which has been successfully
treated with electroconvulsive therapy. Following his most recent
discharge 2 years ago, he had been living independently and working at his trade of commercial illustrator. Two weeks ago he noted
the lethargy and loss of interest in work that usually heralds the onset of an episode of depression . . . "

• Support your best diagnosis. This means that the material you
feature should reflect the diagnostic criteria (DSM-IV-TR, in North
America) for the diagnosis you think most likely. Let's say, for example,
that your patient has symptoms of both depression and psychosis (in
DSM terms, major depressive episode, severe, with psychotic features
and with melancholic features). You believe that melancholia with psychosis is the most likely diagnosis, so the history of the present illness
should emphasize the finding that your patient is never psychotic except during a profound depression. This is not to say that you should
try to hide ambiguities or evidence of competing diagnoses. But your
write-up should, insofar as is consistent with the data, form a picture in
which history, mental status, and diagnosis are mutually supportive
portions of a consistent whole.

• If the story is complicated, try to disentangle it. One way to accomplish this is to leave until later details that don't support your best
diagnosis. Perhaps this less relevant information can be included later
in the personal and social history. You could also present distinct
(though possibly intersecting) themes as separate paragraphs in your
history of the present illness. After describing your patient's depressive
illness, which was actually the cause of his hospitalization, you might
continue as follows:

"In addition to his depression, Mr. Turner has also had a problem
with cross-dressing. This began at about the age of 6 . . . "

• Edit your material. If you have just sat through an hour-long interview and read an old chart as thick as the Chicago Yellow Pages, you may
have learned far more than most readers will need to know. To boil down
your material, you can summarize previous treatment in a line or two, cat-
egorize hospitalizations (so many for mania, so many more for depression), and list symptoms of a typical episode. This saves your reader from
multiple repetitions of essentially identical information.

"At that time [of his first episode of depression] he first noticed lethargy and lack of interest in his work as a commercial illustrator.

Over the next few weeks he became increasingly anorectic, lost 10 pounds, and suffered insomnia that caused him to get up and pace the floor early each morning. This symptom pattern has been repeated during subsequent episodes."

As Platt and McMath (1979) have noted, "The present illness should be an elaboration of these primary data, not a saga of medical care."

• Include significant negatives. When investigating various areas of clinical interest, you asked many questions to rule in or out certain disorders. Some of the negative answers helped you choose the most likely diagnosis on a differential list. Such answers are called *significant* (or *pertinent*) *negatives;* they should be reported in your history of the present illness, along with the important positive answers:

"Although Mr. Leeborg said that he felt severely depressed in the week since he lost his job, he denied insomnia, loss of appetite, and lack of interest in sex."

• Report your findings in plain language. Your readers may include people who are unaccustomed to the sometimes perplexing jargon of the mental health field. Short sentences and active verbs will demonstrate the clarity of your thinking. Avoid abbreviations other than those commonly used in professional journals.

• The patient is a person, not a "case." Many clinicians consider it bad form to refer to patients as "this manic" or "this schizophrenic." Always strive to refer to your patient as "this person" or "this patient with schizophrenia." Such wording helps to preserve the reader's feeling for the humanity of your patient.

Personal and Social History

Childhood through Adult Life

To keep things orderly, you should adhere as closely as you can to chronological sequence when you present this information. Begin with birth and early childhood, and proceed through education, military experience (if any), sexuality, marriage, work history, legal history, and religion. You can use either a paragraph or outline style; the former will be more convenient if you dictate, the latter if you handwrite or keyboard your information.

In this section, strive to present a reasonably complete picture of your patient's background. Even so, you should generally omit data already covered in the history of the present illness. Edit out the anecdotes and trivial details with which patients invariably illustrate their life stories. You should include pertinent negatives, such as the absence of childhood sexual abuse in a patient you suspect of somatization disorder or borderline personality disorder. Also include important past positives, such as previous drug or alcohol misuse, that you might have omitted from the history of the present illness because they no longer affect your patient's life.

Family History

Although it is properly a part of the patient's own life story, family history is traditionally reported in a separate paragraph. Perhaps we do this to emphasize the biological and environmental effects families can have on the development of the adult individual. Include the data you have obtained for physical as well as mental disorders. When reporting the latter, be sure to include not just the diagnosis, but also whatever data you have obtained that would substantiate (or refute) that diagnosis. For example:

> "Although Mrs. Garwaith's father had been diagnosed as having schizophrenia, he had twice been treated in hospital and released, apparently recovered and able to resume the demanding occupation of singing waiter. These details suggested a diagnosis of mood disorder."

If the patient was adopted or if the family history is completely negative, say so and move on.

Medical History

Mention any operations, major medical illnesses, current and recent medications, and hospitalizations for reasons not related to mental health. List any allergies, especially to drugs. If there are none, say so—this information may assume importance, should drug therapy become an issue for your patient. If you have not already done so, mention any habits such as the use of tobacco or alcohol.

Review of Systems

Mention any positive responses to your questioning about past or present physical problems. If somatization disorder has been a consideration in the differential diagnosis, list the symptoms you scored positive in that disorder's specialized review of systems (see Appendix B for details).

Mental Status Examination

For many patients, much of the mental status exam will be normal and can therefore be covered briefly. The order in which you report the various areas is not as important as the fact that you mention each, if only to show that you have considered them all. In describing your patient's mental status, keep in mind which details would be needed to support or refute the diagnoses included in your differential diagnosis. You should report not only positive information, but also the important negatives that allow you to place diagnoses higher or lower in your differential listing.

Describe the patient's general appearance and clothing; contrast apparent age with stated age. Be sure to mention all aspects of affect. If type of affect is unremarkable, "about medium" will do as a descriptor, but also mention lability and appropriateness. When you are trying to describe abnormalities, don't use general terms such as "bizarre" or "peculiar," which carry none of the flavor of the patient's behavior or appearance. Instead, take the trouble to choose words and phrases that are truly descriptive: Instead of "The patient's clothing was strange," say, "The patient was dressed in a tutu and body stocking hand stitched from old flour sacking."

Remember that written mental health records are legal documents. They can be subpoenaed by attorneys and requested by patients themselves, so make sure that your tone and wording will withstand scrutiny. Avoid jokes, complaints, and any other comments that should be kept private. If you need to express an opinion that could be considered pejorative, qualify the statement by admitting that this is your inference:

"He *appeared* to be intoxicated . . . "

"Her manner *seemed* seductive . . . "

Under flow of thought, be sure to mention any abnormalities of association, as well as rate and rhythm of speech. Use examples with direct quotes, both to show the flavor of the patient's speech and to provide a baseline for judging later change.

The findings you report under content of thought will generally mirror what you have already mentioned in the history of the present illness. You should also mention all the other possible contents of thought that were not present. Whereas many patients have no content of thought that is psychopathological, all (except those who are completely mute) do say something. Whatever it is, you should describe it briefly:

> "The patient's content of thought largely concerned his past infidelities and the fact that his wife was about to leave him. He expressed no delusions, hallucinations, obsessions, or phobias."

When your patient has language deficits, state what they are, but also give an example of what you mean:

> "Although Mrs. Treat was able to comprehend simple instructions and spoke with good fluency, she demonstrated a naming aphasia: She could not name the clip and point of a ballpoint pen, and she called my wristwatch 'a time thingy.' "

In reporting cognitive abilities, it is not sufficient simply to mention that the patient was "normal" or "intact." You should note what tests you made, the responses given, and how you interpret the responses. How far off were any incorrect responses? Do circumstances mitigate the errors? For example, if your patient could not recall a name, a color, and a street address after 5 minutes, can this be explained on the basis of poor concentration due to depression? Was abstracting ability impaired? If so, what was the test you used, and what was the response? In reporting serial sevens, note the number of mistakes and the rapidity with which the calculations were done. Did the patient use finger counting as an aid to this calculation?

In reporting insight and judgment, you will usually have to make an interpretation (such as excellent, good, fair, or poor), but be sure to cite your reasoning:

> "Miss Rafael's insight seemed poor in that, despite her clearly manic symptoms, she denied ever being ill a day in her life. However, her judgment was fairly good: She did agree to remain in hospital 'for tests.' She even said that she might resume taking her lithium."

RECORDING YOUR DIAGNOSIS

In North America, the standard for psychiatric diagnosis has been each successive edition of the *Diagnostic and Statistical Manual of Mental Disorders* (DSM) of the American Psychiatric Association. Much of the rest of the world uses the *International Classification of Diseases* (ICD) in one of its many iterations. The DSM, devised by committees of experts and strongly grounded in empirical research, specifies that each patient be assessed in five areas. Each area, called an *axis*, contains information to help describe the patient's current mental health status. The first three of these areas contain the actual diagnostic information:

• Axis I includes the major clinical syndromes; most mental health patients will have at least one Axis I diagnosis. These syndromes include the depressions, psychoses, anxiety disorders, substance use disorders, and other clinical entities that mental health clinicians so typically diagnose and treat. If more than one diagnosis is appropriate, include them all, but list first that which was mainly responsible for the current evaluation.

• Axis II comprises the personality disorders and mental retardation. It helps you maintain sight of long-standing characteristics that define the person you have interviewed. If the diagnosis that occasioned the current evaluation is on Axis II, it should be followed by the words *principal diagnosis*.

• Axis III comprises all physical diagnoses that contribute to your understanding of the patient—for example, asthma, diabetes, obesity, and temporal lobe epilepsy.

• Axis IV is a place to indicate the psychosocial stresses that during the past year may have caused or affected the patient's mental condition, or might materially affect treatment. Table 3 lists the types of stressors that may be noted. You should write down the exact stressor responsible, not the category.

• Axis V, the Global Assessment of Functioning, rates the patient's overall functioning. Two ratings can be made: one that is current, and one that describes the highest level of functioning during the past year. The scale runs from 100 (superior) to 1 (lowest), and is given in Table 6.

The ICD does not maintain a separate axis for personality disorders, but it is similarly grounded in research and the opinions of experts.

FORMULATION

In the case formulation, you attempt to synthesize all that has been learned about the patient's past so as to point the way toward a better future. There are several reasons for preparing a formulation:

To focus your thinking about the patient
To summarize the logic behind your diagnoses
To identify future needs for information and treatment
To present a brief summary of the patient

A number of formats can be used; some of them are so involved that they risk presenting again all the material you have just covered. The method presented here combines the advantages of brevity, completeness, and simplicity.

Of the various sections of the formulation, the two most important are the differential diagnosis and the contributing factors. They contain the original thinking you will do in putting together all the material you have gathered.

A sample formulation, presented piecemeal, follows.

Brief Recapitulation

Following some minimal identifying data, state the symptoms and course of the patient's present illness as based on the facts in the history of the present illness and the mental status examination. Draw from all parts of your report as needed:

> "Mrs. Juneau is a 27-year-old married woman with two previous hospitalizations for a psychosis that has been previously called schizophrenia. For 3 weeks she has stayed in her room, fasting and 'preparing for the end of the world,' which she says she has caused. Her husband brought her to the hospital when he became concerned about her weight loss."

Differential Diagnosis

Each of the possible diagnoses in your differential listing is presented with the principal arguments for and against it. Include Axis I and Axis II diagnoses.

> "*Cognitive psychosis with delusions.* History of head trauma 8 years ago."

> "*Substance use.* She drank heavily during her two psychotic episodes, but has never continued drinking once the psychosis has resolved."

> "*Depression.* Mrs. Juneau feels sad, hopeless, and guilty for some unspecified sin she committed before she was married. She is anorectic, has been nearly sleepless, and has had a 10-pound weight loss.

"*Schizophrenia*. She is delusional now; during a previous episode she has believed that she was put on earth to save the Jews.

Best Diagnosis

State the diagnosis you favor, why you have chosen it, and the authority (the current edition of either DSM or ICD). Note that your best diagnosis may not be the one highest in the hierarchy. The most notable example of this is that a cognitive disorder, if one is possible, must always be ruled out first, but it frequently is not the most likely diagnosis:

> "Mrs. Juneau is probably in the depressed phase of bipolar I disorder (DSM-IV-TR). Her previous episodes of psychosis resolved completely; her husband reports that even without maintenance medication, she was well between episodes. All of her psychotic symptoms appear to be congruent with her mood at the time. Head trauma was 8 years ago and without sequel, and there are no other indications of organicity. Her misuse of alcohol appears to have occurred only in response to her psychotic episodes, which in retrospect were probably mania with psychosis."

Contributing Factors

Here you describe how the various factors you have identified contributed to the development of your patient's main problems. Where applicable, mention biological, dynamic, psychological, and social factors. Depending on the material you have identified, this section could be long or short:

> "A biological basis for Mrs. Juneau's illness may be seen in the family history: Her mother suffered from recurrent depressions. A psychological precipitant may be the death of her father 2 months ago. Medical expenses from previous episodes may be contributing to the depth of her current depression."

Further Information Needed

Briefly cover the interviews, tests, and records you may need to firm up the diagnosis:

> "Records will be requested from Mrs. Juneau's previous admissions to see whether the symptoms she had then could be those of mania. Consider MRI to rule out sequelae of old head injury."

Treatment Plan

Outline your recommendations for treatment. For Mrs. Juneau they were as follows:

Biological
  Lithium 900 mg/day to prevent recurrence of mania
  Fluoxetine 20 mg/day for depression
  Olanzapine as needed to control psychosis
Psychological
  Psychotherapy, focused on feelings of guilt and grief
Social
  Assistance with financial planning
  (?) Referral to Alcoholics Anonymous
  Education of Juneau family regarding bipolar I disorder

Prognosis

What is the likely outcome for this patient?

> "Mrs. Juneau is expected to recover completely. Prophylactic use of a mood stabilizer may prevent subsequent episodes."

THE ORAL PRESENTATION

A verbal presentation of your interview material generally follows the same pattern as the written report. Usually, it is briefer; in fact, any oral presentation longer than 5 or 6 minutes risks boredom and inattention from your listeners. However, you should present a complete, rounded portrait that demonstrates how well you understand the patient.

You can also demonstrate how well organized you are. For a formal presentation, outline your findings on a small note card. This will speed you through your presentation, jog your memory when needed, and save you the discomfort of flipping back and forth through your patient's chart as you search for items of information.

When you are making an oral presentation, be prepared with your diagnosis and differential diagnosis. You should have clearly in mind the reasons for choosing your best diagnosis; some instructors will ask you to defend it with data and logic.

Chapter 21

Troubleshooting Your Interview

To a degree, every interview has flaws, and every interviewer has troubles. The art of the expert interview lies in compensating for the former and minimizing the effects of the latter. In this chapter, we'll look at some of the problems beginning interviewers often face—or should face, once they become aware of them.

Of course, there are many ways that an initial evaluation can go awry, but the outcome can be affected in only a couple of ways. Rapport with the patient probably least often falls victim to problematic interviewing; if there is one area in which most clinicians succeed, it is forming a good working relationship with their patients. Still, missteps in the interview process do occasionally lead patients to withdraw from treatment.

The other effect of an interview that's run aground involves the information we seek. That is, we clinicians sometimes obtain information that we think is accurate and complete, when it is not. The initial interview is the time when we consciously try to learn the pertinent facts about a new patient. Regardless how much we may think we have learned, we tend to form an impression after that first information-gathering phase, whether it lasts just an hour or extends over several sessions. Once we've formed a diagnostic impression, we may find it difficult to revise our first impressions, even in the face of compelling later information.

RECOGNIZING THE TROUBLED INTERVIEW

The good: Most interview situations can be retrieved, once you've figured out what's wrong. The bad: It can be hard to know what's wrong. Here are some signals that could tip you off:

During the Interview

Even while you are talking with the patient, you should be alert for behaviors signaling that an interview is in trouble.

- The patient becomes quiet, quarrelsome, or critical. Most interactions with patients start out well enough; along the way, though, something occasionally happens to sour a patient on the process. The evidence lies in a change in the patient's manner. One who was at first cooperative and talkative may begin to argue about your seemingly noncontroversial statements. Another, initially loquacious, may stop offering spontaneous comments or may begin responding to open-ended questions with single syllables or even grants.
- Although a patient who glances around the room may be attending to hallucinations, it is more likely that this patient has lost interest in your conversation and would like to do something different. I've even known patients who bolted from the room, leaving the interview unfinished. Any signal of inattention is important: Without the patient's active participation, any information you obtain isn't likely to be robust, let alone accurate.
- You get contradictory answers to repetitions of essentially the same question.
- You find that you cannot think of questions to ask that will pin down an important part of the differential diagnosis.
- Your patient continually asks you to repeat your questions.
- *You* want to get up and leave the room.

After the Interview

Once your patient has departed, evidence from your data may tell you that something is awry.

- You find that you have omitted important data points.
- The patient declines to make another appointment.
- Information you've just gathered contradicts data from old charts or collateral sources.
- Your information speaks only to one item in the differential diagnosis.
- You've learned a lot about baseball, but little about the patient's history.
- You haven't learned enough about the patient's feelings.
- You haven't raised issues critical to every interview: sex, substance use, suicidal ideas.

HOW TO DETERMINE WHAT'S WRONG

The following interview diagnostic steps can help you determine what's wrong. Even if you haven't encountered any of the issues I've mentioned above, I recommend taking the fearless first step once in a while, anyway. After all, the most insidious error of all is the one that isn't called to your attention.

Make a Recording

Of course, you can only tape-record an interview with your patient's express written permission, but that seldom presents a barrier. You can explain that you are trying to learn more about the interviewing process, and that recording an interview will give you a better feel for your patients' needs. I wouldn't feel at all backward about admitting—at your level of experience or at mine—that you would like to learn what you need to learn. In my experience, only a small minority of patients will decline permission to be recorded.

A small recorder placed unobtrusively between the two of you on your desk will do the job nicely. If the room is relatively quiet (there are no loud sounds from the hallway and the heating system is well behaved), you should be able to pick up both your voices without difficulty. In the event that there is too much ambient noise in the room, a pair of Radio Shack lapel microphones joined by a "Y" connector will yield instant clarity.

A video recording would be even better—if you can mount the camera so that it shows both your patient and you. (For sound clarity, you'll also need microphones not mounted on the camera.) You will be interested not just in the patient's appearance, but in your own facial expressions and other items of body language. Do you frown, squint, look bored, or roll your eyes? Or just fail to smile an encouragement from time to time? Do you maintain eye contact, or do you spend all your time fussing with your notes? The tool in Appendix E can give some additional structure to your self-assessment.

Do Some Witnessed Interviews

As powerful as your own audio or video recording can be, you can multiply its effectiveness with a little outside help. For generations, the witnessed interview has been a standard means of determining a psychiatrist's fitness for board certification. By begging for some time from a colleague, you can get the same benefits for yourself—without the live-or-die trauma that board candidates suffer. Of course, you could have your consultant sit in with you while you interview a live patient, but that would require a lot of hassle in coordinating the schedules of three people, not to mention the problem for your patient of having someone else physically in the room while you are doing an evaluation. It's generally better to use one of the recordings we have just talked about as the basis for a discussion with your local expert on interviewing. (Be sure your patient agrees that another clinician can have access to the material.)

However, finding an appropriate consultant presents one or two problems of its own. A good choice would be someone you know well enough to ask a favor of, but not *too* well. You need a clinician who will be willing to tell you exactly what's wrong, without worrying too much about offending you. (Candor has much to recommend it in a consultant, so try to get someone you know will be frank with you.) Ask someone with a lot of experience interviewing, preferably someone who teaches—perhaps a teacher from your training program, even if you have already graduated. You really need someone who will take the time to listen to (or watch) an entire interview and give you a half-hour or so of feedback on your style. It might even be a clinician of a discipline different from your own; the experience and the perspective are what you're after, not some arbitrary theoretical stance. Such a person is worth a lot to you, especially if you have been experiencing difficulty with many of your interviews.

WHAT YOU'LL LEARN (AND WHAT TO DO ABOUT IT)

Besides forcing you to confront your verbal tics (it's painful, trust me), the methods described above can reveal difficulties across the spectrum of interview behaviors we've discussed. Here are a few that could show up; the page numbers will take you to the sections of this book that discuss the behaviors you should be practicing.

• *Scope of interview too limited.* It is easy to focus on one or two central questions—severe mood disorder and psychosis come to mind— and leave unexplored issues that might seem more peripheral, but are important anyway. Two examples are marital/family problems resulting from substance use, and personality issues, which can complicate just about any major diagnosis. Free speech is one way to ensure wide coverage. Page 19.

• *Insufficient follow-up of cues.* You risk error if you don't explore hints your patient drops. Let's say that your patient mentions in passing, "I was pretty much running wild those years Dad was gone from the family." You might well pursue what the patient means by "running wild," obtaining a lot of information pertinent to conduct disorder and childhood learning difficulties. But will you remember to ask why Dad was out of the family? Whatever you learn—divorce, a jail sentence, admission to a mental hospital, running away with the babysitter—could be important for your diagnosis. Page 52.

• *Inadequate use of open-ended questions.* When you do identify an area for further exploration, the questions you use can prove critical to the amount and quality of the information you obtain. If you hear about being "abused as a child," you might ask a dozen questions about who hit your patient, when, and under what circumstances, and never learn that your patient was suffering from both physical and sexual abuse. As your expert consultant could tell you, a better approach would be first to ask some open-ended question, on the order of "Please tell me more about that." That way, you'd avoid prematurely closing off an important area of inquiry. As a bonus, open-ended questions would be more likely to reveal something about the emotional consequences of these experiences. It is a common fault for interviewers to become so intent on nailing down certain information that they neglect utterly to give patients enough scope to freely divulge their foremost concerns. I see this especially early in interviews, when there isn't enough (or any) time allotted for free speech. Pages 53 and 61.

• *Inappropriate probing.* However, once you've gotten to know what's foremost in your patient's mind, you'll need specific information about these areas of concern. With poorly chosen probes (questions that are too long, too vague, or phrased in the negative), you could bog down in a mire of trivia or get lost down a rhetorical blind alley. "Why . . . " questions invite speculation that may get you exactly nowhere. Instead, focus on probes that encourage precision, brevity, and accuracy. Page 55.

• *Inadequate control of the interview.* A loquacious or hostile patient can reduce your rapport and the amount of information you obtain. Of course, this won't often be a problem; most patients try to cooperate. But your taped interview could make you instantly aware that occasionally, certain patients with character or behavior quirks will fight you for the driver's seat. If you lose that battle, you may find yourself at a destination miles from where you need to be—knowing, perhaps, quite a lot about the patient's disrespectful son-in-law or a spouse's drinking, and too little about the patient's own fears or foibles. Page 110.

• *Poor rapport.* By the time you come to the end of your recording, you should have a pretty good idea of how well you've connected with your patient. You'll know whether you sound warm, whether you respond with interest to features of the story, and whether you express concern when you hear about issues that especially trouble your patient. If you have any doubts, ask your consultant, who can be a lot more objective about a sensitive issue such as this one. Pages 25 and 114.

• *Ignoring the patient.* OK, for the most part *ignoring* is too strong a term. But an initial interview may come to grief because the clinician, so intent on obtaining the needed information, pays too little attention to the patient's needs. The result: As time wears on, the patient becomes more and more restive, and finally bolts from the room before the interview can be completed. Then the bottom line might be no further chance at an interview with this—or perhaps any other—clinician. How much more satisfactory it is to watch for the little signs of increasing concern: jiggling of a leg, twisting of fingers, decreasing eye contact, or increasing hesitation before replying. A timely "It looks to me like you are feeling uncomfortable; how would you like to proceed?" could save the interview, and probably your relationship with this patient. Page 188.

• *No real plan for the interview.* Early in my career, a clinician who had just failed his boards approached me for help. A single practice interview told me that this psychiatrist had gotten though training without ever learning how to obtain the data necessary to support a diagnosis. This clinician needed to use a semistructured interview like that in Appendix D, at least until he was familiar enough with the routine to do without the training wheels. (I hasten to point out that even today, I too use parts of a semistructured interview once in a while, to remind me to inquire into the fine points of a diagnosis or details of a social history.) Page 327.

• *Your excessive talking.* If your recording reveals that you spend a lot of time talking—perhaps asking complicated questions and then having to explain what you mean—you won't be getting the maximum information out of your first interview. Nonverbal encouragements can help; so can carefully formulating your questions. Pages 36 and 55.

• *Negative countertransference.* Sometimes you just don't like a particular patient (or type of patient). Your recorded interview can reveal (perhaps better to your consultant that to you) how your speech and body language reject this patient. This is something that can affect any interviewer, even one who has been at it a long time. But most experienced clinicians learn to put aside their feelings long enough to get the information they need for diagnosis; later on, if necessary, they can refer such a patient for continuing care. It might help you get past some of your feelings if you practice with a colleague playing the role of this sort of patient. Even recognizing your attitude can go a long way toward helping you disguise feelings that, though perfectly normal and understandable, are not acceptable in the context of a mental health evaluation. Page 27.

- *A matter of misunderstanding.* Of course, the patient may not be paying attention, but could it be that your use of clinical jargon creates confusion? Or perhaps you and the patient come from different cultures or speak with different accents. This problem, which nearly every clinician faces at least occasionally, can often be dealt with by frankly discussing your differences and working hard to lower the fences between you. Even when one of you speaks the other's language relatively well, an interpreter may sometimes be useful. Page 30.

- *Time running out.* I almost wrote, "Not managing your time well," but that isn't always the case. Sometimes the story is too complex, the patient comes in late, or the time allotted is too brief to cover completely all the major areas of a mental health history. Then you'll just have to schedule additional evaluation time; getting on with treatment recommendations without as complete a database as possible has, well, little to recommend it. Page 7.

- *Playing favorites with diagnoses.* Here's an actual example, too often repeated: Based on information from the patient's internist, a clinician decides on a diagnosis of major depression and begins antidepressant therapy—drug therapy happens to be this clinician's special area of expertise. Later, when a consultant suggests that this patient could have a form of somatization disorder, the treatment doesn't change. The pattern of the patient's actual symptoms, not your expectations, should determine your diagnosis. Pages 83 and 223.

- *Leaping to conclusions.* There are innumerable areas where this can be a problem, but let's mention one specifically: making a family history diagnosis. The questions you do or don't ask about a relative who was diagnosed with schizophrenia—At what age? What were the symptoms? How long did they last? Did the relative ever recover?—can turn your thinking in the wrong direction about your patient. It's an even slipperier slope if you simply accept a previous clinician's diagnosis of your new patient. Your recorded interview may reveal that you haven't independently verified conclusions relayed to you from patients, relatives, or old records. Page 84.

- *Neglected differential diagnosis.* A clinician forgot to pull together a differential diagnosis that encompassed all the possibilities, no matter how unlikely. As a result, the patient's depression was treated conventionally, without considering the cause that eventually proved at fault: an endocrine disorder. Page 223.

 • *Unfamiliarity with diagnostic criteria.* To nail a diagnosis, the first thing you need is nails. In the case of mental health diagnoses, that means having more than a nodding acquaintance with the current criteria for the various psychoses, anxiety disorders, mood disorders, substance misuse problems, and other likely major mental conditions. That way, you don't forget to ask questions that will allow a firm, accurate diagnosis. Page 274.

 • *Slighting personal and social history.* It is a mistake when general physicians and surgeons don't obtain information pertaining to a patient's personal background; when a mental health professional commits such an error, it has the potential for calamity. Sure, in the chase for symptoms of mania or anxiety disorders, it's easy to forget the quiet issues such as childhood religious background or success in school. Nevertheless, this material can have consequences for diagnosis and treatment, and it is certainly a part of getting to know the patient as a whole person. Page 70.

 • *Ignoring red flags.* The many varied signs and symptoms that could tip you off to a diagnosis may include a hint of childhood abuse, a family history of mania, or a suggestion of drug use. Of course, red flags often turn into red herrings that don't provide material important to a diagnosis, but you'd hate to be the clinician who overlooks one that proves decisive. Page 151.

 • *Leaving feelings out.* Of course it shouldn't ever happen, but of course it sometimes does. In the rush to obtain all the facts of the history, you forget to ask how the patient feels about a given situation, or even about seeing a mental health clinician. This is especially likely in the case of a person who doesn't like to talk about feelings or isn't in touch with them much at all. Page 59.

 • *Tolerating vagueness.* A vague patient is a frustrating patient, as long experience has made me all too aware. Confronted with someone whose speech wanders, it is tempting to relax and let it wash over you. If that's been your reaction to some patients, you've probably come away with less in hand than you need for an accurate diagnosis. Closed-ended questions and repeated requests for precision can help. Page 200.

 • *Neglecting collateral sources.* A good 10% of the time, I learn something about a patient that makes me wonder, "Is the impression I'm receiving correct?" But so often, the press of time seduces us into accepting what appears to be the case, without making use of collateral information. Quite frankly, that's where the marriage and family therapists have the advantage: They always obtain their information from more than one source—a self-correcting process that other clinicians can but envy. Page 181.

There are many other difficulties you could encounter; they are limited only by the number of patients you evaluate. Using one of the methods described earlier, you should be able to learn the source of the problem and, using material from *The First Interview*, figure out an appropriate remedy.

Summary of the Initial Interview

Information	*Process*
Openings and Introductions	
Introduce yourself	Your initial goals
Explain your role in patient's care	Teach respondent role to patient
Outline time, goals of interview	Help patient feel comfortable
Chief Complaint	
Ask why patient came for treatment	Request for chief complaint is directive but open ended
Free Speech	
Allow several minutes for patient to amplify on reasons for coming	Early part of interview is nondirective
Listen for areas of clinical interest	Establish rapport
Difficulty thinking (cognitive disorders)	Adjust your demeanor to patient's needs
Substance use	Monitor your feelings
Psychosis	Show your positive affect clearly
Mood disorders (depression and mania)	Use language patient can comprehend
Anxiety, avoidance behavior, and arousal	Don't criticize patient or others
Physical complaints	Maintain appropriate distance
Social and personality problems	Don't talk about yourself
Summarize presenting problems before moving on	Call patient by title and last name
	Encourage flow with silent encouragements
	Maintain eye contact
	Nod or smile when appropriate
	Verbal encouragements
	"Yes" or "Mm-hmm"
	Repeat patient's own word or words
	Ask for more information
	Re-request information if patient doesn't respond at first
	Briefly summarize

Information	*Process*
	Reassure patient when indicated
	Must be factual, believable
	Use body language
	Correct any misconceptions about physical, mental symptoms

History of the Present Illness

Describe symptoms	Establish the need for truth
Type	It's for patient's benefit and for
Onset and sequence	yours
Severity	Reassure about confidentiality: "If
Frequency	you can't discuss something,
Duration	don't lie; just ask to talk about
Context	something else"
Stressors	General principles
Vegetative symptoms	Restate what patient says to be
Sleep	sure you understand
Appetite and weight	Don't phrase questions in the
Diurnal variation	negative
Previous episodes	Avoid asking double questions
When?	Encourage precision
What symptoms?	Keep questions brief
Recovery complete?	Watch for new leads
Previous treatment	Use terms patient can understand
Type	Probe for details
Compliance	Use direct questions
Wanted effects	Avoid "Why . . . " questions, as a
Side effects	rule
Hospitalizations	Limit to one to two confrontations,
Consequences of illness	late in session:
Marital and sexual	"Help me to understand"
Social	Mix open- and closed-ended requests
Legal	Open-ended increase validity
Job (disability payments?)	Closed-ended increase information
Interests	Elicit feelings best with
Discomfort	Uninterrupted speech
Feelings about symptoms, behavior	Open-ended questions—"Could
Negative and positive	you tell me more about that?"
How does patient cope with	Direct requests for feelings—"Tell
feelings?	me about your depression"
Defense mechanisms	Also obtain feelings with:
Acting out	Express concern or sympathy—"I'd
Denial	feel angry, too"
Devaluation	Reflection of feelings—"You must
Displacement	have felt frantic"
Dissociation	Watch for emotional cues in voice,
Fantasy	body language—"You looked sad
Intellectualization	just now"
Projection	Interpretations—"Sounds like the
Repression	way you felt as a child"

Information	*Process*
Splitting	Analogy—"Did you feel this way
Reaction formation	when your mother died?"
Somatization	Reduce excessive emotionality
Explore areas of clinical interest	Speak softly yourself
	Closed-ended questions
	Redirect comments that change
	topic
	Re-explain what information you
	need
	Ask whether patient understands
	what you want to know
	Break off interview only as last
	resort

Personal and Social History

CHILDHOOD AND GROWING UP	Take charge of interview
Where was the patient born?	Encourage shorter answers with
Number of siblings and sibship	nods and smiles
position	Directly state when you need to
Reared by both parents?	know about something different,
How did parents get along?	but . . .
Did patient feel wanted as a child?	Make an empathic comment first
If adopted:	Raise a finger to interrupt
What circumstances?	Stop taking notes
Extrafamilial?	If steps above don't work:
Health as a child?	Be direct: "We'll have to move on"
Education	Use more closed-ended questions
Last grade completed	Use multiple-choice questions
Scholastic problems?	Transition to new topics
Activity level?	Use patient's own words
School refusal?	Acknowledge an abrupt transition:
Behavior problems in school?	"Let me change the subject,
Suspension or expulsions?	now"
Sociable as child?	Watch for distortion
Age dating began?	Record significant negatives
Sexual development	
Hobbies? Interests?	
	DEALING WITH RESISTANCE
	Do not allow yourself to become
LIFE AS AN ADULT	angry
Living situation	Switch from discussing facts to
Currently with whom?	feelings
Where?	Reject the behavior, accept the
Finances	person
Ever homeless?	Use verbal and nonverbal
Support network	encouragements
Family ties	Focus on patient's interests
Agencies help out?	Express sympathy
Marital	Reassure patient: Feelings are normal
Number of marriages	Emphasize need for complete
Age at each	database

Information	Process
Problems with spouse?	Name the emotion you suspect
Number of children, age, and sex	patient is having
Stepchildren?	If patient is silent, obtain nonverbal
Work history	response first
Current occupation	Focus on less affect-laden model of
Number of jobs lifetime	patient's behavior
Reasons for job changes	If confrontation is used:
Ever fired? Why?	nonjudgmental, nonthreatening
Military	Last resort: Delay the question
Branch, years of service	
Highest rank attained	RISKIER TECHNIQUES
Disciplinary problems?	Offer an excuse for unfavorable
Combat experience?	information: "All that stress
Legal problems ever?	probably made you want to
Civil	drink"
History of violent behavior	Exaggerate negative consequences
Arrests	that didn't happen: "Nobody
Underlying feelings	died, did they?"
Religion: Which? Different from	Induce patient to brag
childhood?	"Any activities for which you could
How religious now?	have been arrested, but
Leisure activities	weren't?"
Clubs, organizations	
Hobbies, interests	
Sexual preference and adjustment	"Please tell me about your sexual
Learning about sex: details	functioning"
First sexual experiences	
Nature	
Age	
Patient's reaction	
Current sexual preference	
Current practices: details	
Pleasures	
Problems	
Birth control methods	
Extramarital partners	
Paraphilias?	
Sexually transmitted diseases?	
Abuse?	Lead into questions of abuse
Childhood molestation	carefully:
Rape	"Were you ever approached for
Spouse abuse	sex?"
	Avoid terms *abuse* and *molestation*
Substance misuse	Assume that all adults will drink
Type of substance	some
Years of use	Ask about past as well as current use
Quantity	
Consequences	
Medical problems	
Loss of control	
Personal and interpersonal	

Information	*Process*
Job	
Legal	
Financial	
Misuse of prescription	
medications?	
Suicide attempts	You can work up to this gradually:
Methods	"Have you ever had any
Consequences	desperate thoughts? Any ideas
Drug or alcohol associated?	of harming yourself?"
Psychological seriousness	
Physical seriousness	
Personality traits	Assess personality by
Evidence of lifelong behavior	Patient's self-report
patterns	Informants
	History of interaction with others
	Your direct observation

FAMILY HISTORY

Mental disorder in close relatives	"Has any blood relative—parent,
Describe parents, siblings, and	brother, sister, grandparent,
patient's relationship with them	child, aunt or uncle, cousin,
Other adults, children in childhood	niece or nephew—ever had any
home	mental illness, including
	depression, mania, psychosis,
	mental hospitalization, severe
	nervousness, substance misuse,
	suicide or suicide attempts,
	criminality?"

MEDICAL HISTORY

Major illnesses	Important for *all* mental health
Operations	workers to obtain
Medications for nonmental problems	
Dose	
Frequency	
Side effects	
Allergies	
To environment	
To medications	
Nonmental hospitalizations	
Childhood physical, sexual abuse?	
Risk factors for AIDS?	
Physical impairments	

REVIEW OF SYSTEMS

Disorders of appetite	Positive responses in these areas have
Head injury	especial relevance to mental
Convulsions	health diagnoses
Unconsciousness	
Premenstrual syndrome	
Specialized review for somatization	See Appendix B
disorder	

Information   *Process*

<u>Mental Status Exam</u>

Appearance
  Apparent age
  Ethnicity
  Body build, posture
  Nutrition
  Clothing: Neat? Clean? Style?
  Hygiene
  Hairstyle
  Body adornments, jewelry?
Alertness: Full? Drowsy? Stupor?
    Coma?
General behavior
  Activity level
  Tremors?
  Mannerisms and stereotypies
  Facial expressions
  Eye contact
  Voice   } Observed while taking history
Attitude toward examiner
Mood
  Type
  Lability
  Appropriateness
  Intensity
Flow of thought
  Word associations
  Rate and rhythm of speech
Content of thought
  Delusions
  Hallucinations
  Anxiety
  Phobias
  Obsessions and compulsions
  Suicide and violence

Orientation: Person? Place? Time?   "Now, I'd like to ask some routine
Language: Comprehension, fluency,   questions ... "
   naming, repetition, reading,
   writing
Memory: Immediate? Short-term?   "How has your memory been? Do
   Long-term?   you mind if I test it?"
Attention and concentration
  Serial sevens
  Count backwards
Cultural information
  Current events
  Five presidents (prime ministers)

Information	*Process*
Abstract thinking	
Proverbs	
Similarities and differences	
Insight	
Judgment	
	Closure
	Summarize findings
	Set next appointment
	"Do you have any questions for
	me?"

Appendix B

Description and Diagnostic Criteria for Selected Disorders

Brief descriptions of the typical symptoms and course are given here for those mental disorders that are not only better studied but, for the most part, common. With the exception of the personality disorders, all of the conditions discussed here are listed on Axis I. At the end of each section I have paraphrased and simplified the DSM-IV-TR criteria, which in the original are often so complicated as to discourage students from using them. For a fuller explanation of diagnostic criteria, see my book *DSM-IV Made Easy*.

I have substituted bullets (•) and checks (✓) for the numbering system in the original criteria. Bulleted criteria are mandatory and must be fulfilled. Checked items are part of a list and are selective—only a certain number of these must be fulfilled to qualify for the diagnoses.

MOOD DISORDERS

Depression is a disorder of mood in which the patient feels abnormally low-spirited, down in the dumps, sometimes melancholic. The patient has sensations of great distress and of mood being out of control, and often has suicidal ideas. Depression can take a number of forms, each of which has been given a name—and sometimes several alternative names. These forms of depression are often overlapping, so that a given patient may actually be classifiable into more than one category. Here I'll give prominent features of the more important varieties of depression.

Major Depressive Episode

A major depressive episode simply means that the patient has depressive symptoms and that they are more severe than if they are due to dysthymia. These patients usually describe themselves as feeling depressed, but sometimes all they can identify is a feeling of irritability or a loss of enjoyment or interest in usually pleasurable activities. In any case, there is a definite change from the patient's previous level of functioning. Depressed patients typically complain of associated symptoms, including increased or decreased appetite, often with consequent gain or loss of weight; increased or decreased sleep; agitation; psychomotor retardation; fatigue or decreased energy; feelings of worthlessness or guilt; trouble concentrating; and thoughts of death, death wishes, and suicidal ideas. Often there is diurnal variation of mood, with a patient feeling better in the morning or at night.

These symptoms may be mild, perhaps resulting in only minor inconvenience; when depression is severe, sometimes to the point of psychosis, melancholia may be diagnosed. Perhaps 25% of depressed patients also have episodes of mania. A major depressive episode can be experienced as a unipolar depression (major depressive disorder, either single episode or recurrent) or as a component of bipolar I or bipolar II disorder.

Abbreviated Criteria for Major Depressive Episode

- Depressed mood or loss of interest or pleasure that represents a change from previous functioning for 2 weeks, plus at least five of the following symptoms:
  - ✓ Depressed mood
  - ✓ Loss of interest or pleasure
  - ✓ Marked weight gain or loss, or change in appetite
  - ✓ Insomnia or excessive sleep
  - ✓ Psychomotor agitation or retardation
  - ✓ Fatigue or loss of energy
  - ✓ Feelings of worthlessness or excessive guilt
  - ✓ Indecisiveness or loss of concentration
  - ✓ Recurring thoughts of death or suicidal ideas or attempt
- The mood disorder is not due to bereavement, medical disease, or substance use.
- The symptoms cause distress or impair functioning.

Melancholia

Because patients and clinicians are unlikely to associate the severe form of depression known as melancholia with a precipitating stressor, it has sometimes been called *endogenous depression.* (Its official DSM-IV-TR designation is major depressive episode with melancholic features.) These patients may have multiple episodes of depression from which they recover completely; they are likely to have relatives who have also suffered from depression. When ill, they take little pleasure in their usual activities and may not cheer up when with people whose company they normally enjoy. They may awaken early in the morning, well before it is time to arise, and they feel worst at that time of day. They may eat little, and they sometimes experience profound weight loss. They may have little insight into the fact that they are ill: Even if they have recovered completely from previous episodes, they may strenuously deny that recovery is a likely outcome. As a result, they are at severe risk for suicide attempt; untreated, perhaps 15% ultimately kill themselves.

Abbreviated Criteria for Melancholia

- When major depressive episode is at its worst, the patient loses all pleasure or feels no better when good things happen.
- The patient has at least three of the following:
  ✓ Depression worse in the morning
  ✓ Early morning awakening
  ✓ Psychomotor retardation or agitation
  ✓ Loss of appetite or weight loss
  ✓ Excessive guilt feelings
  ✓ Different quality of depressed mood from what one would experience at loss of a loved one

Dysthymia

Compared with those of major depression, the symptoms of dysthymia are less severe but last longer. In the past, this disorder has sometimes been called *characterological depression* or *depressive personality.* Dysthymic patients often seem depressed throughout their lives. Although they remain able to work and take care of themselves and their families, typically they don't much enjoy life. They have some of the same symptoms found in major depression and melancholia, but the symptoms are fewer and less severe.

Abbreviated Criteria for Dysthymia

- Depressed mood most days for 2 or more years, with at least two of the following:
  ✓ Appetite decreased or increased
  ✓ Insomnia or excessive sleeping

✓ Low energy or fatigue
✓ Low self-esteem
✓ Poor concentration or indecisiveness
✓ Feelings of hopelessness

- No major depression, but never without symptoms longer than 2 months during the 2 years.
- Symptoms cause clinically important distress or impair functioning.
- Has never had cyclothymia or a manic, hypomanic, or mixed episode.
- Symptoms not caused by a medical condition, substance use, or a psychosis.

Manic Episode

Patients with mania usually have a sudden onset of euphoric or irritable mood that is accompanied by overactivity and excessive speech. They are easily distractible, need less sleep than usual, and become involved in grandiose plans and schemes. As they become sicker, they lose insight, and their judgment deteriorates. They say or do things they later regret: They may become sexually promiscuous, spend money they do not have, or make other problematic decisions. Many drink excessively. They feel abnormally strong or powerful and may become deluded that they have special powers or have a special religious purpose. Most manic patients also have episodes of depression, sometimes alternating regularly with the high phases; this pattern is diagnosed as bipolar I disorder. Even without treatment, most eventually recover completely.

Abbreviated Criteria for Manic Episode

- At least 1 week of euphoria or irritability (less if hospitalization is needed), with at least three of these symptoms:
  ✓ Grandiosity
  ✓ Reduced need for sleep
  ✓ Increased talkativeness
  ✓ Racing thoughts or speech
  ✓ Easy distractibility
  ✓ Heightened activity or agitation
  ✓ Poor judgment (spending sprees, sexual indiscretions)
- Symptoms cause distress, psychosis, hospitalization, or impaired functioning.
- The symptoms aren't caused by a medical illness or by the use of substances.

PSYCHOTIC DISORDERS

The Schizophrenias

Although the schizophrenias are usually spoken of as a singular disease, in reality this category probably includes several different disorders.

Although some of these patients seem perfectly normal before the onset of the actual schizophrenia symptoms, many of them were introverted social loners as children. Many would qualify for a diagnosis of schizotypal or schizoid personality disorder.

The disease process itself usually begins early in life—late teens or early 20s—and develops gradually over a period of many months. There is usually a prodrome during which the individual may become interested in philosophy, religion, or witchcraft; anxiety or perplexity may be the predominant affect. Isolation may increase, and relatives or friends may note various behaviors that are peculiar, although not exactly psychotic.

Gradually hallucinations (most often auditory) begin, becoming ever more insistent; delusions (especially persecutory) usually develop. As the patient becomes preoccupied with inner feelings and experiences, ability to function at work or school falls off. It may be only at this stage that relatives notice a change in the patient. Affect may become blunted, silly, or inconsequential. Thought associations are often loose. Patients can lose impulse control and, when markedly agitated, sometimes become violent. Although orientation is usually retained, insight is typically lost, and judgment is severely impaired. The disorder is chronic: Though treatment with antipsychotic medicine can reduce or eliminate psychotic symptoms, few patients recover to their premorbid levels of functioning.

Patients with schizophrenia are usually given a subtype diagnosis. In *paranoid schizophrenia*, delusions and auditory hallucinations are the prominent symptoms; onset is often at a later age (mid-30s or after) than with the remaining subtypes. In *catatonic schizophrenia*, there are prominent disorders of motion: stupor, negativism, rigidity, excitement, and posturing. Delusions and hallucinations may be present, but these are less prominent than in the paranoid subtype. In *disorganized schizophrenia*, the principal symptoms are marked loosening of associations and flat or inappropriate affect. Patients with *undifferentiated schizophrenia*, though psychotic (they have delusions, hallucinations, incoherent speech, or markedly disorganized behavior), do not obviously fall into any of the previous three categories. Those with *residual schizophrenia* are not currently psychotic but have residual symptoms (see "Duration" in the criteria list below).

Warning: Schizophrenia today has carefully delineated symptoms, so it shouldn't be overdiagnosed. But until a few years ago it was common to see patients with severe depression, mania, personality disorder, or organic psychoses misdiagnosed as having schizophrenia. Patients who for many years have carried the diagnosis of schizophrenia should be periodically reassessed.

Abbreviated Criteria for Schizophrenia

- Symptoms. [DSM-IV-TR refers to these as the "A" criteria.] For most of at least 1 month, the patient has had two or more of the following:
  ✓ Delusions (only one symptom is required if a delusion is bizarre, such as being abducted in a spaceship from the sun)
  ✓ Hallucinations (only one symptom is required if hallucinations are of at least two voices talking to one another or of a voice that keeps up a running commentary on the patient's thoughts or actions)
  ✓ Speech that shows incoherence, derailment, or other disorganization
  ✓ Severely disorganized or catatonic behavior
  ✓ Any negative symptom, such as flat affect, reduced speech, or lack of volition
- Duration. For at least 6 continuous months, the patient has shown some evidence of the disorder. At least 1 month must include the symptoms of frank psychosis mentioned above. During the balance of this time (either as a prodrome or a residual effect of the illness), the patient must show *either* or *both* of the following:
  ✓ Negative symptoms as mentioned above
  ✓ In attenuated form, at least two of the other symptoms mentioned above (example: deteriorating personal hygiene plus an increasing suspicion that people are talking behind one's back)
- Dysfunction. For much of this time, the disorder has materially impaired the patient's ability to work, study, socialize, or provide self-care.
- The duration of any depressive or manic episodes that have occurred during the psychotic phase has been brief.
- This disorder is not directly caused by a general medical condition or the use of substances, including prescription medications.

Delusional Disorder

Patients with delusional disorder have delusions that are not bizarre but don't qualify for other psychotic diagnoses, such as schizophrenia or organic psychosis. Once this illness strikes, it tends to become chronic. There is good preservation of mood and ability to communicate; if employed, these people remain able to work. They do have trouble in the social sphere, however, and members of their families often instigate the referral for treatment. Several distinct types of delusional disorder have been described.

Erotomanic. This is characterized by the belief that someone (often some-

one famous or of higher social station) is in love with the patient. These patients sometimes make the news for following or otherwise harassing public
figures.

Grandiose. These people believe that they have some special ability or insight; they may believe they have invented something of great value. As a result,
they sometimes haunt various government agencies (patent office, police) in an
effort to pursue their plans.

Persecutory. The patient (or a close associate) is being intentionally
cheated, drugged, followed, slandered, or otherwise mistreated.

Jealous. Most often, these individuals believe that a spouse is being
unfaithful—an idea they may pursue by following the spouse or confronting
the supposed lover.

Somatic. These patients often seek medical help for a belief that they have
a foul body odor, parasites, or infestation of insects on or under the skin, or
that some body part is misshapen.

Mixed. The patient has two or more of the themes above in about equal
portions.

Unspecified.

Abbreviated Criteria for Delusional Disorder

- Nonbizarre delusions (that is, they could really happen) of a type listed
  above for at least 1 month.
- The patient has never met the "A" criteria for schizophrenia (except
  that hallucinations of touch or smell may be present if they are related
  to the theme of the delusions).
- Other than as it relates to the delusion, behavior is not peculiar.
- Any mood symptoms have been brief as compared to the duration of
  delusions.
- The disorder is not directly caused by a medical illness or substance
  use.

Substance-Induced Psychotic Disorder

The category of substance-induced psychotic disorder includes all psychoses
caused by misuse of substances. The predominant symptoms are usually hallucinations or delusions, and they can occur during withdrawal or acute intoxication, depending on the drug. Usually the course is brief. Classic examples of
this disorder are alcoholic auditory hallucinosis and the delusional state that
sometimes accompanies chronic amphetamine use. The psychotic symptoms
may be indistinguishable from those of paranoid schizophrenia. Marijuana, cocaine, hallucinogens, inhalants, opioids, phencyclidine (PCP), and sedatives/
hypnotics have also been implicated in these conditions.

Abbreviated Criteria for Substance Induced Psychotic Disorder

- Prominent hallucinations or delusions (don't include hallucinations the patient realizes are caused by substance use).
- These symptoms have developed within a month of substance intoxication or withdrawal, *or* medication use has caused the symptoms.
- Another psychotic disorder doesn't better explain the symptoms.
- They don't occur solely during a delirium.

SUBSTANCE-RELATED DISORDERS

The terminology keeps changing, but the disorders themselves remain the same: alcohol and drug misuse. The early 21st century presents an ever-widening variety of substances, whose use leads to a few common problems that we'll outline in this section. For any of them, the diagnostician must specify the substances responsible.

Abbreviated Criteria for Dependence

- Distress or impairment, as shown in a single 12-month period by three or more of the following:
  - ✓ Tolerance, shown by either of these:
    - ✓ Markedly increased intake of the substance is needed to achieve the same effect, *or*
    - ✓ With continued use, the same amount of the substance has markedly less effect.
  - ✓ Withdrawal, shown by either of these:
    - ✓ The substance's characteristic withdrawal syndrome is present, *or*
    - ✓ The substance (or one closely related) is used to avoid or relieve withdrawal symptoms.
  - ✓ The amount or duration of use is often greater than intended.
  - ✓ The patient repeatedly tries without success to control substance use.
  - ✓ The patient spends much time obtaining or using the substance.
  - ✓ The patient reduces important activities because of substance use.
  - ✓ The patient continues use despite knowing that the substance has probably caused physical or psychological problems.

Abbreviated Criteria for Intoxication

- Reversible syndrome due to recent use of or exposure to a substance.
- Maladaptive behavioral or psychological changes during or shortly after using the substance.
- The syndrome is not caused by a medical illness or a different mental disorder.

ALCOHOL INTOXICATION

- Behavioral or psychological changes that include inappropriate sexuality or aggression, lability of mood, impaired judgment, and impaired functioning.
- At least one of the following:
  - ✓ Slurred speech
  - ✓ Incoordination
  - ✓ Unsteady gait
  - ✓ Nystagmus
  - ✓ Impaired attention or memory
  - ✓ Coma or stupor

AMPHETAMINE INTOXICATION

- Behavioral or psychological changes that include blunted affect, hypervigilance, interpersonal sensitivity, anger, anxiety or tension, changes in sociability, stereotyped behaviors, impaired judgment, and impaired functioning.
- Shortly after using, at least two of the following:
  - ✓ Slowed or rapid heart rate
  - ✓ Dilated pupils
  - ✓ Raised or lowered blood pressure
  - ✓ Chills or sweating
  - ✓ Nausea or vomiting
  - ✓ Weight loss
  - ✓ Psychomotor agitation or retardation
  - ✓ Muscle weakness, shallow or slowed breathing, chest pain, or heart arrhythmias
  - ✓ Coma, confusion, dyskinesias, dystonias, or seizures

CAFFEINE INTOXICATION

- Shortly after using, at least five of these:
  - ✓ Restlessness
  - ✓ Nervousness
  - ✓ Excitement
  - ✓ Insomnia
  - ✓ Red face
  - ✓ Increased urination
  - ✓ Gastrointestinal upset
  - ✓ Muscle twitching

✓ Rambling speech
✓ Rapid or irregular heartbeat
✓ Periods of tirelessness
✓ Increased psychomotor activity

CANNABIS INTOXICATION

- Behavioral or psychological changes that include anxiety, euphoria, impaired judgment, social withdrawal, and the sensation that time has slowed down.
- Within 2 hours of using, at least two of the following:
  ✓ Red eyes
  ✓ Increased appetite
  ✓ Dry mouth
  ✓ Rapid heart rate

COCAINE INTOXICATION. Identical to amphetamine intoxication (see above).

HALLUCINOGEN INTOXICATION

- Behavioral or psychological changes that include anxiety, depression, ideas of reference, fear of becoming insane, persecutory ideas, impaired judgment, and impaired functioning.
- Perceptual changes (depersonalization, derealization, illusions, hallucinations, synesthesias, and subjective intensification of experience).
- Shortly after use, two or more of these:
  ✓ Dilated pupils
  ✓ Rapid heart rate
  ✓ Sweating
  ✓ Irregular heartbeat
  ✓ Blurred vision
  ✓ Tremors
  ✓ Incoordination

INHALANT INTOXICATION

- Behavioral or psychological changes that include apathy, assertiveness or belligerence, impaired judgment, and impaired functioning.
- Two or more of these:
  ✓ Dizziness
  ✓ Nystagmus

✓ Poor coordination
✓ Slurred speech
✓ Unsteady walking
✓ Lethargy
✓ Diminished reflexes
✓ Psychomotor retardation
✓ Blurred or double vision
✓ Tremors
✓ Generalized muscle weakness
✓ Stupor or coma
✓ Euphoria

OPIOID INTOXICATION

- Behavioral or psychological changes that include euphoria leading to apathy, depression, anxiety, psychomotor agitation or retardation, impaired judgment, and impaired functioning.
- Constricted pupils (or dilation due to brain damage following a severe overdose) and one or more of the following:
  ✓ Drowsiness or coma
  ✓ Slurred speech
  ✓ Impaired memory or attention

PCP INTOXICATION

- Behavioral or psychological changes that include assault, belligerence, impulsivity, agitation, unpredictability, impaired judgment, and impaired job or social functioning.
- Within an hour (less, if PCP is snorted, smoked, or used intravenously), two or more of these:
  ✓ Nystagmus
  ✓ Rapid heartbeat or high blood pressure
  ✓ Numbness or decreased response to pain
  ✓ Trouble walking
  ✓ Trouble speaking
  ✓ Rigid muscles
  ✓ Coma or seizures
  ✓ Abnormally acute hearing

SEDATIVE, HYPNOTIC, OR ANXIOLYTIC INTOXICATION. Identical to alcohol intoxication (see above).

Abbreviated Criteria for Withdrawal

- A syndrome specific to a substance develops when someone who has used it frequently and for a long time stops or markedly reduces its intake.
- This syndrome causes clinically important distress or impairs work, social, or other functioning.
- This syndrome is neither the result of a medical illness nor better explained by a different mental disorder.

ALCOHOL WITHDRAWAL (UNCOMPLICATED)

- Two or more of the following develop:
  - ✓ Autonomic overactivity (sweating or rapid heartbeat)
  - ✓ Worsened tremor of hands
  - ✓ Insomnia
  - ✓ Nausea or vomiting
  - ✓ Short-lived hallucinations or illusions (visual, tactile, or auditory)
  - ✓ Increased psychomotor activity
  - ✓ Anxiety
  - ✓ Grand mal seizures

AMPHETAMINE WITHDRAWAL

- Dysphoric mood and two or more of the following:
  - ✓ Fatigue
  - ✓ Unpleasant, vivid dreams
  - ✓ Hypersomnia or insomnia
  - ✓ Increased appetite
  - ✓ Increased or reduced psychomotor activity

COCAINE WITHDRAWAL Identical to amphetamine withdrawal (see above).

HALLUCINOGEN PERSISTING PERCEPTION DISORDER (FLASHBACKS)

- After stopping use of a hallucinogen, at least one of the symptoms of perception that occurred during intoxication recurs. These could include flashes of color, trails of images, afterimages, halos, macropsia, micropsia, geometric hallucinations, and false peripheral perception of movement.

NICOTINE WITHDRAWAL

- Four or more of the following:
  - ✓ Dysphoria or depression
  - ✓ Insomnia
  - ✓ Anger, frustration, or irritability
  - ✓ Anxiety
  - ✓ Trouble concentrating
  - ✓ Restlessness
  - ✓ Slowed heart rate
  - ✓ Increased appetite or weight

OPIOID WITHDRAWAL

- Three or more of these:
  - ✓ Dysphoria
  - ✓ Nausea or vomiting
  - ✓ Aching muscles
  - ✓ Tearing or runny nose
  - ✓ Dilated pupils, piloerection, or sweating
  - ✓ Diarrhea
  - ✓ Yawning
  - ✓ Fever
  - ✓ Insomnia

SEDATIVE, HYPNOTIC, OR ANXIOLYTIC WITHDRAWAL   Identical to alcohol withdrawal (see above).

COGNITIVE DISORDERS

Cognitive disorders are behavioral or psychological abnormalities that are associated with temporary or permanent brain dysfunctions. The cause can be an abnormality of brain structure, chemistry, or physiology; it is not always known. Cognitive disorders are recognized by impairment in four main areas: intellectual functioning, judgment, memory, and orientation. Patients may also have abnormalities of mood and impulse control. Most such conditions can be broadly categorized as either delirium or dementia.

Delirium

Delirium usually begins acutely. Patients cannot focus or maintain their attention and are easily distractible; they may have either increased or decreased motor activity. Their thought processes slow down; they have trouble solving problems and reasoning. Visual hallucinations may confuse them so that they cannot tell whether they are dreaming or awake. They may accept these hallucinations as reality, thereby experiencing anxiety or fear; sometimes they attempt to run away. All symptoms may worsen at night—a phenomenon called *sundowning*. Later recall for the foregoing symptoms may be spotty or nil.

The causes of delirium include endocrine disorder, infection, brain tumor, cessation of alcohol intake, drug toxicity, vitamin deficiency, fever, seizures, liver or kidney disease, poisons, and the effects of surgical operations. Often multiple causes contribute to a single episode. Delirium tends to begin acutely and to fluctuate in intensity. Usually short-lived, it resolves once the underlying condition has been relieved.

Abbreviated Criteria for Delirium

- Reduced level of consciousness, as well as difficulty focusing, shifting, or sustaining attention.
- Cognitive change (deficit of language, memory, orientation, perception) that a dementia cannot better explain.
- These symptoms develop rapidly (hours to days) and tend to vary during the day.
- History, physical examination, or laboratory data suggest that medical illnesses or substance use (or some combination) has directly caused the condition.

Demontia

The cardinal feature of dementia is loss of memory, beginning with recent memory and, as the dementia worsens, involving more remote memories. Patients with dementia show loss of ability to think and to remember that is severe enough to interfere with work and social life. Dementias may be transient, but more often they persist and progress, often to the point that patients show impaired judgment and abstract thinking. Severely demented patients may not recognize family members; sometimes they get lost in their own homes. Failure of judgment and of impulse control can lead to loss of the social graces, as shown by making crude jokes or by inattention to personal hygiene. Use of language is usually spared until late in the disease.

Onset is usually insidious, and the misconceptions (hallucinations or illusions) so common in delirium are often absent, especially early in the process. Usually an organic cause can be identified. A few causes (subdural hematoma, normal-pressure hydrocephalus, hypothyroidism) can be successfully treated, leading to full recovery from the dementia symptoms. Causes include primary diseases of the central nervous system, such as Alzheimer's disease, Huntington's disease, multiple sclerosis, and Parkinson's disease; infectious diseases, such as neurosyphilis and AIDS; vitamin deficiencies; tumors; trauma; and various diseases of liver, lungs, and the endocrine and cardiovascular systems. Dementias are found mainly in older patients, and the course is usually one of chronic deterioration.

Abbreviated Criteria for Dementia

- Impaired memory (can't learn new information or can't recall information previously learned), *plus*
- At least one of the following:
  - ✓ Aphasia (problems using language)
  - ✓ Apraxia (trouble carrying out motor activity despite intact motor functioning)
  - ✓ Agnosia (despite intact sensory functioning, the patient fails to recognize or identify objects)
  - ✓ Impaired executive functioning (problems abstracting, organizing, planning, or sequencing information)
- Each of these symptoms impairs work or social functioning.
- The decline in mental functioning begins gradually and worsens steadily.
- These impairments don't occur solely during a delirium, and they aren't better explained by another Axis I disorder, such as depression or schizophrenia.
- There is evidence of cause by substance use or a medical illness (including Alzheimer's disease).

Amnestic Disorder

The most common cause of amnestic disorder is chronic alcohol use with resultant vitamin B_1 (thiamine) deficiency; in such cases, the condition is popularly known as *Korsakoff's psychosis*. Patients with amnestic disorder rather suddenly lose short-term memory, sometimes to the extent that they cannot recall events that took place scant minutes earlier. Remote memory is usually less involved. Many patients confabulate information spontaneously or in response to prompting ("Didn't I see you in the bar last night?"). Recovery can occur, although chronicity is more the rule.

Abbreviated Criteria for Amnestic Disorder

- Impaired memory (inability to learn new information or to recall information previously learned).
- These symptoms materially impair functioning, and they represent a decline in the patient's previous level of functioning.

- These symptoms don't occur solely during a delirium or dementia.
- There is evidence of cause by substance use or a medical illness.

ANXIETY DISORDERS

Warning: Many mentally ill patients have anxiety symptoms as a part of their over-all complaints. It is important not to let anxiety symptoms, which may be presenting complaints of many patients, obscure underlying diagnoses that may be more important for diagnosis and treatment. In this regard, be especially alert for the presence of depressive syndromes and substance-related disorders.

Generalized Anxiety Disorder

Patients with generalized anxiety disorder seem chronically and unreasonably worried about multiple life circumstances. Some authorities believe that this condition affects as many as 5% of the general population; others hold that it is often misdiagnosed when another, more specific anxiety disorder or some other Axis I or Axis II disorder is responsible for a patient's symptoms. When present, it usually starts in early adulthood; women are affected about twice as often as men. It may be encountered especially in the practices of internists and general practitioners.

Abbreviated Criteria for Generalized Anxiety Disorder

- For the majority of days during 6 months, the patient is anxious or worried about several events or activities.
- The patient has trouble controlling these feelings.
- Associated with this anxiety and worry, at least five of the following symptoms are frequently present:
  ✓ Feeling restless, edgy, keyed up
  ✓ Tiring easily
  ✓ Trouble concentrating
  ✓ Irritability
  ✓ Increased muscle tension
  ✓ Trouble sleeping (initial insomnia or restless, unrefreshing sleep)
- Aspects of another Axis I disorder do not provide the focus of the anxiety and worry.
- The symptoms cause distress or impair functioning.
- The disorder is not directly caused by a medical illness or by substance use.
- It does not occur only during a mood disorder, psychotic disorder, posttraumatic stress disorder, or pervasive developmental disorder.

Panic Attack and Panic Disorder

Panic attacks are discrete episodes of anxiety without identifiable cause. When they occur more than once (or a patient is afraid they will), we say that the patient has panic disorder. Panic disorder affects perhaps 2% of all adults; it has a strong genetic component and may be somewhat more common in women than in men. Although it can start at any age, it usually develops in young adults. It is often associated with agoraphobia.

Abbreviated Criteria for Panic Attack

- Sudden severe fear or discomfort that peaks within 10 minutes.
- During this discrete episode, four or more of the following symptoms occur:
  - ✓ Chest pain or other chest discomfort
  - ✓ Chills or hot flashes
  - ✓ Choking sensation
  - ✓ Derealization (feeling unreal) or depersonalization (feeling detached from self)
  - ✓ Dizzy, lightheaded, faint, or unsteady sensations
  - ✓ Fear of dying
  - ✓ Fear of loss of control or becoming insane
  - ✓ Heart pounding, racing, or skipping beats
  - ✓ Nausea or other abdominal discomfort
  - ✓ Numbness or tingling
  - ✓ Sweating
  - ✓ Shortness of breath or smothering sensation
  - ✓ Trembling

Abbreviated Criteria for Panic Disorder

- The patient has recurrent panic attacks that are not expected.
- For a month or more after an attack, the patient has had one or more of the following:
  - ✓ Ongoing concern that there will be more attacks
  - ✓ Worry as to the significance of the attack or its consequences (for health, control, sanity)
  - ✓ Change in behavior, such as doing something to avoid or combat the attacks
- The panic attacks are not directly caused by a medical condition or by substance use.
- They are not better explained by another anxiety or mental disorder.

Agoraphobia

Agoraphobia originally meant "fear of the marketplace," but it now comprises fears of being any place where escape might be difficult or help might not be available. The patient is therefore unable to leave home or needs a companion to do so, or suffers discomfort when away from home. Relatively uncommon (perhaps 1 in 200 adults), agoraphobia is more common in women. Often it begins early in life following a panic attack or a traumatic event. Most patients with agoraphobia also have panic attacks. Agoraphobia that occurs by itself is diagnosed as agoraphobia without history of panic disorder.

Abbreviated Criteria for Agoraphobia

- The patient has anxiety about being in a place or situation from which escape is difficult or embarrassing, or where help might not be available if a panic attack occurred.
- The patient:
  ✓ Avoids these situations or places (restricting travel), *or*
  ✓ Endures them with distress (a panic attack might occur), *or*
  ✓ Requires a companion when in the situation.
- Other mental disorders don't explain the symptoms better.

Obsessive–Compulsive Disorder

Obsessive–compulsive disorder is a well-studied illness that begins in the teens or 20s and often persists lifelong. It is characterized by ideas or impulses that come unbidden into the patient's awareness, accompanied by anxiety or dread. These feelings are experienced as foreign (ego-alien), silly, or irrational, and the patient tries to resist having them. The main compulsive patterns include handwashing, cleaning, and compulsive checking to be sure that some action (such as turning off the stove) has in fact been accomplished. Symptoms of depression are common.

Abbreviated Criteria for Obsessive–Compulsive Disorder

- The patient has obsessions or compulsions or both.
  ✓ Obsessions. The patient must have all of the following:
    - Recurring, persisting thoughts, impulses, or images inappropriately intrude into awareness and cause marked distress or anxiety.
    - These ideas are not just excessive worries about ordinary problems.

- The patient tries to ignore or suppress these ideas or to neutralize them by thoughts or behavior.
- There is insight that these ideas are products of the patient's own mind.

✓ Compulsions. The patient must have all of the following:
  - There is a need to repeat physical behaviors (checking, handwashing) or mental behaviors (counting things, silently repeating words).
  - These behaviors occur as a response to an obsession or in accordance with strict rules.
  - These behaviors seek to reduce distress or to prevent something that is dreaded.
  - These behaviors either are not realistically related to the events they are supposed to counteract or are clearly excessive for that purpose.
- During some part of the illness, the patient recognizes that the obsessions or compulsions are unreasonable or excessive.
- The obsessions and/or compulsions cause severe distress, take up more than an hour per day, or interfere with the patient's usual routine or functioning.
- If the patient has another Axis I disorder, the content of obsessions or compulsions is not restricted to it.
- The symptoms are not directly caused by a medical illness or by substance use.

Posttraumatic Stress Disorder

Posttraumatic stress disorder is a modern term comprising what was formerly called *shellshock* in soldiers and the reactions of civilians to rape or any major naturally occurring or human-made calamity, such as earthquakes and airplane crashes. Three major features characterize this syndrome: (1) persistent reliving of the traumatic event through dreams or waking thoughts, (2) avoiding human relationships or reminders of the event, and (3) symptoms of hyperarousal. Development of symptoms may be delayed for weeks or years, and they often fluctuate over time; their severity is usually proportional to the intensity of the traumatic event. The condition is more likely to occur in children, elderly persons, and those who are socially isolated.

Abbreviated Criteria for Posttraumatic Stress Disorder

- The patient has experienced or witnessed an unusually traumatic event that has both of these elements:
  - The event involved actual or threatened death or serious physical injury to the patient or to others, *and*
  - The patient felt intense fear, horror, or helplessness.

- The patient repeatedly relives the event in at least one of the following ways:
  - ✓ Intrusive, distressing recollections (thoughts images)
  - ✓ Repeated, distressing dreams
  - ✓ Through flashbacks, hallucinations, or illusions, feeling or acting as if the event were recurring
  - ✓ Marked mental distress in reaction to cues that evoke the event
  - ✓ Physiological reactivity (rapid heartbeat, elevated blood pressure) in response to these cues
- The patient repeatedly avoids the trauma-related stimuli and has numbing of general responsiveness, as shown by three or more of the following:
  - ✓ Tries to avoid thoughts, feelings, or conversations concerned with the event
  - ✓ Tries to avoid activities, people, or places that recall the event
  - ✓ Cannot recall an important feature of the event
  - ✓ Exhibits marked loss of interest or participation in activities important to the patient
  - ✓ Feels detached or isolated from other people
  - ✓ Is restricted in ability to love or feel other strong emotions
  - ✓ Feels life will be brief or unfulfilled (lack of marriage, job, children)
- The patient has at least two of the following symptoms of hyperarousal that were not previously present:
  - ✓ Insomnia (initial or interval)
  - ✓ Irritability
  - ✓ Poor concentration
  - ✓ Hypervigilance
  - ✓ Increased startle response
- The symptoms above have lasted longer than 1 month.
- These symptoms cause distress or impair functioning.

ANOREXIA NERVOSA

Patients with anorexia nervosa feel they are overweight when they are not. As a result, they severely limit food intake to the point of severe weight loss, malnutrition, and (in females) the cessation of normal menses. They may abuse diuretics and laxatives; sometimes they will vomit to maintain low weight. Severe symptoms can lead to death. This disorder is relatively common (up to 0.5%) among young females; recent information suggests that it occurs about one-tenth that often in young males.

Abbreviated Criteria for Anorexia Nervosa

- Refusal to maintain a minimum body weight (at least 85% of expected weight).
- Despite being underweight, the patient intensely fears becoming fat.
- Self-perception of the body is abnormal, as shown by at least one of the following:
  - Unduly emphasizes weight or shape in self-evaluation
  - Denies seriousness of low weight
  - Has a distorted perception of own body shape or weight
- Due to weight loss, a female patient has missed at least three consecutive periods.

SOMATIZATION DISORDER

Affecting perhaps 1% of adult women (rare in men), somatization disorder is characterized by multiple somatic complaints. Suspect it in any woman who presents a complicated or vague history; responds poorly to treatment; is dramatic, demanding, or seductive; has a family history of personality disorder; was abused sexually as a child; misuses substances; or has depression with unusual features. Many of these patients attempt suicide. This diagnosis is often overlooked even by mental health professionals.

Abbreviated Criteria for Somatization Disorder

- Starting before age 30, the patient has many physical complaints occurring over several years.
- The patient has sought treatment for these symptoms, or they have materially impaired work, social, or personal functioning.
- The patient has at some time experienced at least eight symptoms from the following list, distributed as noted. These symptoms need not be concurrent.
  - *Pain symptoms* (four or more) related to different sites (such as head, abdomen, back, joints, extremities, chest, or rectum) or body functions (such as menstruation, sexual intercourse, or urination).
  - *Gastrointestinal symptoms* (two or more, excluding pain), such as nausea, bloating, vomiting (not during pregnancy), diarrhea, intolerance of several foods.
  - *Sexual symptoms* (at least one, excluding pain), including indifference to sex, difficulties with erection or ejaculation, irregular menses, excessive menstrual bleeding, vomiting throughout all 9 months of pregnancy.

- *Pseudoneurological symptoms* (at least one), including impaired balance or coordination, weak or paralyzed muscles, lump in throat or trouble swallowing, loss of voice, retention of urine, hallucinations, numbness (to touch or pain), double vision, blindness, deafness, seizures, amnesia or other dissociative symptoms, loss of consciousness (other than with fainting). None of these is limited to pain.
- For each of the symptoms above, one of these conditions must be met:
  - ✓ Physical or laboratory investigation determines that the symptom cannot be fully explained by a general medical condition or by substance use, including medications and drugs of abuse.
  - ✓ If the patient does have a general medical condition, the impairment or complaints exceed what you would expect based on history, laboratory findings, or physical examination.
- The patient doesn't consciously feign the symptoms for material gain (malingering) or to occupy the sick role (factitious disorder).

PERSONALITY DISORDERS

Currently, 10 personality disorders are recognized in DSM-IV-TR (more are waiting in the wings for inclusion); they are divided into three clusters. Of these 10, 5 have been reasonably well studied and therefore have greater validity than the rest. These 5, which are further described below, are italicized in the following outline. In all personality disorders, the attitudes and behaviors are present from early adult life and are experienced in a variety of situations

Cluster A comprises patients who can be described as withdrawn, cold, suspicious, or irrational. Cluster A includes paranoid, *schizoid*, and *schizotypal* personality disorders.

In Cluster B are patients who tend to be dramatic, emotional, and attention-seeking; their moods are labile and often shallow. They often have intense interpersonal conflicts. Cluster B includes *antisocial*, *borderline*, histrionic, and narcissistic personality disorders.

Patients in Cluster C tend to be anxious and tense, often overcontrolled. This cluster includes avoidant, dependent, and *obsessive–compulsive* personality disorders.

Schizoid Personality Disorder

Schizoid personality disorder usually begins in childhood or teens. These patients relate poorly to others and show a restricted emotional range. Typically they are lifelong loners who feel little need to associate with other people. They appear unsociable, cold, and seclusive, and they may succeed at solitary jobs that others find difficult to tolerate. These patients may daydream excessively, become attached to animals, and often do not marry. However, they do retain contact with reality unless they develop schizophrenia.

Abbreviated Criteria for Schizoid Personality Disorder

- Isolation from social relationships and restricted emotional range in interpersonal settings, as shown by at least four of the following:
  - ✓ Rejects close relationships, including family
  - ✓ Prefers solitary activities
  - ✓ Has little interest in sexual activity with another person
  - ✓ Enjoys few activities, if any
  - ✓ Other than close relatives, has no close friends or confidants
  - ✓ Does not appear affected by criticism or praise
  - ✓ Is emotionally cold, detached, or bland
- These symptoms do not occur solely in the course of another psychotic disorder (such as schizophrenia), a mood disorder with psychotic features, or a pervasive developmental disorder.
- They aren't directly caused by a medical illness.

Schizotypal Personality Disorder

Because they have magical thinking, ideas of reference, illusions, or unusual mannerisms or dress, patients with schizotypal personality disorder can seem quite odd. Despite their odd behaviors, many marry and work, though they may get along poorly with others and sometimes decompensate under stress. They may eventually develop schizophrenia, and their relatives are at increased risk for that disorder.

Abbreviated Criteria for Schizotypal Personality Disorder

- Isolation and discomfort with social relationships, as well as cognitive or perceptual distortions and peculiar behavior, as shown by at least five of the following:
  - ✓ Ideas of reference (not delusional)
  - ✓ Behavior is influenced by odd beliefs or magical thinking inconsistent with subcultural norms (may include marked superstitions, belief in telepathy)
  - ✓ Unusual perceptions or bodily illusions (e.g., "I felt like O. J. Simpson was right there in the room with me")
  - ✓ Odd speech (vague, excessively abstract, impoverished)
  - ✓ Paranoid or suspicious ideas
  - ✓ Affect that is constricted in range or inappropriate to the topic (e.g., silly, aloof, unresponsive)

✓ Odd behavior or appearance

✓ Other than close relatives, no close friends or confidants

✓ In social situations, marked anxiety that is not reduced by familiarity; this is associated with paranoid fears rather than negative self-judgments

- Does not occur only in the course of schizophrenia or another psychotic disorder, a mood disorder with psychotic features, or a pervasive developmental disorder.

Antisocial Personality Disorder

Although patients with antisocial personality disorder often seem charming personally, from an early age (before 15) they cannot follow society's rules. This behavior affects nearly every life area. There may be substance use, fighting, lying, and criminal behavior of any conceivable sort: theft, violence, confidence schemes, and child and spouse abuse. These patients may glibly claim to have guilt feelings, but they do not appear to feel genuine remorse for their behavior. Although they may complain of multiple somatic problems and will occasionally make suicide attempts, the manipulative nature of all their interactions with others makes it difficult to decide whether their complaints are genuine.

Warning: It is important not to make this diagnosis if antisocial behavior occurs only in the context of substance use. Although these patients often have a childhood marked by incorrigibility, delinquency, and school problems such as truancy, fewer than half the children with this sort of background eventually develop the full adult syndrome. Therefore, this diagnosis should never be made before age 18.

Abbreviated Criteria for Antisocial Personality Disorder

- Conduct disorder before age 15: For 12 months or more, the patient repeatedly violated rules, age-appropriate societal norms, or the rights of others, as shown by at least three of the following:

  Aggression against people or animals

  ✓ Frequent bullying or threatening

  ✓ Often starting fights

  ✓ Using a weapon that could cause serious injury (gun, knife, club, broken glass)

  ✓ Physical cruelty to people

  ✓ Physical cruelty to animals

  ✓ Theft with confrontation (armed robbery, extortion, mugging, purse snatching)

  ✓ Forcing sex upon someone

Property destruction
- ✓ Deliberately setting fires to cause serious damage
- ✓ Deliberately destroying the property of others (except fire setting)

Lying or theft
- ✓ Breaking into a building, car, or house belonging to someone else
- ✓ Frequent lying or breaking promises for gain or to avoid obligations ("conning")
- ✓ Stealing valuables without confrontation (burglary, forgery, shoplifting)

Serious rule violation
- ✓ Beginning by age 12, frequent staying out at night against parents' wishes
- ✓ Running away from parent overnight twice or more (once if for an extended period)
- ✓ Frequent truancy by age 12

- Since age 15, has shown disregard for the rights of others in a variety of situations by at least three of the following:
  - ✓ Repeatedly behaves in ways that are grounds for arrest, whether arrested or not
  - ✓ Lies, uses aliases, or cons others for gain or gratification
  - ✓ Is impulsive or does not plan ahead
  - ✓ Exhibits irritability and aggression that lead to recurrent physical fights or assaults
  - ✓ Recklessly disregards safety of self or others
  - ✓ Shows irresponsibility by repeated failure to sustain employment or honor financial obligations
  - ✓ Lacks remorse for own injurious behavior (shows indifference or rationalizes)
- The patient is currently at least 18 years old.
- Antisocial behavior does not occur solely during a manic episode or schizophrenia.

Borderline Personality Disorder

Patients with borderline personality disorder often appear to be in a crisis of mood behavior or interpersonal relationship. Often feeling empty and bored, they attach themselves strongly to others and then become intensely angry or hostile when they believe that they are being ignored or mistreated by those upon whom they feel dependent. They may impulsively try to harm or mutilate themselves. Although these patients may experience brief psychotic episodes, these episodes resolve so quickly that they are seldom confused with the endogenous psychoses. Intense, rapid mood swings, impassivity, and unstable interpersonal relationships make it difficult for these patients to achieve their full potential socially at work or in school.

Warning: Borderline personality disorder is a diagnosis frequently applied to patients who have other disorders that are more pressing from the standpoint of treatment. In the 21st century, it may still be the condition we most overdiagnose.

Abbreviated Criteria for Borderline Personality Disorder

- Unstable impulse control, interpersonal relationships, moods, and self-image, as shown by at least five of these:
  - ✓ Frantic attempts to prevent abandonment, whether real or imagined (don't include self-injurious or suicidal behaviors, covered below)
  - ✓ Unstable relationships that alternate between idealization and devaluation
  - ✓ Identity disturbance (severely distorted or unstable self-image or sense of self)
  - ✓ Potentially self-damaging impulsiveness in a least two areas, such as binge eating, reckless driving, sex, spending, substance use (again, don't include suicidal or self-mutilating behaviors, listed separately below)
  - ✓ Self-mutilation or suicidal thoughts, threats, or other behavior
  - ✓ Severe reactivity of mood, creating marked instability (mood swings of intense anxiety, depression, irritability that last a few hours to a few days)
  - ✓ Chronic feelings of boredom or emptiness
  - ✓ Anger that is out of control or inappropriate and intense (demonstrated by frequent temper displays, repeated physical fights, or feeling constantly angry)
  - ✓ Brief paranoid ideas or severe dissociative symptoms related to stress

Obsessive–Compulsive Personality Disorder

Patients with obsessive–compulsive personality disorder have a lifelong tendency to be rigid and perfectionistic, often to the point that their resulting indecisiveness, preoccupation with detail, scrupulosity, and insistence on doing things their way interfere with their effectiveness in work or social situations. They may have trouble expressing affection; often they seem quite depressed, and this depression may wax and wane, sometimes to the point that it becomes severe enough to drive them into treatment. Sometimes these people are stingy; they may be savers, refusing to throw away even worthless objects they no longer need.

Abbreviated Criteria for Obsessive–Compulsive Personality Disorder

- Preoccupation with control, orderliness, and perfection overshadow qualities of efficiency, flexibility, and candor, as shown by at least four of these:
    - ✓ Becomes preoccupied with details, lists, order, organization, rules, or schedules to such an extent that the purpose of the activity is lost ("can't see the forest for the trees")
    - ✓ Allows perfectionism to interfere with completing a task
    - ✓ Exhibits workaholism (works to exclusion of leisure activities)
    - ✓ Is excessively, even for patient's own cultural or religious background, overly conscientious, inflexible, or scrupulous about ethics, morals, or values
    - ✓ Saves items of no real or sentimental value
    - ✓ Won't cooperate or delegate tasks unless others agree to do things the patient's way
    - ✓ Is stingy toward self and others; hoards money against future needs
    - ✓ Is rigid and stubborn

Appendix C

Sample Interview, Written Report, and Formulation

INTERVIEW WITH PATIENT

The patient, a man who appears to be in his late 20s, is dressed in a hospital gown over chino pants and a white shirt, buttoned to the top. He sits in a straight-backed chair, seldom gazing at the interviewer. His nose and lips are swollen and bruised, and there is a large cut under his right eye. His facial expression is immobile; he doesn't smile once throughout the interview. His words are occasionally slightly mumbled. The interviewer's voice is warm and quiet.

> INTERVIEWER: (*Shakes hands with the patient.*) Good morning. My name is Dr. _____.
>
> PATIENT: Hi.
>
> INTERVIEWER: I want to thank you for helping us out today with this demonstration interview.
>
> PATIENT: It's OK.
>
> INTERVIEWER: I'll probably take notes from time to time, just to remind me of questions I might want to ask. Now, can you tell me a little bit about what sort of difficulty brought you here?
>
> PATIENT: Um—hopelessness, despair, nowhere to go but to the heavens.
>
> INTERVIEWER: Nowhere but to the heavens. Does that mean that you were thinking about dying?
>
> PATIENT: Thinking?—Wanting!
>
> INTERVIEWER: Wanting to die. Can you tell me a bit more about that?

Of course, "Tell me more about that" is the classic, open-ended request for the patient to elaborate further on what was just said.

PATIENT: Well, I'm thinking, an option is either to hurt someone or hurt myself. And I don't like hurting anyone, and so I'd rather hurt myself.

INTERVIEWER: I see.

PATIENT: And I don't want to live. You can die if you have, like, cancer, but not when you have your head so screwed up. So you have to live with that.

INTERVIEWER: Yes.

PATIENT: They don't call that terminal, they call that . . . "oh, well!"

INTERVIEWER: So, did you actually make some kind of a suicide attempt?

PATIENT: Oh, yeah! The voices said, "Jump, now's the time." I took all my clothes off; I figured, "You won't be needing these." And they all stopped, all the vehicles stopped, so I ran across the street and then—that's the last thing I remember, seeing a truck in the distance going faster than everyone else. I went for it.

INTERVIEWER: So you headed right for the truck.

With several responses so far, the interviewer's contributions have largely been made to facilitate more speech on the part of the patient. The principle of free speech is largely preserved.

PATIENT: Fast truck. I remember being in the ambulance, someone beating on me, telling me to wake up.

INTERVIEWER: So you were actually hit by the truck, do you think?

PATIENT: That's what they say, yeah, and by the looks of it.

INTERVIEWER: Yeah, it looks like you got beaten up a little bit. And then you remember being in the ambulance . . .

Notice the "Yeah" in the last speech—not at all the usual style of this interviewer, who is probably unconsciously trying to make a connection by using speech a little more in tune with the patient's own. Throughout the interview, this interviewer uses words the pa tient can understand; there is little in the way of medical jargon that might confuse the patient or inhibit the formation of rapport.

PATIENT: For a split second, while they were beating on me.

INTERVIEWER: Well, how does it seem to you now? I mean, you tried to kill yourself—and here you are, not dead.

PATIENT: It seems. Well, in the hospital I thought I was dead. I was in this white room. It was like the waiting area before Heaven. I was in the waiting area; it was just some room.

INTERVIEWER: Uh-huh.

PATIENT: And now, I think, I might still be in a waiting area.

INTERVIEWER: I see.

PATIENT: You guys will help with that?

INTERVIEWER: Well, I suspect that nobody here is going to help you die.

A direct answer is better than an evasion. However, a still better response would have been on the order of the classical "I can't do that, but I can do this"—for example, "We'll do all we can to help you want to live."

PATIENT: Oh.

INTERVIEWER: Do you still want to die?

PATIENT: (*Nods.*)

INTERVIEWER: You said that you'd been feeling hopeless. How long had that been?

Note that the interviewer often picks up on the patient's own words to turn the conversation in another direction.

PATIENT: Years.

INTERVIEWER: Uh-huh. Has it been worse recently?

PATIENT: Oh, yeah. I was hopeless once in a while. It wasn't every day. Since last summer.

INTERVIEWER: Since last summer. So that's how many months now?

PATIENT: Seven.

An apparent attempt to roughly assess the patient's orientation to time and ability to calculate.

INTERVIEWER: Uh-huh. Had you been having other feelings? Like, had you felt worthless?

PATIENT: Oh, yeah.

INTERVIEWER: Do you have any idea why?

PATIENT: Well, I tried to get jobs, thinking that might work.

INTERVIEWER: Yes.

PATIENT: Can't get one.

Thus far, the interviewer has identified three areas of clinical interest to investigate: psychosis (the voices), mood disorder, and social difficulties. There may be more to come.

INTERVIEWER: Do you feel pretty much the same throughout the day, or is one time of day better for you than another?

PATIENT: Best is at night, right when I go to bed.

INTERVIEWER: So when you go to bed at night, that's better somehow. Has your sleep been pretty good?

PATIENT: Here [in the hospital] it has.

INTERVIEWER: How about normally . . . what sort of trouble do you have with your sleep?

A less careful interviewer might move on to some other topic, rather than pinning the patient down on the subject of his sleep prior to hospitalization. I wonder, though, about using the term "normally"—just what time frame would that seem to indicate? It might be better to specify the time frame as "just before you were admitted."

PATIENT: I'd wake up every hour, grinding my teeth.

INTERVIEWER: Mm-hmm. When you wake up, do you think about things?

PATIENT: Yeah.

INTERVIEWER: What sorts of things?

PATIENT: "What am I going to do?"

INTERVIEWER: Uh-huh. Do you sleep pretty soundly in the morning, then?

PATIENT: Not until recently.

INTERVIEWER: Uh-huh. Do you wake up really early, before it's time to get up, and then you don't get back to sleep at all?

Better would be the open-ended "What sort of trouble were you having?"

PATIENT: Yeah. I'm saying, "Why did I wake up so early?"

INTERVIEWER: Do you feel rested when you sleep?

PATIENT: Yeah.

INTERVIEWER: You do feel rested.

PATIENT: But I feel pretty rested when I don't sleep. It's weird, it seems I don't need sleep.

INTERVIEWER: How's your appetite?

PATIENT: Good. Here it is.

INTERVIEWER: How about before you came in?

PATIENT: Not good.

INTERVIEWER: Has your weight changed any?

PATIENT: Yeah. I lost 10 pounds. I don't know about now; I might have gained weight.

INTERVIEWER: Mm-hmm. Over what period of time did you lose 10 pounds?

Throughout this interview, you'll note that the clinician uses a lot of verbal encouragements—"uh-huh" and its variants—as a clear but minimally intrusive way to indicate that the patient's message is being received and that the information flow should continue, without directing the flow in any way. What the written record cannot show is the use of nods, smiles, eye blinks, and other nonverbal methods that encourage with no intrusion at all. To improve readability, I've cut out about half the nondirective verbal encouragements the interviewer actually does use.

PATIENT: About a week.

INTERVIEWER: So that's pretty rapid. You weren't eating much. Not interested in food?

PATIENT: Not much.

INTERVIEWER: Were you interested in other things?

PATIENT: Nope. Well, I had a girlfriend who has a kid. I was interested in him.

INTERVIEWER: You're interested in your girlfriend's child.

PATIENT: He's a nice boy. I helped him.

INTERVIEWER: And at the time you made your suicide attempt, were you maintaining your interest pretty much in that child?

PATIENT: Yeah, but she didn't want me around.

INTERVIEWER: She didn't want you. What about things like reading or watching television—was your interest good there?

PATIENT: No.

INTERVIEWER: Could you keep your mind on things?

PATIENT: Yeah, television, if I did watch it. That's about it. (*Pause*) But not for long periods.

If the interviewer were to move on too quickly to the next topic, the overall impression of this patient's ability to focus his concentration would be somewhat different.

INTERVIEWER: Just for a short time? Like, about how long?

PATIENT: Half-hour.

INTERVIEWER: So you couldn't watch a full-hour show and retain it.

PATIENT: Without thinking about something.

INTERVIEWER: Would you find that when people were around who you liked, that took your mind off feeling bad?

PATIENT: Yeah.

INTERVIEWER: That would help. How long would it help for?

PATIENT: Until I realized what was going on with me.

INTERVIEWER: So that would be just, like, for a few minutes it would distract you?

Objection, Your Honor—leading the witness! Much better would be "How long would it usually distract you?"

PATIENT: Yeah.

INTERVIEWER: OK. Did you feel guilty about things?

PATIENT: Yeah.

INTERVIEWER: What sorts of things?

PATIENT: That I put myself in this position. I could have avoided it by certain decisions I made. But now it's too late.

INTERVIEWER: Mm-hmm. Do you feel that you're deserving to die?

PATIENT: Yeah.

INTERVIEWER: Do you feel like you're deserving to be punished?

PATIENT: Yeah, in a way.

INTERVIEWER: Mm-hmm.

PATIENT: I know a lot of people do it, but I knew better.

INTERVIEWER: You knew better. A lot of people do . . . do what?

Again the interviewer is picking up on the patient's previous speech, this time with elaboration. It's a method of verbal encouragement that can guide the conversation without appearing to be excessively controlling.

PATIENT: Similar things to what I do.

INTERVIEWER: Uh-huh. The things that you feel guilty about. Can you tell me what some of those are?

PATIENT: Like spending money on drugs. Staying in hotel rooms instead of spending it on apartments or food.

INTERVIEWER: Mm-hmm.

PATIENT: Bills.

INTERVIEWER: Right. And what sort of drugs have you been having a problem with?

PATIENT: Heroin and cocaine.

INTERVIEWER: Has this been for quite a long time?

PATIENT: Couple of years.

INTERVIEWER: How much of a heroin habit have you had?

PATIENT: I'd say a half gram a day.

INTERVIEWER: And how much would that cost you?

PATIENT: Twenty bucks. And 20 bucks for coke.

INTERVIEWER: And also $20 for cocaine. Well, as habits go, how strong would you say that is?

PATIENT: Do I want it now?

INTERVIEWER: Yeah.

PATIENT: Strong.

This interviewer either isn't sure just how much of a habit half a gram is or wants to give the patient an opportunity to demonstrate some expertise. In any event, asking a patient for an explanation is a good way to ensure that you have the right information. It also helps promote rapport.

INTERVIEWER: So you feel a pretty strong craving right now.

PATIENT: Not really that strong a craving; just probably if I had a lot of money and a place to go, I would probably do it.

INTERVIEWER: You would go out and use drugs again.

PATIENT: 'Cause they make me feel safe.

INTERVIEWER: Back before you were using drugs, how was your mood then?

With two serious problems to consider, the interviewer is trying to learn which one started first. The important reason: to differentiate between a primary mood disorder and one that is secondary to drug use, with their differing treatment implications.

PATIENT: It would depend where I was at, but . . . there was always something missing.

INTERVIEWER: Always something missing, even before you were using drugs.

PATIENT: Yeah. And back in school, I never fit in, really. I mean, I had friends but I didn't fit in.

Another area of clinical interest rears its head: the possibility of personality disorder.

INTERVIEWER: Mm-hmm.

PATIENT: Uncomfortable.

INTERVIEWER: You felt uncomfortable, even with friends. Can you talk about that a little bit more, about that feeling of discomfort?

Even this far into the interview, the interviewer extends an invitation to expand on these feelings. Open-ended probes are the way to develop information about emotions.

PATIENT: Like, you don't want to say the wrong thing or get made fun of. You don't want to do anything that will get you made fun of. So really, you just keep quiet, keep to yourself. And then nothing does happen. You don't get more friends.

INTERVIEWER: So you were always very afraid of making a mistake, of seeming out of place. And that's at least partly because you felt out of place. Has that been true throughout your adult life?

Ordinarily, I recommend against long interviewer speeches. After all, the more an interviewer talks, the less time the patient has to talk. However, occasional summary statements, such as the one just above, can ensure that the interviewer has understood and can help connect with the patient.

PATIENT: (*Nods.*)

INTERVIEWER: What about when you were a kid?

PATIENT: That's the only time when I wasn't afraid, before my parents got divorced. I remember the first day we lived here, my parents said, "There's a kid out there your age—go play with him." I ran out there, pushed him on his tricycle. We became best friends.

INTERVIEWER: And that was when you were how old?

PATIENT: Five.

INTERVIEWER: And did that last clear up until your parents got divorced?

PATIENT: (*Nods.*)

INTERVIEWER: And how old were you then?

PATIENT: Parents got divorced when I was about 7—6, 7.

INTERVIEWER: Did you live with your mom or with your dad then?

PATIENT: My mom, in California, so I missed some school. My other brothers lived with my dad. 'Cause they were going to school.

INTERVIEWER: And was it when you were 7 or so that you started to feel out of place?

PATIENT: I think so. I mean, right from the start, I felt awkward in certain situations. I gradually got it back, then it all went to heck. Then I switched schools and then I got it back again. And then I went to a middle school and lost it all. And never got it back.

INTERVIEWER: You lost it all—what does that mean?

PATIENT: It means all my friends were in a different area than I was, and I had to make all new friends, and I never did.

INTERVIEWER: So you never really got back to where you were.

PATIENT: Yeah, and I just kept it there.

INTERVIEWER: Back then, when you were, say, a teenager, did you feel depressed then?

PATIENT: Mm-hmm.

INTERVIEWER: Was it as depressed as you're feeling now?

PATIENT: No, I thought of suicide, but I'd never do it.

INTERVIEWER: And when was the first time you made a suicide attempt?

PATIENT: Two years ago.

INTERVIEWER: Uh-huh. Was that after you started to use drugs?

This interviewer puts quite a lot of effort into determining the sequence of symptoms— what happened first, followed by what else? This information will prove important in diagnosis and in determining what treatment might help.

PATIENT: (*Nods.*)

INTERVIEWER: And what did you do to yourself then?

PATIENT: I tried to shoot the most heroin I ever did.

INTERVIEWER: You tried to overdose on heroin.

PATIENT: Yeah, and I took some prescription pills.

INTERVIEWER: And obviously that didn't work . . .

PATIENT: Right.

INTERVIEWER: Were you hospitalized then?

PATIENT: Yeah, I woke up 3 days later.

INTERVIEWER: That's quite a long time.

PATIENT: That was the closest.

INTERVIEWER: And have you made any suicide attempts between then and this one?

Have you noticed that the interviewer starts many questions with the word "And?" We all have verbal tics, which can be annoying or helpful to one degree or another, and I would recommend that you analyze your own to see which should be expunged. In this case, the repeated conjunction may actually serve to help tie the interview together while moving it forward.

> PATIENT: Yeah, I took a bunch of over-the-counter sleeping pills. Those things just made my heart go crazy, so I took myself to the emergency [room].
>
> INTERVIEWER: Mm-hmm.
>
> PATIENT: And then I felt myself passing out when I got there. They charcoaled me and that was . . . (*Long pause*)
>
> INTERVIEWER: Well, now, you said that you had been hearing voices. Can you tell me about that?
>
> PATIENT: My head's thinking one thing, and then this voice will sound, like, outside, inside my head, I don't know: "It's OK. Just do it."
>
> INTERVIEWER: By that is meant . . .
>
> PATIENT: Whatever I'm thinking.
>
> INTERVIEWER: Whatever you're thinking. So this voice kind of encourages you.
>
> PATIENT: (*Nods.*)
>
> INTERVIEWER: Does it ever say anything different from that?
>
> PATIENT: It tells me not to do stuff.
>
> INTERVIEWER: Like what?
>
> PATIENT: Like "It's a bad idea right now. Don't do it."
>
> INTERVIEWER: Mm-hmm.
>
> PATIENT: I've always had it.
>
> INTERVIEWER: You've always had this voice. Dating back to when?
>
> PATIENT: When I was a kid. It kept me out of trouble, a lot of times.
>
> INTERVIEWER: I see. Do you think that this voice is an actual person or thing out there somewhere? Or could it be your own conscience or your own thoughts?

Note the forced choice. An open-ended question might have worked better here—for example, " . . . Or could there be some other explanation?"

> PATIENT: I used to think it was my conscience, until recently when it got so strong I can almost see it. And that's when I started thinking it was something else.
>
> INTERVIEWER: Mm-hmm.

PATIENT: My brother died. I swear that has something to do with it.

INTERVIEWER: I didn't understand that.

PATIENT: My brother got murdered. And that had something to do with me not dying.

INTERVIEWER: So you're thinking that—

PATIENT: At the time I was trying to do the heroin overdose, same day I got out of the hospital, my grandfather died.

INTERVIEWER: Wow!

Shorthand for "That's a really heavy load for one person." This sort of response tells the patient that the clinician understands and cares; it is a premier example of one-word rapport building.

PATIENT: It was, like, they had to do a switch. Me for him. It was already safe.

INTERVIEWER: So you think that in some way, your grandfather died so you could live?

PATIENT: (*Nods.*)

INTERVIEWER: That's a pretty big responsibility. How does that make you feel?

PATIENT: Well, he was really sick. And that's the kind of guy he is, so I'm not surprised.

INTERVIEWER: What did he die of?

PATIENT: Old age.

INTERVIEWER: And you said that your brother died—he got murdered.

Good for this interviewer, who remembered to ask about the murdered brother! This may have been facilitated by the note taking mentioned at the outset of the interview.

PATIENT: He was stabbed. And he got only about 2 years.

INTERVIEWER: The person who stabbed him only got 2 years in prison for that. What were the circumstances?

PATIENT: He'd just got out of prison, my brother, and he didn't know where to go, and he was sleeping in the park with bums. And they were cooking, and he went to borrow a bike that wasn't his, to buy beer, and the dude whose bike it was just flipped out—said "Get off my bike," and went after him with a knife.

INTERVIEWER: I see. So your brother had been in prison, for what?

PATIENT: For burglary.

INTERVIEWER: And had he been in a lot of trouble much of his life?

PATIENT: Not really, just alcohol.

INTERVIEWER: Oh, he drank. And was that why he did the burglary—he was intoxicated at the time?

PATIENT: Yeah.

INTERVIEWER: And has anybody else in your family had any drug or alcohol problems?

PATIENT: Yeah, my brother.

INTERVIEWER: Another brother?

PATIENT: Yeah, and then my aunt and uncles.

INTERVIEWER: So you had some aunts and uncles, on your dad's side or—

PATIENT: Mom's side, and then my stepdad.

INTERVIEWER: Was your mother a drinker or a drug user?

PATIENT: Yeah.

INTERVIEWER: Tell me about her.

PATIENT: She would drink and smoke pot.

INTERVIEWER: And is she still alive now?

PATIENT: (*Nods.*)

INTERVIEWER: Is she still drinking?

PATIENT: No.

INTERVIEWER: She got straightened out. How did that happen?

PATIENT: She quit.

INTERVIEWER: Does that make you feel that there's some kind of hope for you?

PATIENT: I quit before. I've had 7 months clean.

INTERVIEWER: Really? That's terrific! When was that?

The compliment is hardly necessary, but in context it seems heartfelt, and perhaps it does help to cement whatever feelings the patient may be forming for the interviewer.

PATIENT: Last year.

INTERVIEWER: And then you just slipped back into it.

PATIENT: I just felt like shit still.

INTERVIEWER: You mean, even though you were clean and sober, you still felt very depressed.

PATIENT: Uh-huh. Hopeless. And I had money.

INTERVIEWER: Were you working at that time?

PATIENT: No, but I had $6,000 in the bank.

INTERVIEWER: Really! Wow. And that didn't help you to feel any better.

PATIENT: Nope.

INTERVIEWER: Even though you were not using, not drinking, you still felt terribly depressed.

PATIENT: (*Nods.*)

INTERVIEWER: And were you thinking about killing yourself then?

PATIENT: (*Nods.*)

INTERVIEWER: Do you think you felt about as bad then as you do now?

PATIENT: (*Nods.*) Yup.

INTERVIEWER: Well, I was asking about your relatives. I heard about your brothers and your mom. What about your dad—was he a drinker or a drug user?

PATIENT: My stepdad.

INTERVIEWER: What about your biological father?

PATIENT: He did that stuff, but he quit. But when I was growing up, he was a drinker.

INTERVIEWER: I see. What kind of work did he do?

PATIENT: He was a sales manager.

INTERVIEWER: And do you have any kind of a relationship with him now?

PATIENT: Now, more so than I did. I didn't for a while.

INTERVIEWER: Mm-hmm. And what about your mom—do you see her?

PATIENT: (*Nods.*)

INTERVIEWER: How do you and she get along?

PATIENT: Pretty good, for the most part.

INTERVIEWER: You know your brother died at one point, and your grandfather died, and I'm sure that you felt bad when those events happened. Can you compare how you feel now, with your depression, to the way you felt when they died?

PATIENT: When my brother died, I felt relief for him. He was lucky; he didn't have to go through that crap any more. Same with my grandpa, 'cause he was in pain. So my depression [compared to] that—I wish I could be with them.

INTERVIEWER: So the way you feel now, it's quite different from how you felt when they died. Is that correct?

An important summary statement—to try to characterize the type and degree of depression now, as compared with how people feel when a loved one dies.

PATIENT: Yeah.

INTERVIEWER: And do you still feel now that you wish you were dead?

PATIENT: Yes.

INTERVIEWER: You said that you hoped that somebody here would help you to die. Does that seem like a realistic hope to you?

PATIENT: I don't see why not; they do it for people with cancer. My brain has cancer.

INTERVIEWER: Your brain has cancer—what do you mean by that?

PATIENT: Cancerous thoughts.

INTERVIEWER: Cancerous thoughts. Well, suppose that with medication or some other treatment, your brain could get over these cancerous thoughts?

PATIENT: Yeah, well, that would be something else.

INTERVIEWER: That would be something different.

PATIENT: Kind of works with heroin. The thing with heroin, it just shuts the cancerous thoughts down. But it doesn't make you feel better. I don't want to hang out with anyone. I just like to sit in a room and watch TV, and the cancerous thoughts be shut down. And that's why I do that.

INTERVIEWER: Does it seem to you that when you use heroin, it's to shut down some of these really bad, negative thoughts that you have?

PATIENT: Exactly.

INTERVIEWER: You mentioned that you heard these voices. Have you ever had any other experiences that most people don't have?

Good use of transition—picking up on the patient's own words and using that as a bridge to other questions about mental phenomena.

PATIENT: Uh, no.

INTERVIEWER: Do you see visions, for instance?

PATIENT: Yeah.

INTERVIEWER: Tell me about that.

PATIENT: I see visions of me hanging.

INTERVIEWER: Hanging, like by a rope, you mean?

PATIENT: See visions of me smashing my car into a brick wall. I see visions of me jumping off the train platform, right into the train.

INTERVIEWER: Are those visions something that you can actually see, just the way you see me now? Or is it more like something that's played on your mental mind's screen?

PATIENT: No, I see it.

INTERVIEWER: You can actually see it. You see it as clearly as you see me?

PATIENT: Yeah.

INTERVIEWER: And have you ever had the feeling or thoughts that people were plotting against you in some way or another, trying to harm you?

PATIENT: No.

INTERVIEWER: Spy on you?

PATIENT: Spy on me, yeah.

INTERVIEWER: Tell me about that.

PATIENT: Cops do these things. Try to stop me.

INTERVIEWER: Uh-huh. So you thought that may be the police might be trying to stop you from harming yourself.

PATIENT: Yeah. There's cameras everywhere.

INTERVIEWER: On this ward there are cameras, that's true. What about outside? Do you feel there are cameras everywhere there?

PATIENT: Pretty much. You go to malls, there will be. There's cameras on lights, stoplights.

INTERVIEWER: Has anybody in your family ever had any other mental illnesses besides using drugs or alcohol?

Oops. This would be an excellent point to ask whether the cameras are focusing just on him, or whether they are intended for use on everyone. The latter response would of course evoke far less concern.

PATIENT: (*Shakes head.*)

INTERVIEWER: Depression . . .

PATIENT: Yeah, my stepdad.

INTERVIEWER: Your stepdad.

PATIENT: He did drugs and he quit, and he's been clean for 6 or 7 years. The other day, he had to go home because he's so depressed.

INTERVIEWER: Anybody besides your stepdad?

PATIENT: No.

INTERVIEWER: Anybody in the family with schizophrenia? . . . Any kind of psychosis or craziness? . . . Anybody else who's ever tried to kill himself?

PATIENT: (*Shakes his head "no" to each of the questions above.*)

INTERVIEWER: Let's see, you had two brothers. Any other brothers or sisters?

PATIENT: No.

INTERVIEWER: Are you oldest or—

PATIENT: Youngest.

INTERVIEWER: You're the youngest. How old are you now?

PATIENT: Thirty-one.

INTERVIEWER: Uh-huh. And you mentioned your experiences when you were growing up. How far did you go in school?

PATIENT: All the way . . . high school, graduated. Went to college for a little bit.

INTERVIEWER: And what kind of work have you done?

PATIENT: I've done carpet; I worked in a car wash; delivering pizza. I've worked in warehouses.

INTERVIEWER: Do you like working?

PATIENT: Yeah.

INTERVIEWER: You get a good feeling out of that.

PATIENT: Yeah.

INTERVIEWER: What's the longest job you've held?

PATIENT: Five years.

INTERVIEWER: That's pretty good. What was that?

Another compliment. A good rule is this: Never say anything that is complimentary unless you truly mean it. It sounds as though that is the way this interviewer feels.

PATIENT: Delivering pizza.

INTERVIEWER: And once you leave here, do you think you might try to get another job?

PATIENT: I've been trying, but they don't call me back. That's why I get hopeless.

INTERVIEWER: Yeah. Your brother was in prison at one time. Have you ever had troubles like that?

The interviewer uses previous information as a bridge to a topic that could be sensitive.

> PATIENT: Never.
>
> INTERVIEWER: And you mentioned your girlfriend. Have you ever been married?
>
> PATIENT: No.
>
> INTERVIEWER: Have you had quite a few girlfriends?
>
> PATIENT: Yes.
>
> INTERVIEWER: And has your relationship with women been pretty satisfactory ordinarily?
>
> PATIENT: Yeah.
>
> INTERVIEWER: Sexual satisfaction?
>
> PATIENT: OK.
>
> INTERVIEWER: How about when you're really depressed? Is your interest in sex different when you're really depressed?

Note that this interviewer has delayed for a long time the question about libido when depressed, until it flows more naturally into the conversation and until the patient is maximally used to the interview process.

> PATIENT: Don't do it.
>
> INTERVIEWER: You just don't do it. Not interested? How's your physical health been?
>
> PATIENT: Good.
>
> INTERVIEWER: Have you had any difficulty that has caused you to have an operation?
>
> PATIENT: My back hurts.

But did he ever have an operation? In context, it seems reasonable to assume that he did not, but one goal of interviewing is accuracy.

> INTERVIEWER: Have you ever been unconscious, other than when you were hit by the truck?
>
> PATIENT: (*Shakes head.*)
>
> INTERVIEWER: Have you had other hospitalizations, besides psychiatric?
>
> PATIENT: Just when I was a kid. I fell on my head, from about 8 feet high.
>
> INTERVIEWER: Wow!

PATIENT: I was playing hide-and-seek, and I landed on my head. Cracked both wrists. Got a concussion.

INTERVIEWER: And you were out for how long then?

PATIENT: A split second. But I was dizzy all day long.

INTERVIEWER: I see. Did you recover from that fairly quickly then?

PATIENT: Yeah. I slept that night in the hospital.

INTERVIEWER: Now, I know you've had difficulty with depression for quite some time. Have you had antidepressant treatment of any kind?

PATIENT: Just pills.

INTERVIEWER: What kind of pills have you had?

PATIENT: Lexapro, Wellbutrin, and Depakote.

INTERVIEWER: And did those seem to make any difference?

PATIENT: Unh-unh.

INTERVIEWER: How long did you take each one of them?

PATIENT: Four months for Lexapro, a month for the Wellbutrin and Depakote.

INTERVIEWER: And why did you stop taking them?

PATIENT: Lexapro was making me tired and upset my stomach. Same with the Depakote and Wellbutrin.

INTERVIEWER: Do you know how much you were taking of each of those?

PATIENT: No.

INTERVIEWER: Was it several pills a day of each?

PATIENT: Yeah. Four Depakotes, and one or two Wellbutrin.

INTERVIEWER: And the Lexapro?

PATIENT: I think it was two.

To try to pin down the adequacy of previous treatment, the interviewer has gone after this information like a terrier after a rat.

INTERVIEWER: And have you had any courses of psychotherapy? . . . Group therapy? . . . Cognitive-behavioral therapy?

PATIENT: (*To each in turn*) No.

INTERVIEWER: Nothing of that sort. Now some people who have depression have the opposite feeling at times, too—where they feel ecstatic or too happy, on top of the world. Has that ever happened to you?

PATIENT: Yeah.

INTERVIEWER: Can you tell me about that?

PATIENT: Like the other day, I had a ticket for not wearing my seat belt. I took a class for 20 bucks—it was a $200 ticket—and they voided the ticket.

INTERVIEWER: That made you feel pretty good.

PATIENT: Yeah. Even though I had nothing in my wallet, [nothing] to eat, and barely any gas.

INTERVIEWER: I see. How long did that up feeling last?

PATIENT: Huh! Five minutes.

INTERVIEWER: Have you ever had up feelings that lasted for days at a time?

PATIENT: No.

INTERVIEWER: Now, are there other important experiences that you've had that you haven't talked about so far?

This is a fishing expedition, designed to provide an opportunity to discuss anything else that might be on the patient's mind. This time it turns up negative, but it's a good idea to cast such a line at least once during every initial interview.

PATIENT: No.

INTERVIEWER: Have you ever had the experience of having thoughts that seem pointless or silly to you, that you'd go back to over and over again?

PATIENT: No.

INTERVIEWER: Do you have any fears or phobias?

PATIENT: Yeah.

INTERVIEWER: Like . . .

PATIENT: Fear of speaking in public, fear of drowning, fear of burning to death, fear of failure, fear of being laughed at.

INTERVIEWER: Do these fears cause you to change your way of life in any way?

PATIENT: Yeah, I avoid it.

INTERVIEWER: So what sorts of things do you avoid?

PATIENT: I avoid meeting new people. I avoid anything that can injure me.

INTERVIEWER: If you have to speak in public, are you able to do it but it's just uncomfortable for you, or do you just not do it at all?

PATIENT: Well, going to school, we never had to do it, in college. But I would have just done it.

INTERVIEWER: So you'd have done it, but you wouldn't have been happy about it.

PATIENT: Or I'd have been bad at it.

INTERVIEWER: Would you ever get panic attacks—where you would feel something awful was about to happen to you, and your heart would beat really fast?

PATIENT: I get those all the time.

INTERVIEWER: Do you get them even now?

PATIENT: Bad. I hate that.

INTERVIEWER: What sorts of thing set them off?

PATIENT: Anything. I can be playing basketball; next thing I know, I feel one coming on. My balls get all cold, weird feelings. I know what it is, I just try to let it go. Gets me light-headed and feel I've got to puke.

INTERVIEWER: How often do those experiences happen?

PATIENT: Depends. Sometimes, when it happens it's like four times, five times a day. Sometimes they don't happen for a month.

INTERVIEWER: Have you ever talked to a doctor about it?

PATIENT: He said I had an anxiety attack. Gave me Xanax.

INTERVIEWER: Did that seem to help?

PATIENT: Yeah.

INTERVIEWER: Of course, there are problems with Xanax, too. People can get kind of used to taking it, and they may *want* to take it.

This response borders on intervention—the clinician is venturing an (albeit tentative) opinion as to the dangers of certain medications. However, there is probably no harm in the context of a patient who has had considerable experience with substance misuse and who has already made several suicide attempts.

PATIENT: It made me tired, though. They'd give me a pill and I'd break it up in fourths.

INTERVIEWER: Are you much of a worrier?

Actually, a comment or bridge would be welcome here—something to indicate that the interviewer understands the importance of the patient's not abusing Xanax. (For that matter, it wouldn't be amiss to make it explicit that the patient hasn't misused Xanax.) In any event, the interviewer might say something like "I think I understand about the Xanax. Let's move on to something else"—and then ask about worries.

PATIENT: Yeah, I worry.

INTERVIEWER: What do you worry about?

PATIENT: Anything . . . what's going to happen next . . . where I'm going to go from here . . . how can I control this . . . anything that's not in my control, I worry.

INTERVIEWER: (*With an "Uh-huh" for each of the worries above*) Have you sought help from organizations like AA or NA for drug use?

PATIENT: Yeah.

INTERVIEWER: And what sort of help has that been?

PATIENT: AA—that's where I got my 7 months clean. I stopped going because there's a lot of new people in there. They were talking about how much drugs they did, and I was like, "I don't want to hear that."

INTERVIEWER: It was a downer for you?

PATIENT: Yeah, it just makes me want to do drugs.

INTERVIEWER: But then you got back into doing drugs.

PATIENT: Yeah.

INTERVIEWER: I was curious about something you said earlier today. You weren't working, but you had $6,000 in the bank. I'm wondering how that could be.

PATIENT: I got in a car accident. The settlement was $6,000.

INTERVIEWER: I see. And, did you spend that fairly quickly then?

PATIENT: Couple of months.

INTERVIEWER: On drugs?

PATIENT: Drugs and hotel rooms, 'cause I had nowhere to live.

INTERVIEWER: Well, good. I think I have a pretty good understanding of what's happened with you. Now I'd like to change directions and ask you a couple of quiz questions, if I could. What is the date today?

This transition is an explicit notice that the interviewer has the information needed and wants to move on.

PATIENT: (*States date, month, and year correctly.*)

INTERVIEWER: And where are we right now?

PATIENT: (*Answers correctly.*)

INTERVIEWER: Let's see, did I tell you my name?

PATIENT: Dr. _____.

All interview tests of memory are only approximations, and this one—just the name of the interviewer—is pretty rough. But in conjunction with the patient's evident clarity of thought during the previous 40 minutes or so of interview, the interviewer apparently feels justified in not pursuing the issue of memory in greater detail.

INTERVIEWER: Good. Can you tell me who the president is?

PATIENT: (*With more prompting, names several previous presidents in correct order.*)

INTERVIEWER: I know you've been asked to do things like subtracting sevens from 100. Would you mind doing that now?

PATIENT: Ninety-three.

INTERVIEWER: OK, keep subtracting sevens until you get below 60.

PATIENT: OK, 93, 86, 79, 72, 67 . . . I screwed up already.

INTERVIEWER: (*After a long pause while the patient struggles*) Well, you did great, actually.

PATIENT: Did I?

INTERVIEWER: You got farther than most people do.

PATIENT: I got them right?

The patient shows a touching eagerness for reassurance that he has performed well. It suggests the degree of his dependency. It is fair to give reassurance whenever it is merited, but not when it is obviously in opposition to the facts.

INTERVIEWER: All but the last one. And that finishes the questions I wanted to ask you today. Thank you very much for your time.

This interviewer has obtained a great deal of material pertinent to the diagnosis and treatment of this patient. In 45 minutes, information has been obtained for every one of the eight areas of clinical interest. In addition, we have learned a fair amount (though not nearly enough) about this patient's personal and social background.

All interviews are flawed, however, and this one is no exception. Offhand, I can list half a dozen points that are either covered inadequately or not touched upon at all. How many can you find?

WRITTEN REPORT

Identifying data: This is a repeat psychiatric hospitalization for Marco Carlin, a 30-year-old single white man.

Chief complaint: "Hopelessness, despair, nowhere to go but to the heavens."

Informants: The patient alone.

History of the present illness: Mr. Carlin was admitted to the hospital following a suicide attempt in which a truck hit him while he was running through heavy traffic. He had been experiencing severe depression, characterized by feelings of hopelessness and worthlessness, for about 7 months, building on a longer history of depression that goes back many years. Prior to admission he suffered from insomnia (interval and terminal waking) and poor appetite, with a 10-pound weight loss in 1 week. However, since admission his sleep and appetite have improved. During this 7-month period of severe depression, he maintained interest in television and his girlfriend's child, though his libido has been markedly reduced. His concentration has been somewhat diminished; people he likes distract him only briefly. He admits to guilt feelings and believes he deserves to be punished and to die. He appears to feel worse now than when he experienced the deaths of his brother and his grandfather; for the latter, death was a release. Other than a few minutes' response to a fortunate event, he denies periods of elation.

Past treatment for depression has included Lexapro (4 months on 2 tablets/day), Wellbutrin (1 month on 1 or 2 tablets), and Depakote (1 month on 4 tablets). He has never had cognitive-behavioral therapy, group therapy, or other psychotherapy.

Some of Mr. Carlin's guilt feelings center on his drug use, which has persisted for at least the past 2 years. Spending about $20 a day on heroin and $20 for cocaine, he feels he has had a serious drug use problem. He craves drugs right now and he feels would use drugs again. Heroin shuts down his unacceptable thoughts. He states that he has felt severely depressed even when he is not using drugs or drinking.

Yet another area of concern is auditory hallucinations. He claims that for years ("I've always had it"), he has heard a voice that will say things like "Just do it" and "It's a bad idea right now, don't do it." He says that this voice often helped him when he was a child. He used to consider it the voice of his conscience, but recently it has become so strong that he can "almost see it."

Personal and social history: Even as a child, Mr. Carlin felt that he did not fit in. He felt awkward, repeatedly changing schools and having to make new friends; as a teenager, he felt depressed, though not suicidal. His parents were divorced when he was about 7, after which he lived with his mother in California. His two older brothers lived with his father. He considers that he has a reasonably good relationship with his natural father and with his mother. He graduated from high school and briefly attended college. He has held a variety of jobs, including installing carpet, working in a car wash, and (for 5 years) delivering pizza. He has been out of work lately, however, and has been unsuccessful at finding another job. He has never married, but has had girlfriends. When not depressed, he has no difficulties with sexual satisfaction.

His family history includes numerous relatives who have misused substances, including his biological father, a sales manager who drank earlier in his life. A brother was in prison.

Mr. Carlin's physical health has been good overall. At age 8, the patient struck his head in a fall and was hospitalized overnight for concussion. He complains of back pain, but has had no operations; he takes no medications other than for his mental condition.

Mental status exam: Mr. Carlin still wishes that he were dead and that someone in the hospital would help him die to relieve him of his "cancerous thoughts." He believes this is a reasonable expectation. He has seen clear visual hallucinations of himself hanging by a rope, smashing his car into a brick wall, or jumping off a train platform. Although he denies persecutory ideas, he admits to some feelings that the police may be spying on him—the evidence is that there are cameras everywhere. He is oriented for person, place, and time; his fund of knowledge (presidents) is good; and his remote memory and retention/recall are unimpaired. His concentration is reasonably good; he subtracted serial sevens with one error.

Although he did not bring up these issues spontaneously, he admits to some fears (drowning, failure, burning to death, speaking in public, being laughed at). As a result, he says that he avoids people and situations that could injure him, but he admits that if he were called on to speak to an audience, he'd probably go ahead and do it. He denies obsessional ideas, but admits to panic attacks.

Impression

Axis I: Diagnosis deferred

1. Mood disorder
   Depression secondary to head trauma
   Substance-induced mood disorder with depressive features
   Major depressive disorder, recurrent, possibly with dysthymia
   Bipolar I disorder
   Bipolar II disorder

2. Substance misuse
   Cocaine abuse
   Heroin abuse
   Cocaine and/or heroin dependence

3. Possible anxiety disorder
   Social phobia
   Generalized anxiety disorder
   Panic disorder with agoraphobia

4. Possible psychosis
   Substance-induced psychotic disorder
   Major depressive disorder, severe, with psychotic features
   Schizophrenia

Axis II: Diagnosis deferred
   Possible personality disorder not otherwise specified, with avoidant and
      schizoid traits

Axis III: Recently hit by truck

Axis IV: Currently unemployed

Axis V: Global Assessment of Functioning
   15 current
   70 (highest past year)

FORMULATION

Summary

This 30-year-old single white man was admitted to the hospital following his attempt at suicide by being hit on the highway by a moving truck. He has had depression of varying degrees dating back to about age 7; his depression has been
complicated in recent years by the use of cocaine and heroin. He has been
treated with several medications, largely to no avail. He has recently been unemployed and is currently homeless.

Differential Diagnosis

Depression. Major depression is supported by the presence of numerous criteria
and a history of repeated suicide attempts. Mr. Carlin states that his depression
antedates his use of drugs and persists even when he is not using drugs. The
long-standing depressive symptoms argue for coexisting dysthymia.

Psychosis. Mr. Carlin does not have sufficient "A" criteria for a diagnosis of
schizophrenia, and there is something less than compelling about his auditory
hallucinations. His symptoms seem insufficiently mood-congruent for major
depression with psychosis. The amount of recent substance use seems insufficient for a substance-induced psychosis. Nonetheless, he should be observed
carefully for further emerging symptoms of psychosis.

Substance misuse. Although it is unclear from this interview whether he has
actual substance dependence, it almost doesn't matter. It is obvious that his
substance use has been enough to interfere with his life; it may underlie his current depression.

Anxiety disorder. The patient has admitted to symptoms of several different anxiety disorders. There is insufficient information to make any firm diagnosis; indeed, his responses to questions suggest that he may have been overly compliant with the interview process.

Personality disorder. Some sort of Axis II diagnosis is supported by this patient's possible overcompliance with interview questions and long history of drug use. Diagnosis deferred for now, in light of Axis I possibilities above.

Best Diagnosis

The most pressing diagnosis to address at present is major depressive disorder, along with abuse (at minimum) of cocaine and heroin.

Contributing Factors

Family history (father, brother) is strongly implicated in Mr. Carlin's substance misuse. Divorce of parents when the patient was young may have contributed to mood disorder. Substance use and depression may exacerbate one another.

Further Information Needed

In addition to prior medical records and the impressions of other clinicians, interviews with parents may help to disentangle the threads of Mr. Carlin's depression and substance use, as well as to resolve the questions concerning possible anxiety disorder(s) and psychosis. Subsequent interviews should reveal additional details not covered already, including the means of his current support, religious history, and military service.

Treatment Plan

> Further trials on antidepressant medication
> Psychotherapy (perhaps cognitive-behavioral therapy) directed at feelings of depression
> Twelve-Step program for substance misuse
> Referral for assistance with housing and employment

Prognosis

If the diagnosis of major depression is accurate and the patient responds to medication and cognitive-behavioral therapy, it might provide a platform from which to succeed in managing his substance use. On the other hand, if his substance use cannot be brought under control, management of his depression could prove very difficult. The prognosis is complicated by the possibility of an Axis II disorder.

Appendix D

A Semistructured Interview

For decades, clinicians have used structured and semistructured interviews to gather health care data. These instruments are more effective than traditional freewheeling interviews at producing accurate principal diagnoses and at uncovering secondary diagnoses. For example, one study found that the Structured Clinical Interview for DSM (SCID) identified five times more clinical diagnoses than were documented in the patients' charts. On the other hand, structured instruments can reject unwarranted clinical diagnoses; a structured interview study of homeless patients found fewer cases of antisocial personality disorder than did traditional clinical methods.

I've written this appendix not to replace your free-flowing interview but to help you cover the ground necessary for the most complete diagnosis possible. Although the questions will provide you with the material to make your diagnoses, they won't score themselves. For example, you'll have to evaluate whether your depressed patient has major depressive disorder, bipolar depressive episode, dysthymia, melancholia, or seasonal mood disorder. You will have to elicit details at many points; in a fully structured interview that a technician could administer, that work would be done for you. This guide is intended for mental health care professionals who already have a grounding in mental disorders.

I've written out screening questions (**boldface**) twice: just below, where you can copy them for ready reference; and again at the beginning of each diagnostic set. (There is some evidence that asking all the stem questions first helps discourage a tendency to say "no" once the person discovers that positive answers lead to further questioning.) If you get negative answers to a set of screens, you can skip the follow-up questions and move on.

The last two sections contain no screens, but don't pass them by. They will remind you of the tremendous breadth of information you need about your patient's background, personality, feelings, and general behavior.

ALL SCREENS

A1. Was there ever a time when you felt unusually down, depressed, or sad most of the day?

A2. Was there ever a time when you felt that most of the time you didn't enjoy your usual activities or take pleasure from them?

B1. Have you ever had a time when you felt the opposite of depressed—you felt unreasonably happy, euphoric, "on cloud nine"?

B2. Did you ever have a time when you (or others) noticed that you were unusually cross, irritable, or cranky?

B3. Has there been a time when you were much more active than is normal for you?

C1. Have you ever have an attack or spell when you suddenly felt anxious, fearful, or extremely uneasy?

C2. Have you ever had a sudden attack or spell when you felt faint, you felt you couldn't breathe, or your heart seemed to race?

D1. Have you had fears or phobias related to anything? Examples: animals (such as spiders, dogs, snakes); blood, needles, or injections; heights; airplane travel; being closed in; thunderstorms; blushing; eating in public; speaking, singing, or playing a musical instrument before an audience.

D2. Have you had anxiety about being in a place or situation (such as a store or the movies)—a place that you'd have trouble escaping from, or where there might be no help available if you had a panic attack?

E1. Have you ever had ideas or thoughts that keep coming back to you—thoughts that you try to resist but cannot?

E2. Do you ever experience physical behaviors that you feel you have to perform over and over, such as handwashing, checking the stove, or counting things?

F1. Have you ever had a traumatic, stressful experience that you found you kept on reliving or having to avoid?

G1. Do you worry a great deal of the time?

G2. What do you worry about?

H1. Have you ever had experiences like seeing visions or hearing voices that other people couldn't see or hear?

H2. Do you ever taste things or smell things that other people cannot, or feel things on your skin or in your body that other people cannot?

J1. Have you ever felt that people were spying on you, talking behind your back, or working against you in some other way?

J2. Have you ever felt you had some sort of a special mission in life—perhaps a divine purpose or calling?

J3. Have you had some other seemingly strange experience you couldn't explain or account for?

K1. Have you ever used alcohol or street drugs?

K2. Have you ever taken prescription or over-the-counter medication in a way that was different from the recommendation or prescription?

K3. Have you ever felt you drank or used drugs to excess?

K4. Have other people ever expressed concern about your drinking or drug use?

L1. How has your memory been? I'd like to test it, if that's OK.

L2. Has there ever been a period in your life that you couldn't remember later?

L3. Did you ever find yourself in a strange location and couldn't remember how you got there?

M1. Has your general health always been good?

M2. Have you had much medical attention for different conditions?

N1. Have you ever felt fat when people said you were too thin?

N2. Did you ever make yourself throw up because you felt so full?

N3. Do you ever go on eating binges, when you rapidly eat far more than normal?

P1. Have you ever felt or feared that there was something terribly wrong with you physically—that you had a serious medical illness or condition that doctors couldn't identify?

Q1. Have you ever felt that there was something about your body or your appearance that wasn't right—something that other people didn't seem to recognize?

R1. Do you easily become angry?

S1. Do you ever behave impulsively?

S2. Do you ever do things like pull out strands of your hair, or become destructively aggressive, or steal from stores, or set fires?

T1. Do you gamble?

U1. Has any blood relative—by which I mean a parent, brother, sister, grandparent, child, aunt, uncle, cousin, niece, or nephew—ever had symptoms like yours?

U2. Has any of these relatives had any mental illness, including depression . . . mania . . . psychosis . . . schizophrenia . . . nervousness . . . severe anxiety . . . mental hospitalization . . . suicide or suicide attempt . . . substance misuse or alcoholism . . . or a history of criminal behavior? [Pause for response between illnesses.]

MOOD DISORDERS

A1. Was there ever a time when you felt unusually down, depressed, or sad most of the day?

A2. Was there ever a time when you felt that most of the time you didn't enjoy your usual activities or take pleasure from them?

If "yes" to either:

    Did you feel that way most days?

    How long did these periods last?

    How many such periods have you had?

    Do you feel that way now?

    Did you ever completely recover from such a period of sadness?

    How severe is/was the experience—did it affect your work, your home life, or your social life?

    Have you ever been treated for depression? If so, details?

    Were you hospitalized?

    During a typical period of depression:

        Does your appetite go down?

        Do you lose weight? If so, how much?

        Does your sleep change? If so, up or down? Does it affect you most days?

        Do you tend to awaken very early in the morning and be unable to get back to sleep?

        Do you usually feel better in the morning or in the evening, or is there no difference?

        Do you feel slowed down or speeded up? If either, is it usually enough that other people can notice?

        Do you feel unusually tired or lacking in energy? If so, is this true most days?

        Do you feel worthless or more guilty than warranted about something—not just about feeling sick? If so, is this true most days?

    Are you indecisive, or do you have trouble focusing your concentration? If either, is this true most days?

    Do you think about dying?

        If so, how often does this thought occur to you?

    Do you consider suicide?

        If so, please tell me about that.

    Have you ever made a suicide attempt?

        If so, when? How?

        Physically/medically serious?

        Psychologically serious?

    When you are depressed, do your arms or legs feel heavy, rather like lead?

    When you are depressed, do you ever feel so bad that you hear or see things that others cannot see or hear? If so, details?

    When you are depressed, do you ever think that you deserve to feel this bad, or that other people are trying to harm you or work against you in some other way? If so, details?

When you are depressed, have you felt that things were hopeless or there was no use?

When you are depressed, do you feel better when something good happens (for example, when you are with friends or if you get a raise)?

When you are depressed, do you feel different than you would when, say, someone close to you died?

When you are depressed, do you lose your sense of pleasure in almost everything?

Do you tend to become depressed at a particular season of the year? If so, details?

Are you the sort of person who usually (not just when depressed) feels highly sensitive to rejection?

B1. Have you ever had a time when you felt the opposite of depressed—you felt unreasonably happy, euphoric, "on cloud nine"?

B2. Did you ever have a time when you (or others) noticed that you were unusually cross, irritable, or cranky?

B3. Has there been a time when you were much more active than is normal for you?

If "yes" to any of these three:

How long did this period last?

How many such periods have you had?

Do you feel that way now?

Did you ever completely recover from such a period of excessive happiness?

How severe is/was the experience—that is, did it affect your work, your home life, or your social life? If so, in what way?

Were you given treatment in any way for such a period? If so, details?

Were you hospitalized?

During such periods:

Do you feel like you have special strengths or powers others don't have (such as having telepathy or reading minds), or that you were a special or exalted person (for example, Jesus or a movie star)? If so, details?

During such periods, how is your sleep? Details?

If sleep during these periods is less than normal: Do you feel you need less sleep than usual?

During such periods, do you talk more than usual, or do others claim that you do?

During such periods, do your thoughts seem to race from one thing to another?

During such periods, do you (or others) notice that you are more easily distractible than usual?

During such periods, do you feel speeded up in your activity level, or
do others say that this is the case?

During such periods, do you make more plans than you normally
would?

During such periods, how is your sex drive?

What about your judgment during such periods—do you think it is
impaired in any way? Here's what I mean:

Do you spend money you later wished you hadn't?

Do you get into legal scrapes?

Do you pursue sex relations in a way that isn't normal for you?

Do you ever think you hear or see things that others can't see or
hear? If so, details?

Do you feel spied upon or persecuted or that other people are trying to harm you or work against you in some other way? If so,
details?

ANXIETY DISORDERS

**C1. Have you ever have an attack or spell when you suddenly felt anxious,
fearful, or extremely uneasy?**

**C2. Have you ever had a sudden attack or spell when you felt faint, you felt
you couldn't breathe, or your heart seemed to race?**

If "yes" to either:

How many such attacks have you had?

How often do they occur, on average?

How long do these attacks last?

How severe is/was the experience—enough to affect your work, your
home life, or your social life?

Have you ever been treated for such an episode? If so, details?

Were you hospitalized?

During these attacks, have you ever had any of these sensations:

Chest pain or other chest discomfort?

Chills or hot flashes?

Choking?

Feeling that things were unreal or that you were detached from yourself?

Feeling dizzy, lightheaded, faint, or unsteady on your feet?

Fear of dying?

Fear that you would lose control or become insane?

Heart pounding, racing, or skipping beats?

Nausea or other abdominal discomfort?

Numbness or tingling?

Sweating?

Shortness of breath or smothering sensation?

Trembling?

D1. Have you had fears or phobias related to anything? Examples: animals (such as spiders, dogs, snakes); blood, needles, or injections; heights; airplane travel; being closed in; thunderstorms; blushing; eating in public; speaking, singing, or playing a musical instrument before an audience.

If "yes," ask for each feared stimulus:

How often has this fear occurred?

How many episodes have you had?

Does this sort of fear seem unreasonable or out of proportion to you?

Does this fear cause you to avoid the situation?

Does it interfere with your usual routine or social, work, or personal functioning?

Have you ever had treatment for it?

D2. Have you had anxiety about being in a place or situation (such as a store or the movies)—a place that you'd have trouble escaping from, or where there might be no help available if you had a panic attack?

If "yes":

Do you therefore sometimes avoid stores or the movies (or the other places)?

If you do go into one of these situations, do you feel anxious when you are there?

Do you ever take a companion to help you if you should have a panic attack while away from home?

E1. Have you ever had ideas or thoughts that keep coming back to you— thoughts that you try to resist but cannot?

If "yes":

How often do these ideas occur?

Do you try to resist or suppress these ideas/thoughts?

Do they come from your own mind, or does it seem that they are imposed on you from somewhere outside you?

E2. Do you ever experience physical behaviors that you feel you have to perform over and over, such as handwashing, checking the stove, counting things?

If "yes":

Do these behaviors occur in response to an obsessional idea?

Do they make you follow strict rules when carrying them out?

Do they prevent something bad from happening?

Do they reduce your distress?

Do they *cause* severe distress?

How much time do they take up?

Do they interfere with your usual routine or with work, social, or personal functioning? If so, details?

F1. Have you ever had a traumatic, stressful experience that you found you kept on reliving or having to avoid?

If "yes":

What was the event?

When did it occur?

Did it cause a sense of severe fear, horror, or helplessness?

Have you had any experiences that caused you to relive the event:

Intrusive thoughts or images?

Flashbacks, hallucinations, illusions, or feeling as if the event was recurring?

Cues that symbolize or resemble the event, causing you marked distress?

Physiological events (such as rapid heartbeat, raised blood pressure) in response to these cues?

Have you repeatedly tried to avoid the stimuli that remind you of the trauma? If so, in which of these ways:

Have you tried to avoid feelings, thoughts, or conversations that remind you of the event?

Have you tried to avoid activities, people, or places that remind you of the event?

Have you been unable to recall any important features of the event? If so, which?

Have you lost interest in activities that are important to you? If so, which ones?

To what degree?

Have you felt isolated from other people?

Have you felt you've lost the ability to feel love or other strong emotions?

Have you felt that your life would be brief or unrewarding—such as a lack of marriage, job, or children?

Have you had any of the following symptoms that weren't present before the event:

Insomnia?

Irritability?

Trouble concentrating?

Excessive vigilance (such as frequently scanning the surroundings for signs of danger)?

Increased startle response?

G1. Do you worry a great deal of the time?

C2. What do you worry about?
> If patient lists three or more worries:
>> Do you have trouble controlling these worries?
>> How many days a month do you think you worry about these matters?
>> For how many months have you had worries like this?
>> Did it lead to trouble with your job, your family life, or your personal life?
> When you worry:
>> Do you have feelings of being restless, edgy, or keyed up?
>> Do you get tired easily?
>> Do you have trouble concentrating?
>> Do you feel irritable?
>> Do you have increased muscle tension?
>> Do you have trouble sleeping?

PSYCHOTIC DISORDERS

H1. Have you ever had experiences like seeing visions or hearing voices that other people couldn't see or hear?

H2. Do you ever taste things or smell things that other people cannot, or feel things on your skin or in your body that other people cannot?
> If "yes" for voices:
>> How lifelike are they? Do they sound as real as my voice does now?
>> Do they seem to come from inside your head or somewhere outside?
>> When did you start hearing them?
>> Are they male or female?
>> Whose voices are they?
>> How many voices do you hear?
>>> If more than one voice, do they ever talk with one another?
>>> Do they ever talk together about you?
>> How often do the voices occur?
>>> If every day, how often each day?
>> Do they tell you what to do?
>> Do you ever follow their commands?
> If "yes" for visual material:
>> Can you see them as clearly as you see me now?
>> When do you see them?
>>> If every day, how often each day?
>> When did you start seeing them?
> If "yes" for tastes, smells, or tactile sensations:
>> Please describe these sensations.

How often do you experience them?
   If every day, how often each day?
What are you doing when you experience them?
When did you start having them?
For all hallucinations:
   What do you think causes these experiences to occur?
   Could there be any connection between these experiences and drug or alcohol use?
   Have you had any physical illness that could help account for these experiences?

J1. Have you ever felt that people were spying on you, talking behind your back, or working against you in some other way?

J2. Have you ever felt you had some sort of a special mission in life—perhaps a divine purpose or calling?

J3. Have you had some other seemingly strange experience you couldn't explain or account for?

[If patient needs additional information: Here are some examples of the sort of thing I mean:

Have you ever felt that people could hear your unspoken thoughts or read your mind?

Have you ever felt that someone on TV or the radio was sending messages that were meant for you alone?

Have you ever thought that someone from outside could put thoughts into your mind or take them out?

Have you ever felt that you've done something so awful that you deserve punishment for it?

Have you ever felt that you were someone famous, or that you had abilities or powers that other people don't have?]

If "yes" to any of the three questions above:

Specifically, what have you noticed?

How long have you had these experiences?

Who or what do you think has been responsible for these events?

How have you tried to combat them?

Has anyone close to you had similar experiences?

Could there be any connection between these experiences and drug or alcohol use?

SUBSTANCE MISUSE

K1. Have you ever used alcohol or street drugs?

K2. Have you ever taken prescription or over-the-counter medication in a way that was different from the recommendation or prescription?

K3. Have you ever felt you drank or used drugs to excess?

K4. Have other people ever expressed concern about your drinking or drug use?

    If "yes" to any of these:

        Which substances?

        How long have you used them?

        Do you use them now?

        Have you ever had withdrawal symptoms when coming off a specific substance?

            Alcohol/sedatives: sweating, rapid heartbeat, tremor, sleeplessness, nausea, vomiting, brief hallucinations or illusions, speeded-up activity, grand mal seizures, anxiety?

            Cocaine/amphetamines: dysphoric mood, fatigue, vivid bad dreams, sleep increased or decreased, increased appetite, activity speeded up or slowed down?

            Opioids: dysphoric mood, nausea, vomiting, aching muscles, tearing, runny nose, dilated pupils, erect hairs, sweating, diarrhea, yawning, fever, sleeplessness?

        Have you ever found yourself having to use increasing amounts of the substance to get the same effect?

        Have you ever found that you've used more of the substance than you meant to?

        Have you tried to control your use of the substance, but found you couldn't?

        Does your substance use occupy a lot of your time—getting it, using it, or recovering from its effects?

        Have you found that your substance use has caused you to abandon important work, social, or leisure activities such as home life, getting together with friends?

        Has your substance use caused you distress or impaired your functioning?

          If so, how?

        Have you continued to use the substance, even though you knew that it was probably causing you to have physical or psychological problems?

        Has substance use ever caused you not to fulfill major obligations, such as attending school, going to work, or taking care of children?

        Have you used substances even when doing so was physically dangerous—such as driving a vehicle?

        Has substance use caused you to have legal problems?

          If so, how many, and when?

        Has substance use ever caused you to have social or interpersonal problems?

          If so, did you continue to use the substance anyway?

DIFFICULTY THINKING (COGNITIVE DISORDERS)

L1. **How has your memory been? I'd like to test it, if that's OK.**
Repeat back to me [a name, a color, a street address]
What's the date today?
Who is the current president? Name the one just before. And the three
 before that person.
Please subtract 7 from 100. Now 7 from that. Good, and keep going until
 you get below 60.

L2. **Has there ever been a period in your life that you couldn't remember
later?**
If so, please tell me about it.
How often has this happened?

L3. **Did you ever find yourself in a strange location and couldn't remember
how you got there?**
If so, please tell me about it.
How often has this happened?

What were those three items I asked you to repeat a few minutes ago?

Alternative: Screen with the Mini-Mental State Exam (see p. 148).

PHYSICAL COMPLAINTS

M1. **Has your general health always been good?**
M2. **Have you had much medical attention for different conditions?**
If "yes" to the first or "no" to the second:
 What illnesses have you had? Details?
 Have you had other medical conditions?
 Use of medications?
Now I'd like to ask about some symptoms people often experience. Have
 you ever had:
 Pain symptoms, such as these:*
 Head pain (other than headache)?
 Abdominal pain?
 Back pain?
 Pain in your joints?

---

*To count as positive, each symptom must have:
 1. Not been fully explained by a general medical condition or substance use; *and*
 2. Caused impairment or caused the patient to seek treatment; *and*
 3. Exceeded the discomfort or impairment you'd expect for any medical condition that seems related.

    Pain in your arms or legs?
    Chest pain?
    Rectal pain?
    Pain with menstruation?
    Pain with sexual intercourse?
    Pain on urination?
Gastrointestinal symptoms, such as these:*
    Nausea?
    Abdominal bloating?
    Vomiting (other than during pregnancy)?
    Diarrhea?
    Intolerance of several foods?
Sexual symptoms, such as these:*
    Indifference to sex?
    Difficulties with erection or ejaculation?
    Irregular menses?
    Excessive menstrual bleeding?
    Vomiting throughout all 9 months of pregnancy?
Pseudoneurological symptoms, such as these:*
    Impaired balance or coordination?
    Weak or paralyzed muscles?
    Lump in throat?
    Trouble swallowing?
    Loss of voice?
    Retention of urine?
    Hallucinations?
    Numbness (to touch or pain)?
    Double vision?
    Blindness?
    Deafness?
    Seizures?
    Amnesia?
    Other dissociative symptoms?
    Loss of consciousness (other than fainting)?

N1. Have you ever felt fat when people said you were too thin?
N2. Did you ever make yourself throw up because you felt so full?
    If "yes" to either:
    When was it?
    Is this still the case?
    What did you weigh then?
    How tall were you then?
    Were you afraid of gaining weight?
    Did you exercise a lot to lose weight?

Did you ever use laxatives to lose weight?

At that time, how did your body look to you? Thin, fat, or about right?

How important was your body weight or shape to you then?

If patient is female: During this time, did your periods stop?

    If so, for how long?

N3. Do you ever go on eating binges, when you rapidly eat far more than normal?

If "yes":

How often does this occur?

At these times, do you feel you've lost control of your eating?

To keep from gaining weight, do you ever use laxatives? Use diuretics? Throw up? Fast? Exercise a lot?

P1. Have you ever felt or feared that there was something terribly wrong with you physically—that you had a serious medical illness or condition that doctors couldn't identify?

If "yes":

Please describe your symptoms.

How long have they lasted?

What disease or condition are you afraid of?

Q1. Have you ever felt that there was something about your body or your appearance that wasn't right—something that other people didn't seem to recognize?

If "yes":

Do you spend a lot of time thinking about this problem, or trying to deal with it?

What steps have you taken to remedy it?

IMPULSE CONTROL DISORDERS

R1. Do you easily become angry?

If "yes":

In what sorts of situations do you become so angry?

Do you become so angry that you lose control?

As a result, do you ever destroy property? If so, how often?

As a result, do you ever assault another person? If so, how often?

S1. Do you ever behave impulsively?

S2. Do you ever do things like pull out strands of your hair, or become destructively aggressive, or steal from stores, or set fires?

If "yes" to any:

Do you feel a sort of tension just before performing any of these activities?

Do you feel gratification, pleasure, or relief during or after the activity?

T1. Do you gamble?
>   If "yes":
>   How often?
>   Have you ever felt that you gambled excessively—that it was out of control?
>   Do you find that gambling preoccupies you—that you spend a lot of time figuring out how to get money to gamble, or reliving your past gambling experiences, or planning new gambling ventures?
>   Have you ever needed to put more money into play to achieve the same excitement?
>   Have you tried to control your gambling and couldn't?
>>   If so, how?
>>   How many times has this happened?
>   Have you felt restless or irritable when trying to control your gambling?
>   Do you ever gamble as an escape from your problems or to cope with depressed or anxious moods?
>   Have you ever gambled to try to recoup your losses?
>   Have you ever lied to conceal how much you've lost gambling?
>   Have you ever had to rely on other people for money to cover your gambling debts?
>   Have you ever used money that wasn't yours to gamble with?
>   Has gambling ever put at jeopardy a job, an important relationship, or a chance for your career or education?

FAMILY HISTORY

U1. Has any blood relative—by which I mean a parent, brother, sister, grandparent, child, aunt, uncle, cousin, niece, or nephew—ever had symptoms like yours?

U2. Has any of these relatives had any mental illness, including depression ... mania ... psychosis ... schizophrenia ... nervousness ... severe anxiety ... mental hospitalization ... suicide or suicide attempt ... substance misuse or alcoholism ... or a history of criminal behavior? [Pause for response between illnesses.]
>   For any positive response:
>   What were this person's symptoms?
>   How old was the patient at the time?
>   Do you know what treatment was given?
>   What happened to this person? [Possibilities might include recovery, continued illness but functioning in society, inability to work, repeated or chronic hospitalization.]

CHILDHOOD THROUGH ADULT LIFE

Childhood

Where were you born?
How many brothers and sisters did you have?
Were you the oldest, youngest—which number in the list?
Were you reared by both parents?
How did your parents get along?
  If they fought, what about?
  If they divorced or separated, how old were you then?
With whom did you live?
If you were adopted, how old were you at the time?
  Do you know what the circumstances behind the adoption were?
How was your health as a child?
How far did you go in school?
  Were you ever held back in school?
  Any behavior or disciplinary problems in school?
  Any truancy?
  Were you ever suspended or expelled?
Did you have many friends as a child?
What interests and hobbies did you have as a child?
Outside of school, did you have legal or disciplinary problems?
  If so, did you ever steal things?
  Set fires?
  Deliberately destroy the property of others?
  Behave cruelly toward people or animals?
  Run away from home overnight?

Adult Life

Are you married?
  If so, number of times, and your age each time?
  How did early marriage(s) end—divorce, death of spouse?
With whom do you live now?
Number of children, ages?
Do you have any stepchildren?
  If so, how many?
  How is your relationship with them?
What is your current occupation?
Number of jobs lifetime?
  Reasons for job changes?
  Were you ever fired? Why?
If you are not working now, what is your current means of support?

Any military service?
   If so, which branch?
   Number of years?
   Highest rank attained?
   Combat experience?
   Disciplinary problems in military?
How important is religion to you now?
   What is your current religious affiliation?
   Is it different from the religion of your childhood?
   If so, what made you change?
What are your current leisure activities?
   Clubs, organizations?
   Hobbies, interests?
When did you first learn about sex?
What were the circumstances?
How old were you when you began dating?
How old were you at your first sexual experience?
   What was its nature?
   How did you feel about it?
Can you tell me about your current sexual interests?
Have there ever been sexual practices or experiences that troubled you?
Were you ever abused as a child?
   Sexually?
   Physically?
As an adult, were you ever raped or sexually abused? If so, details?

SOCIAL AND PERSONALITY PROBLEMS

The following questions will elicit information about how patients view themselves and interact with others. In most cases, the answers will not allow you to make a firm diagnosis; you will need to obtain further information from other resources.

What sort of a person do you think you are?
What do you like most about yourself?
What do you like least about yourself?
Do you have many friends, or are you more of a loner?
How well do you get along with your [husband/wife/partner]?
Do you have any problems in getting along with members of your family?
Do you avoid any of your relatives because of difficulties getting along?
Any difficulties with friends?
Have you had any interpersonal problems at work?

Do you tend to be suspicious of people's motives, or are you more a trusting sort of person?

Do you like being the center of attention, or are you more comfortable staying in the background?

Are you usually comfortable being by yourself, or do you find you need the presence of other people?

Have you ever done something that turned out to be poor judgment? What was it?

Have you ever had some sort of legal difficulty? If so, details?

Have you ever been arrested? Spent time in jail? If so, details?

Have you ever done something that could have gotten you into legal difficulties, but you were never found out?

When you do [these behaviors], do you tend to feel sorry afterward?

Do you feel that other people would like to deceive, exploit, or harm you? If so, examples?

Do you feel that your friends or acquaintances are disloyal to you? If so, examples?

Do you tend to bear grudges? If so, examples?

Do you prefer to do things by yourself? If so, examples?

Does criticism or praise affect you much? If so, examples?

Are you a superstitious person? If so, examples?

Do you believe in the supernatural, such as telepathy, black magic, mind reading? If so, examples?

Are your relationships with other people usually long-lasting? If so, examples?

Does your mood tend to be pretty stable, or are you more of an up-and-down sort of person? If so, examples?

Do you tend to describe yourself as feeling "empty"? If so, examples?

Do you feel angry much of the time or frequently lose your temper or get into fights? If so, examples?

Do you like being the center of attention? If so, examples?

Do you feel that you are easily influenced by the opinions of other people? If so, examples?

Do you often have fantasies about yourself as achieving vast success, ideal love, power, brilliance? If so, examples?

Do you often feel that you deserve special treatment or consideration? If so, examples?

Is it hard for you to identify with the feelings of other people? If so, examples?

Do you fear embarrassment or disapproval so much that you avoid new activities or interactions with other people? If so, examples?

In new relationships, do you often feel inadequate? If so, examples?

Do you feel you need a lot of advice and reassurance when making every-day decisions? If so, examples?

Does the fear that you'll lose support make it hard for you to disagree with others? If so, examples?

Do you get so preoccupied with details that you sometimes lose sight of the purpose of what you are doing? If so, examples?

Do you regard yourself as being especially stubborn? If so, examples?

Would you say that you are a perfectionist? If so, examples?

Appendix E

Assessing Your Interview

All patients, and therefore all interviews, are different. Instructors also vary in the emphasis they place on the several aspects of the initial interview. However, there are many aspects that most clinicians agree are crucial for the typical interview. These aspects include factual material, as well as items that contribute to the process of obtaining information. They are listed in this appendix, where a rough numerical value is assigned to each.

You can score your own interview from a tape recording, or have a colleague do it for you while you are interviewing. The overall score and subsection scores should help you plan where to expend additional effort. The scoring system used has been adapted and extended from articles by Maguire and associates (Appendix F).

For each section below, score 0 if the rated behavior or item of data was not observed or covered at all. Score the maximum number of points if the item was covered completely (as judged from the patient's case notes in chart), or if the desired behavior was consistently present. Give proportional credit for partial answers or behaviors.

The maximum score is 200 points. For a beginner, any score above 140 is acceptable, although advanced interviewers should average much higher.

Mental status data are not included in this self-assessment, which was designed to evaluate only the historical and interactive portions of the initial interview.

1. *Initiating the interview* (10 points)

Interviewer	No	Yes
a. Greets the patient	0	1
b. Shakes hands	0	1
c. Mentions patient's name	0	1
d. Mentions own name	0	1
e. Explains status (training?)	0	1
f. Indicates where to sit	0	1
g. Explains purpose of interview	0	1
h. Mentions time available	0	1
i. Mentions note taking	0	1
j. Asks whether patient is comfortable	0	1

2. *History of present illness* (58 points)

Interviewer asks about	No								Yes
a. Main complaint(s)	0	1	2	3	4	5	6	7	8
b. Onset of problems	0		1		2		3		4
c. Stressors	0		1		2		3		4
d. Key events in course of illness	0		1		2		3		4
e. Current medication									
1. Name or description	0			1					2
2. Dose	0			1					2
3. Wanted effects obtained	0			1					2
4. Side effects noted	0			1					2
5. Duration of effect	0			1					2
f. History of previous episodes									
1. Type	0		1		2		3		4
2. Similarity to present episode	0		1		2		3		4
3. Previous treatment	0		1		2		3		4
4. Outcome of treatment	0		1		2		3		4
g. Effects of illness on work	0		1		2		3		4
h. Effects of illness on family	0		1		2		3		4
i. Patient's feelings about problems	0		1		2		3		4

3. *Medical history* (10 points)

Interviewer asks about

	No		Yes
a. Relevant data on physical illness	No		Yes
b. Allergies to medications	0	1	2
c. Operations	0	1	2
d. Previous hospitalizations	0	1	2
e. Relevant review of systems	0	1	2

4. *Personal and social history* (20 points)

Interviewer asks about

	No		Yes
a. Details of family of origin	0	1	2
b. Education	0	1	2
c. Marital history	0	1	2
d. Military history	0	1	2
e. Work history	0	1	2
f. Sexual preference and adjustment	0	1	2
g. Legal problems	0	1	2
h. Current living situation	0	1	2
i. Leisure activities	0	1	2
j. Source of support	0	1	2

5. *Family history of mental disorder* (6 points)

Interviewer asks about

	No		Yes
a. Symptoms to make diagnosis	0	1	2
b. Response to treatment	0	1	2
c. All first-degree relatives	0	1	2

6. *Screening questions* (26 points)

Interviewer screens for

	No		Yes
a. Depression	0	1	2
b. Panic attacks	0	1	2
c. Phobias	0	1	2
d. Obsessions and compulsions	0	1	2
e. Mania	0	1	2

6. *Screening questions* (cont.)	No				Yes
f. Psychosis	0		1		2
g. Childhood abuse	0		1		2
h. Alcohol/drug abuse	0		1		2
i. Suicidal ideas/attempts	0		1		2
j. History of violence	0		1		2

7. *Establishing rapport* (18 points)

Interviewer	No				Yes
a. Smiles, nods at appropriate times	0	1	2	3	4
b. Uses language patient understands	0	1	2	3	4
c. Responds with feeling, empathy	0	1	2	3	4
d. Maintains eye contact	0		1		2
e. Maintains appropriate distance	0		1		2
f. Appears self-assured and relaxed	0		1		2

8. *Use of interview techniques* (44 points)

Interviewer	Poor				Good
a. Explores verbal leads to new material	0	1	2	3	4
b. Controls flow of interview while allowing patient scope for response	0	1	2	3	4
c. Clarifies uncertainties to obtain complete information	0	1	2	3	4
d. Makes smooth transitions; if abrupt, they are pointed out	0	1	2	3	4
e. Avoids use of jargon	0	1	2	3	4
f. Asks brief, single questions	0	1	2	3	4
g. Does not repeat questions already asked	0	1	2	3	4
h. Uses open, nondirective questions	0	1	2	3	4
i. Facilitates patient's replies verbally and nonverbally	0	1	2	3	4
j. Encourages precise answers (dates, numbers where appropriate)	0	1	2	3	4
k. Seeks out and sensitively handles emotionally loaded material	0	1	2	3	4

9. *Ending the interview* (8 points)

Interviewer	No		Yes
a. Warns that interview is nearly over	0	1	2
b. Gives brief, accurate summary	0	1	2
c. Solicits questions from patient	0	1	2
d. Makes a concluding statement of appreciation, interest	0	1	2

Appendix F

Bibliography and Recommended Reading

BOOKS

American Psychiatric Association. (2000). *Diagnostic and statistical manual of mental disorders* (4th ed., text rev.). Washington, DC: Author. [Indispensable for a thorough understanding of current diagnostic thinking.]

American Psychiatric Association. (2006). *Practice guidelines for the treatment of psychiatric disorders.* Arlington, VA: Author. [Includes *Psychiatric evaluation of adults* (2nd ed.).]

Cannell, C. E., & Kahn, R. L. (1968). Interviewing. In G. Lindzey & E. Aronson (Eds.), *The handbook of social psychology* (2nd ed., pp. 526–595). Reading, MA: Addison-Wesley.

Cormier, L. S., & Nurius, P. S. (2003). *Interviewing and change strategies for helpers* (5th ed.). Pacific Grove, CA: Thomson/Brooks/Cole. [Massive, detailed textbook for all mental health professionals, but especially slanted toward psychologists and social workers. Material on different types of therapy, as well as interviewing strategies.]

Ekman, P. (2001). *Telling lies: Clues to deceit in the marketplace, politics, and marriage* (3rd ed.). New York: Norton. [A great deal of information about lying and its detection.]

Gill, M., Newman, R., & Redlich, F. C. (1954). *The initial interview in psychiatric practice.* New York: International Universities Press. [Classic description of interviewing style that focuses on the patient's needs and capabilities.]

Leon, R. L. (1989). *Psychiatric interviewing: A primer* (2nd ed.). New York: Elsevier. [This volume covers much of the same material as *The first interview.* The author explicitly favors a nondirective approach to gathering information.]

MacKinnon, R. A., & Yudofsky, S. C. (1986). *The psychiatric evaluation in clinical practice.* Philadelphia: Lippincott. [Only the first third of this book concerns clinical interviewing. The balance is given over to clinical laboratory testing, personality tests, and rating scales. The section on psychodynamic case formulation provides some information not readily available else-where.]

Morrison, J. (2006). *DSM-IV made easy: The clinician's guide to diagnosis* (updated ed.). New York: Guilford Press. [A learner's guide to the increasingly complex and lengthy *Diagnostic and statistical manual of mental disorders*, now updated for DSM-IV-TR.]

Morrison, J. (2007). *Diagnosis made easier.* New York: Guilford Press. [Step by step, this new book helps the reader make sense of the interview material.]

Othmer, E., & Othmer, S. C. (2002). *The clinical interview using DSM-IV-TR.* Washington, DC: American Psychiatric Press. [Encyclopedic in its coverage, this book adheres strictly to the DSM-IV-TR format.]

Shea, S. C. (1998). *Psychiatric interviewing: The art of understanding* (2nd ed.). Philadelphia: Saunders. [Long-winded and occasionally pretentious, it nevertheless introduces a great deal of relevant material.]

Simms, A. (1988). *Symptoms in the mind.* London: Baillière Tindall. [A British text that contains more in the way of current mental health terminology and definitions than any other I have seen.]

Sullivan, H. S. (1954). *The psychiatric interview.* New York: Norton. [An early, classical description of how to do an initial interview.]

ARTICLES

Note: For purposes of the comments, the following articles are listed chronologically within author groups, rather than alphabetically by author.

Sandifer, M. G., Hordern, A., & Green, L. M. (1970). The psychiatric interview: The impact of the first three minutes. *American Journal of Psychiatry, 126,* 968–973. [Half of all observations made by interviewers in this study were made within the first 3 minutes of an experimental interview. These data can sometimes have a decisive impact on diagnosis.]

Maguire, G. P., & Rutter, D. R. (1976). History-taking for medical students. 1: Deficiencies in performance. *Lancet, ii,* 556–560. [Senior medical students showed significant deficiencies in taking histories. These included avoidance of personal issues, use of jargon, lack of precision, failure to pick up on cues, needless repetition, poor clarification, failures of control, inadequate facilitation, and inappropriate question style (leading or complicated questions).]

Maguire, P., Roe, P., Goldberg, D., Jones, S., Hyde, C., & O'Dowd, T. (1978). The value of feedback in teaching interviewing skills to medical students. *Psychological Medicine, 8,* 695–704. [In a randomized trial, feedback (video, audio, or ratings of practice interviews) led to greater ability to obtain relevant, accurate facts. Only the video and audio groups also showed improved technique.]

Maguire, P., Fairbairn, S., & Fletcher, C. (1986). Consultation skills of young doctors. I: Benefits of feedback training in interviewing as students persist. *British Medical Journal, 292,* 1573–1576. [Young physicians who had ei ther been given feedback training by video or allotted to conventional teaching in interview skills were followed up 5 years later. Both groups had improved since graduation, but "those given feedback training had maintained their superiority in the skills associated with accurate diagnosis." The authors conclude that feedback training should be given to all students.]

Platt, F. W., & McMath, J. C. (1979). Clinical hypocompetence: The interview. *Annals of Internal Medicine, 91,* 898–902. [House officers in internal medicine had problems with initial interviews. These include poor rapport, inadequate data base, failure to formulate hypotheses, excessive control of interview (patients complained of not being listened to), and acceptance of patients' reports of lab data or interpretations of what another health care provider said, rather than the primary data of symptoms. Examples are given.]

Rutter, M., & Cox, A. (1981). Psychiatric interviewing techniques: I. Methods and measures. *British Journal of Psychiatry, 138,* 273–282. [The introductory article in this series. The series of seven articles by these authors is a landmark in the study of interview technique. These studies are based on interviews with mothers of child psychiatry patients and compare four interviewing styles that have been recommended by experts. Although the research they report has not been replicated, the findings are so logical and the methodology so impeccable that they strike the reader as received truth. These articles provide much of the basis for this manual.]

Cox, A., Hopkinson, K, & Rutter, M. (1981). Psychiatric interviewing techniques: II. Naturalistic study: Eliciting factual material. *British Journal of Psychiatry, 138,* 283–291. [This article demonstrates that "a directive style with specific probes and requests for detailed descriptions" produced facts of better quality than did an approach that was more freestyle. Informants talked more when interviewers talked less and used more openended questions. Double questions led to confusion, but multiple-choice questions sometimes were helpful.]

Hopkinson, K., Cox, A., & Rutter, M. (1981). Psychiatric interviewing techniques: III. Naturalistic study: Eliciting feelings. *British Journal of Psychiatry, 138,* 406–415. [Several techniques were found to facilitate expression of emotion. These included "a low level of interviewer talk with few interruptions, a high rate of open rather than closed questions, direct requests for feelings, interpretations and expressions of sympathy."]

Rutter, M., Cox, A., Egert, S., Holbrook, D., & Everitt, B. (1981). Psychiatric interviewing techniques: IV. Experimental study: Four contrasting styles. *British Journal of Psychiatry, 138,* 456–465. [The authors taught two interviewers to use any of four interviewing styles: (1) A "sounding board" style used minimal activity; (2) "active psychotherapy" tried to explore feelings and elicit emotional linkages and meanings; (3) a "structured" style used active cross-questioning; (4) a "systematic exploratory" style combined high use of both fact- and feeling-oriented techniques.]

Cox, A., Rutter, M., & Holbrook, D. (1981). Psychiatric interviewing techniques: V. Experimental study: Eliciting factual material. *British Journal of Psychiatry, 139*, 29–37. [This paper reports data on the study described just above. The authors conclude that "it is desirable to begin clinical diagnostic interviews with a lengthy period with little in the way of detailed probing and in which informants are allowed to express their concerns in their own way." Systematic questioning is essential to elicit good-quality facts. "Better data were obtained when interviewers were sensitive and alert to factual cues and chose their probes with care."]

Cox, A., Holbrook, D., & Rutter, M. (1981). Psychiatric interviewing techniques: VI. Experimental study: Eliciting feelings. *British Journal of Psychiatry, 139*, 144–152. [A variety of interview styles can be used to elicit feelings from patients. Gathering good factual information is entirely compatible with eliciting feelings.]

Cox, A., Rutter, M., & Holbrook, D. (1988). Psychiatric interviewing techniques: A second experimental study: Eliciting feelings. *British Journal of Psychiatry, 152*, 64–72. [Expression of emotions was maximized when interviewers used "active" techniques, such as interpretation, reflection of feelings, and expression of sympathy. This was especially true if the informant's "spontaneous rate of expression was relatively low."]

OTHER ARTICLES USED IN THE PREPARATION OF THIS BOOK

Booth, T., & Booth, W. (1994). The use of depth interviewing with vulnerable subjects. *Social Science and Medicine, 39*, 415–423.

Britten, N. (2006). Psychiatry, stigma, and resistance. *British Medical Journal, 317*, 963–964.

Budd, E. C., Winer, J. L., Schoenrock, C. J., & Martin, P. W. (1982). Evaluating alternative techniques of questioning mentally retarded persons. *American Journal of Mental Deficiency, 86*, 511–518.

Eisenthal, S., Koopman, C., & Lazare, A. (1983). Process analysis of two dimensions of the negotiated approach in relation to satisfaction in the initial interview. *Journal of Nervous and Mental Disease, 171*, 49–53.

Eisenthal, S., & Lazare, A. (1977). Evaluation of the initial interview in a walk-in clinic. *Journal of Nervous and Mental Disease, 164*, 30–35.

Folstein, M. F., Folstein, S. E., & McHugh, P. R. (1975). Mini-Mental State: A practical method for grading the cognitive state of patients for the clinician. *Journal of Psychiatric Research, 12*, 189–198.

Hamann, J., Leucht, S., & Kissling, W. (2003). Shared decision making in psychiatry. *Acta Psychiatrica Scandinavica, 107*, 403–409.

Harrington, R., Hill, J., Rutter, M., John, K., Fudge, H., Zoccolillo, M., et al. (1988). The assessment of lifetime psychopathology: A comparison of two interviewing styles. *Psychological Medicine, 18*, 487–493.

Jellinek, M. (1978). Referrals from a psychiatric emergency room: Relationship of compliance to demographic and interview variables. *American Journal of Psychiatry, 135*, 209–212.

Jensen, P. S., Watanabe, H. K., & Richters, J. E. (1999). Who's up first?: Testing for order effects in structured interviews using a counterbalanced experimental design. *Journal of Abnormal Child Psychology, 27*, 439–445.

Kendler, K. S., Silberg, J. L., Neale, M. C., Kessler, R. C., Heath, A. C., & Eaves, L. J. (1991). The family history method: Whose psychiatric history is measured? *American Journal of Psychiatry, 148*, 1501–1504.

Koenigs, M., Young, L., Adolphs, R., Tranel, D., Cushman, F., Hauser, M. (2007). Damage to the prefrontal cortex increases utilitarian moral judgments. *Nature, 446*, 908–911.

Lovett, L. M., Cox, A., & Abou-Saleh, M. (1990). Teaching psychiatric interview skills to medical students. *Medical Education, 24*, 243–250.

Meyers, J., & Stein, S. (2000). The psychiatric interview in the emergency department. *Emergency Medicine Clinics of North America, 18*, 173–183.

Pollock, D. C., Shanley, D. E., & Byrne, P. N. (1985). Psychiatric interviewing and clinical skills. *Canadian Journal of Psychiatry, 30*, 64–68.

Rogers, R. (2003). Standardizing DSM-IV diagnoses: The clinical applications of structured interviews. *Journal of Personality Assessment, 81*, 220–225.

Rosenthal, M. J. (1989). Towards selective and improved performance of the mental status examination. *Acta Psychiatrica Scandinavica, 80*, 207–215.

Stewart, M. A. (1984). What is a successful doctor–patient interview?: A study of interactions and outcomes. *Social Science and Medicine, 19*, 167–175.

Torrey, E. F. (2006). Violence and schizophrenia. *Schizophrenia Research, 88*, 3–4.

Wissow, S. L., Roter, D. L., & Wilson, M. E. H. (1994). Pediatrician interview style and mothers' disclosure of psychosocial issues. *Pediatrics, 93*, 289–295.

Index

In this index, definitions are indicated by the use of *italics* and main discussions of certain topics by **boldface**.